Physical Activity and Educational Achievement

A growing body of research evidence suggests that physical activity can have a positive effect on educational achievement. This book examines a range of processes associated with physical activity that are of relevance to those working in education – including cognition, learning, memory, attention, mood, stress and mental health symptoms – and draws on the latest insights from exercise neuroscience to help explain the evidence.

With contributions from leading scientists and educationalists from around the world, this book cuts through the myths to interrogate the relationship between physical activity and educational achievement in children, adolescents and young adults in a variety of cultural and geographical contexts. Examining both the benefits and risks associated with physical activity from the perspectives of exercise science and educational psychology, it also looks ahead to ask what the limits of this research might be and what effects it might have on the future practice of education.

Physical Activity and Educational Achievement: Insights from Exercise Neuroscience is fascinating reading for any student, academic or practitioner with an interest in exercise science and education.

Romain Meeusen is Head of the Department of Human Physiology at the Vrije Universiteit Brussel, Belgium.

Sabine Schaefer is Head of the Department of Motion Science, Motor Science and Cognition, Saarland University, Germany.

Phillip Tomporowski is a Professor of Kinesiology at the University of Georgia, USA.

Richard Bailey is Senior Researcher at the International Council of Sport Science and Physical Education (ICSSPE) based in Berlin, Germany.

T0175031

ICSSPE Perspectives
The Multidisciplinary Series of Physical Education and Sport Science

By publishing Perspectives, ICSSPE aims to facilitate the application of sport science results to practical areas of sport by integrating the various sport science branches. In each volume of Perspectives, expert contributions from different disciplines address a specific physical education or sport science theme, which has been identified by a group of leading international experts.

ICSSPE Editorial Board Members

Kari L. Keskinen
Pedro Ferreira Guedes de Carvalho
Carl R. Cramer
Rosa López de D´Amico
Keith Gilbert
John Nauright
Karin Volkwein
Filip Mess
Wolfgang Baumann
Detlef Dumon
Katrin Koenen

Also available in this series:

Physical Activity and Educational Achievement

Insights from Exercise Neuroscience

Edited by Romain Meeusen, Sabine Schaefer, Phillip Tomporowski and Richard Bailey

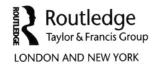

Routledge
Taylor & Francis Group

LONDON AND NEW YORK

First published 2018 by Routledge

2 Park Square, Milton Park, Abingdon, Oxfordshire OX14 4RN
52 Vanderbilt Avenue, New York, NY 10017

Routledge is an imprint of the Taylor & Francis Group, an informa business

First issued in paperback 2019

British Library Cataloguing-in-Publication Data
A catalogue record for this book is available from the British Library

Library of Congress Cataloging in Publication Data
A catalog record for this book has been requested

ISBN: 978-1-138-23497-0 (hbk)
ISBN: 978-0-367-23351-8 (pbk)

Typeset in Sabon
by Swales & Willis Ltd, Exeter, Devon, UK

Contents

Contributors

Editors

Richard Bailey is an internationally recognized authority on physical activity and human development. His academic qualifications are in Physical Education, Philosophy, and Psychiatry. Richard has been a Full Professor at several universities, including holding the Founding Chair in Sport and Education at the University of Birmingham, in the UK. He now works as Senior Researcher at the International Council of Sport Science and Physical Education (ICSSPE), the world umbrella body for sport, sport science and physical activity. He is a prolific author and blogger, including columns on physical activity and learning for *Psychology Today* and sport for the *Huffington Post*. Richard has worked with many national and international organizations, including the United Nations Educational, Scientific and Cultural Organization, Organisation for Economic Co-operation and Development, the World Health Organization, the International Olympic Committee (IOC), sportscoachUK, Die Deutsche Gesellschaft für Internationale Zusammenarbeit, the Professional Golfers Association, English Premier League, Sport England, and the English, Scottish, German, South African and Korean governments. He has directed studies that have influenced policy and practice around the world. He directed the English Talent Development for Schools programme, the IOC-funded Sport in Education worldwide study, and the sportscoachUK-funded Participant Development Review. More recently, he was the key contributor to the Nike-led Designed to Move initiative, and he is consultant for Nike's global physical activity programme.

Romain Meeusen is head of the Human Physiology Research Group at the Vrije Universiteit Brussel, Belgium. His research interest is focused on exercise and the brain in health and disease, exploring the influence of neurotransmitters on human performance, training and rehabilitation. Recent work is on thermoregulation, neurogenesis, cognition, nutrition in health and disease. He teaches on exercise physiology, training and coaching and sports physiotherapy. Romain has published about 550 articles and book chapters in peer-reviewed journals and 21 books on sport physiotherapy, and given lectures at more than 900 national and international conferences. He is past President of the Belgian Society of Kinesiology, the Belgian Federation of Sports Physiotherapy and the Society of Kinesiology, Belgium. He is former Board member of the European College of Sport Science (2000–2013), and of the American College of Sports Medicine (ACSM) (2010–2013). In 2006 he gave the president's lecture at the annual meeting of the ACSM. In 2009 he received the Belgian Francqui Chair at the Université Libre de Bruxelles on Exercise and the Brain. He is also holder of two named lecturing chairs at the Vrije Universiteit Brussel. He is director of the Human Performance lab of the Vrije Universiteit Brussel, where he works with several top athletes, and is scientific advisor of the Lotto Cycling Institute (Lotto-Soudal professional cycling team).

Sabine Schaefer studied psychology at the Free University in Berlin, Germany, where she received her PhD in 2005, with a thesis entitled 'Concurrent Cognitive and Sensorimotor Performance: A Comparison of Children and Young Adults'. After her dissertation, she worked as a research scientist at the Max Planck Institute for Human Development in Berlin. In 2015, she accepted a position as assistant professor for exercise psychology at the University of Leipzig. As of April 2016, she is professor for exercise science with a focus on motor and cognitive functioning at Saarland University. Her research focuses on the interplay of cognition and motor performances across the lifespan. In age-comparative studies, she has shown that older adults often have pronounced performance decrements when performing a cognitive and a motor task simultaneously, whereas children occasionally profit from such dual-task situations. Her research has also focused on cognitive and fitness interventions in old adults.

Phillip Tomporowski is a professor in the Department of Kinesiology at the University of Georgia, USA. He serves as Director of the Cognition and Skill Acquisition Laboratory and Principal Investigator of a U.S. Department of Education 21st Century Community Learning Center grant, the Physical Activity and Learning Program. Tomporowski and his colleagues mentor and guide a core of graduate and undergraduate students who provide physical activity, reading and mathematics enrichment programmes to elementary-aged children. He is an Associate Editor for the *Translational Journal of the American College of Sports Medicine*.

Authors

Serge Brand is research psychologist and psychotherapist at the University of Basel (Switzerland) Psychiatric Clinics (UPK), with special emphasis on patients with major depressive disorders, anxiety disorders, sleep disorders and stress-related disorders such as posttraumatic stress disorder. Further, his current position is adjunct professor at the Faculty of Psychology, Faculty of Medicine, at the Department of Sport, Exercise and Health of the University of Basel, and at the Kermanshah University of Medical Sciences, Kermanshah, Iran. Recently, Serge established a tight and productive collaboration with Markus Gerber and Uwe Pühse (Department of Sport, Exercise and Health of the University of Basel) to investigate the influence of physical activity in patients suffering from psychiatric disorders such as major depressive disorders and sleep disorders. Further, Serge's research interests focus on mental toughness, physical activity, sleep, biopsychological processes such as brain-derived neurotrophic factor and cortisol in patients with mood disorders, multiple sclerosis and autism spectrum disorder. More recently, Serge has also been focusing on topics of evolutionary psychology such as mate choice, the Dark Triad and romantic love.

Henning Budde, PhD, is a Professor for Sport Science and Research Methodology at the Medical School Hamburg, Germany, as well as at the Physical Activity, Physical Education, Health and Sport Research Centre, Sports Science Department at the Reykjavik University, Iceland and at the Lithuanian Sport University in Kaunas. In 2014 he finished his *Habilitation*, the highest academic degree in Germany, at the Humboldt University in Berlin. His research interest lies in the field of exercise neuroscience with a research focus that relates to the neurobiological effects of exercise on the brain and how the brain induces movements. He has published over 70 articles in peer-reviewed journals. As a teacher, he is interested in how these findings can be implemented in school settings.

Anna Bugge, PhD, is an Assistant Professor at the Center of Research in Childhood Health (RICH) in the Department of Sport Science and Clinical Biomechanics at the University of Southern Denmark. She earned her PhD in epidemiology from the same institution, and her MS from the Department of Nutrition, Exercise and Sports at the University of Copenhagen, Denmark. Her research has focused on the effects of physical activity on metabolic health and, in recent years, also on mental health, academic achievement and cognitive abilities. She has been involved in several large-scale, school-based intervention studies, and her research has been funded by both national and private health foundations and the Danish Ministry of Education.

Darla M. Castelli, PhD, is a Professor of physical education and health education pedagogy in the Department of Kinesiology and Health Education at the University of Texas at Austin, USA. Dr Castelli is the director of the Kinetic Kidz Lab where she studies the effects of physical activity on motor and cognitive performance in school-aged children and emerging adults. She is also interested in the relationship between metabolic risk factors and cognition and how physical activity can reverse its effects. She recently received a Graduate Teaching Award and is a Joe R. and Teresa Long Endowed Faculty Fellow. You can visit her webpage at www.edb.utexas.edu/education/.

Andy Daly-Smith has been a Senior Lecturer in Physical Activity, Exercise in Health for 11 years at Leeds Beckett University, UK. He is currently studying toward a PhD on exercise and cognition in obese children. Andy has a Master's degree in Sport and Exercise Science and a Postgraduate Certificate in Higher Education and is a Senior Fellow of the Higher Education Academy. His research focuses on two key themes: active ingredients in promoting physical activity and evaluating the effect of physical activity on physiological and psychosocial outcomes. Currently, in addition to his PhD, Andy is collaborating on projects in the following areas: active lesson implementation, evaluation of a primary school pedometer-based intervention on physical activity and cognition, and a process and impact evaluation of an active lessons intervention in secondary school. Andy is a founding member of the Yorkshire and Humber Physical Activity Knowledge Exchange, a multi-stakeholder partnership focused on improving the physical activity within the region.

R. Davis Moore is an expert on health behaviours and psychophysiological health. He holds degrees in psychology and exercise science from the University of Georgia, USA, and bio-behavioural science from the University of Illinois. He was also a research fellow at the University of Montreal, Canada, before moving to the University of South Carolina, where he is currently an assistant professor in the Department of Exercise Science and the Institute for Mind and Brain. Davis currently directs the Concussion and Health Neuroscience Laboratory, where he conducts research on the benefits of health behaviours on psychophysiological development, as well as the deleterious effects of sport-related concussion on brain and psychological health. He is a prolific author and regularly presents across North America and Europe. Through his research, Davis aims to improve public health by promoting the brain and body health of future generations.

Greta Defeyter took her first degree in Psychology at the University of Essex, UK. After completing an Economic and Social Research Council-funded PhD she began working as a Senior Research Officer at the University of Essex. She moved to Northumbria University in 2003 and became a Professor of Psychology in 2013. Greta is currently Director of Healthy Living at Northumbria University. She has an excellent reputation for her research with premier sports clubs and schools and she has led over 200 projects involving children and young people, examining the effects of various interventions on cognition. In addition to numerous international publications on cognitive child development her research has been highly commended by the Joseph Rowntree Foundation and she received a British Psychological Fellowship in 2014. Greta has received significant funding from the Economic Social Research Council, the Wellcome Trust, Public Health Englan, the British Academy, local authorities and industry.

Danusa Dias Soares received her PhD from the Department of Physiology and Biophysics at Universidade Federal de Minas Gerais, Brazil (2003), working with the serotonergic system and fatigue mechanisms during exercise. During her PhD she did an internship at INSERM U471 in Bordeaux, France (2002), where she worked with the serotonergic system and different models of stress. Danusa is a Full Professor of Exercise Physiology at Universidade Federal of Minas Gerais, where she has been teaching since 1994. She did her postdoctoral research on exercise, nutrition and the brain at Vrije Universiteit Brussel, Belgium (2014–2015). Danusa is currently the coordinator of the Exercise Physiology Laboratory (LAFISE) at Universidade Federal of Minas Gerais, where she is continuing her research on monoaminegic systems (serotonin and dopamine) and exercise and on nutritional manipulation on brain function and exercise.

Eric S. Drollette is an expert on developmental neurocognitive kinesiology. Eric's research background includes investigating the effects of physical activity interventions and acute exercise effects on higher-order cognitive processing, academic achievement and memory in developing children. His academic qualifications are in Kinesiology with a doctoral degree from the University of Illinois at Urbana-Champaign, USA. He currently holds a position as a postdoctoral research fellow at the Beckman Institute for Advanced Science and Technology. He recently accepted an Assistant Professor position at the University of North Carolina Greensboro where he will continue his research and aim to increase public health concerns regarding maladaptive health trends in paediatric populations and to promote early intervention as a means of improving cognitive health and functioning in today's youth.

Avery D. Faigenbaum is a Full Professor in the Department of Health and Exercise Science at the College of New Jersey, USA. His research interests focus on paediatric exercise, resistance training and preventive medicine. He is a Fellow of the American College of Sports Medicine and of the National Strength and Conditioning Association, and serves as Associate Editor of *Pediatric Exercise Science* and the *Journal of Strength and Conditioning Research*.

Karsten Froberg is Associate Professor of the Exercise Epidemiology Research Unit, Centre of Research in Childhood Health (RICH), Department of Sports Science and Clinical Biomechanics at the University of

Southern Denmark. Karsten is also Visiting Professor at the University of Rome 'Foro Italico'. He is a highly qualified researcher and university teacher in the area of childhood physical activity and health. His experience has been acquired from assignments at national and international universities, university colleges and sport organisations. He is an experienced supervisor of students at bachelor, master and PhD levels, and has acted as external examiner and official opponent in connection with masters' and PhD theses and dissertations, including serving as a national examiner for candidates for lectureships at teacher training colleges. He has worked as an international scientific consultant and been an invited speaker and chair at many national and international scientific conferences. To date, he is the author or co-author of 176 scientific papers.

Guido Fumagalli is Full Professor of Pharmacology at the Medical School of the University of Verona, Italy. His recent work has been on stem cells in brain disorders and on motor skills development. He has been dean of the Faculty of Sport Science, Provost for research and is now director of the Research Center on Child Motor Development of the University of Verona.

Markus Gerber is an internationally recognized researcher in the area of physical activity, stress and health across the lifespan. His academic qualifications are in physical education, sport and health psychology. Markus is currently a Professor in Sport and Psychosocial Health at the Department of Sport, Exercise and Health of the University of Basel, Switzerland. His main research interests focus on the potential of physical activity to protect against the negative health outcomes associated with chronic stress, physical activity in patients with mental disorders, physical activity counselling and promotion of behaviour skills, school-based and workplace health promotion, sleep and mental toughness. He has written over 100 academic papers and has published several books.

Marios Goudas is a Professor in the Department of Physical Education and Sport Science at the University of Thessaly, Greece. His research focuses on motivation, self-regulation and life skills programmes in physical education and sport.

Charles H. Hillman, PhD, is a Professor at Northeastern University, USA, where he currently holds appointments in the Department of Psychology and the Department of Health Sciences. He directs the Cognitive and Brain Health Laboratory, which has the mission of understanding the role of health behaviours on brain, cognition and academic performance to maximize health and well-being, and promote the effective functioning of individuals across the lifespan. Dr Hillman has published more than 140 refereed journal articles and ten book chapters, co-edited a text entitled *Functional Neuroimaging in Exercise and Sport Sciences* (Springer, 2012), and authored a monograph in the *Monographs of the*

Society for Research in Child Development. He has served on an Institute of Medicine of the National Academies committee entitled 'Educating the Student Body: Taking Physical Activity and Physical Education to School', and is a member of the 2018 Health and Human Services Physical Activity Guidelines for Americans Advisory Committee.

Anita Hökelmann studied Sport Science at the University of Leipzig, Germany, and has been working for many years as a sport scientist and professor in the field of motor control, motor learning and motor behaviour in sport at the Otto von Guericke University of Magdeburg. She is mainly interested in technical compositional types of sports, such as dancing, gymnastics, figure skating and diving.

Erin K. Howie is an Assistant Professor of Exercise Science in the Department of Health, Human Performance, and Recreation at the University of Arkansas in Fayetteville, Arkansas, USA, and an Adjunct Research Fellow in the School of Physiotherapy and Exercise Science at Curtin University in Perth, Western Australia. She received her PhD in Exercise Science from the University of South Carolina in May 2013. Her research interests generally include the promotion and measurement of physical activity in children, particularly the effects of physical activity on educational outcomes, implementation analysis of physical activity interventions and the influence of mobile technology on children's activity, movement and behaviour.

Lena Hübner studied sports science at Bielefeld University, Germany, and since 2015 has been research associate at the Institute of Human Movement Science and Health at Chemnitz University of Technology, Germany, in the working group Sports Psychology (with focus on Prevention and Rehabilitation). She is interested in the association between physical activity (chronic as well as acute exercise) and motor learning in older adults.

Jacob J. Kay is a doctoral student with particular interests in physical activity, cognition and brain health. He holds a Master's degree in psychology from the University of Wisconsin-Milwaukee, USA, and is currently working toward his PhD in Exercise Science at the University of South Carolina with an emphasis on rehabilitation. Jacob works primarily in the Concussion and Health Neuroscience Laboratory under the direction of Dr R. Davis Moore, where he conducts research on the psychophysiological benefits of exercise, and on advancing the assessment, management and rehabilitation of concussive injuries. For his dissertation, Jacob aims to investigate the benefits of graded physical activity and mindfulness training for individuals with post-concussion syndrome.

Thomas Klotzbier studied at the Institute for Sports and Movement Science at the University of Stuttgart, Germany, and has been working there for four years. In addition to didactic training in the soccer-specific area he brings with him a wealth of practical experiences from his background as a former soccer player. He further teaches an introductory course in motor learning and control as a set of principles and guidelines for students who aspire to become practitioners in various professions. In his current doctoral thesis he deals with motor–cognitive interferences across the entire lifespan and with different populations, in relation to sport performance as well as to a rehabilitative context. Thanks to his involvement in various science-oriented projects and studies, he was also able to gain worthwhile experience in the areas of Parkinson's disease, dementia and developmental coordination disorder; this has enabled him to lecture on motor learning and control theories in an application-oriented manner.

Kristel Knaepen, PhD, graduated as Master in Rehabilitation Science and Physiotherapy at the Vrije Universiteit Brussel, Belgium, in 2005, magna cum laude. From 2006 to 2008 she worked, respectively, at the Department of Rehabilitation Research and the Department of Movement Education and Sports Training of the Vrije Universiteit Brussel, Belgium. In 2008, she started working on the Automated Locomotion Training using an Actuated Compliant Robotic Orthosis (ALTACRO) project (http://altacro.vub.ac.be/), connecting human neuroscience and gait rehabilitation robotics, at the Department of Human Physiology of the Vrije Universiteit Brussel. In 2012, she joined the FP7 European project CYBERLEGs (www.cyberlegs.eu/), furthering her research on neurophysiology and human–robot interaction during walking. She received her PhD in Rehabilitation Science and Physiotherapy at the Vrije Universiteit Brussel in 2015. Currently, she holds a post-doc position at the German Sports University Cologne, continuing her research on the neurophysiology of human gait and studying the mechanisms of transfer of physical and cognitive training gains in healthy elderly people. She teaches exercise physiology and basics of neuroscience, has published six papers as first author and nine papers as co-author in peer-reviewed international journals and presented her findings at 19 (inter)national scientific conferences.

Flora Koutsandréou, MA, is a PhD student and researcher at the Medical School Hamburg, Germany. Her research focuses on the effects of different physical activity regimes on cognition, brain activity and steroid hormones.

Sebastian Ludyga is a postdoctoral researcher at the Department of Sport, Exercise and Health at the University of Basel, Switzerland. His research is focused on acute and chronic effects of exercise on cortical activity, event-related brain potentials and executive function in children with and without attention deficit-hyperactivity disorder. Recently, Sebastian Ludyga and his research group published a meta-analysis on the acute effects of moderate aerobic exercise on executive function in different age and fitness groups in *Psychophysiology*. In current projects, he is responsible for the development of short-term and long-term interventions targeting executive functions and cognitive control.

Bryan A. McCullick, PhD, taught PE at elementary, secondary and collegiate levels. At the University of Georgia, USA, he serves as Coordinator of the Health and Physical Education Program in the Department of Kinesiology. Stemming from his strong commitment and concern for quality PE, physical activity and sport instruction for children, his research has targeted issues germane to teacher/coach development and teaching/coaching expertise. A fellow in the Society of Health and Physical Educators (SHAPE) America Research Consortium, McCullick's research has appeared in the *Journal of Sport and Health Science*, *Journal of Teaching in Physical Education* (JTPE), *Research Quarterly for Exercise and Sport* (RQES), *Quest*, *Sport, Education and Society*, *International Journal of Sports Science and Coaching* and *Physical Education and Sport Pedagogy*. Dr McCullick is co-author of the text, *Enhancing Children's Cognition with Physical Activity* (Human Kinetics, 2015). He was an Associate Editor for RQES for 8 years and is on the editorial boards for JTPE, RQES and *Sport Coaching Review*.

Jim McKenna has been Professor of Physical Activity and Health for 11 years and is head of the Active Lifestyles research centre in the School of Sport at Leeds Beckett University, UK. This group centres on exploring responses to physical activity and optimizing the promotion of active living. Currently, he has 150+ peer-reviewed journal publications and numerous substantial grants focused on behaviour change as applied to physical activity and sport/coaching. That work spans individual, group and/or whole communities. Recent work has centred on how sport, especially soccer, can be used to encourage and support positive behaviour change among unreached community groups. Academically, his work draws mainly on positive psychology and neuroscience. His daily work revolves around research contracts, supporting academics and working with PhD students. He is a prize-winning teacher, research supervisor and journal reviewer. He also reviews extensively both for peer-reviewed journals and for respected funding agencies.

Terry McMorris is Emeritus Professor in the Institute of Sport, University of Chichester, UK, and Visiting Professor in the Department of Sport and Exercise at Portsmouth University. He is a former Visiting Professor at the Institute for Sport and Physical Education, University of Edinburgh, and teaches part-time in the Department of Psychology, Northumbria University. Terry originally trained as a schoolteacher and spent 19 years teaching in his home town of Hartlepool. He obtained a Master of Physical Education degree from the University of New Brunswick, Canada, before joining Chichester and then obtaining a PhD from the University of Southampton. He has published widely on the role of exercise, particularly acute exercise, on cognition and edited two books on the subject, one co-authored with Phillip Tomporowski and Michel Audiffren. He has also published books on motor learning and coaching, the latter with Tudor Hale.

Andrew Manley, PhD, is a principal lecturer in Sport and Exercise Psychology at Leeds Beckett University, UK. He is also a registered practitioner psychologist with the Health and Care Professions Council, a chartered sport and exercise psychologist with the British Psychological Society and a senior fellow of the Higher Education Academy. Andrew works with individuals and groups from a range of backgrounds to enhance psychological aspects of participation, performance and well-being. Andrew's primary research examines the impact of specific sources of information (e.g. reputation, clothing) on perception and behaviour within various interpersonal relationships (e.g. coach–athlete, student–teacher, client–practitioner). In addition, Andrew's recent work has explored the potential benefits of commercial technology (e.g. active video games) within three primary contexts: education, physical activity and sports injury rehabilitation.

Eduardo Matta Mello Portugal's Bachelor degree was in Physical Education at Gama Filho University, Brazil. He then achieved a Master of Science degree in Sports and Exercise Science at Rio de Janeiro State University. Currently, he is in the third year of a PhD in Psychiatry and Mental Health at Federal University of Rio de Janeiro and he is working as professor in a university (Faculdade Gama e Souza, Rio de Janeiro). His main interests are understanding how psychoneuroimmunogy mechanism are modulated by different configurations of exercise. He is testing for his PhD on the effects that affective response has in physiological response (i.e. immune system activation) during exercise.

Notger G. Müller is a trained neurologist and Professor at the Medical Faculty of the Otto von Guericke University Magdeburg, Germany, and head of the neuroprotection laboratory at the German Center for Neurodegenerative Diseases (DZNE) in Magdeburg. He is interested in individual differences in cognitive function, mainly attention and working memory, how these functions interact and how they can be enhanced by training.

Patrick Müller received his Master's degree in sports science in 2015 and is currently working on his PhD thesis in Exercise Science at the German Center for Neurodegenerative Diseases (DZNE) in Magdeburg, Germany. His research focuses on neural mechanisms of physical exercise and prevention strategies against neurodegenerative diseases. To understand the mechanisms of neurodegeneration better he is also studying medicine.

Claudia Niemann studied Biology and Physical Education at Free University of Berlin, Germany, and Humboldt University of Berlin. She received her PhD from Jacobs University Bremen in the field of movement and cognitive science in 2015. Recently she has authored and co-authored several articles in international journals on the effect of physical activity on cognitive performance across the lifespan.

Russell R. Pate is a Professor of Exercise Science in the Arnold School of Public Health at the University of South Carolina in Columbia, South Carolina, USA. Dr Pate is an exercise physiologist, receiving his PhD in Exercise Physiology from the University of Oregon in 1974, with more than 30 years' experience studying physical activity and fitness in children and adolescents. He currently serves as Chair of the National Physical Activity Plan Alliance. His research focuses on physical activity measurement, health implications and interventions in children and adolescents. Currently, he is conducting National Institutes of Health-funded research that is examining changes in physical activity as children transition from elementary to high school, studying community-based obesity prevention programmes, disseminating a physical activity intervention in preschools and developing a physical activity self-report instrument for youth.

Daniel M. Pendleton, MS, is a Research Professional at the University of Georgia, USA, in the Department of Kinesiology. His research interests include the effects of physical activity on cognition for young adults and children. He is interested in exercise-induced memory and achievement in children. Danny is also the Senior Project Director for the Physical Activity and Learning After School Program that is funded by the U.S. Department of Education and Georgia Department of Education. Danny also serves as the Lab Coordinator for the Cognition and Skill Acquisition Laboratory. Danny's dedication to research has enabled him to be a part of acute physical activity studies, as well as multi-year and multi-site school year length physical activity studies. Now in his final year of his PhD programme at the University of Georgia, Danny aims to understand more of the effects of physical activity on learning in school-aged children.

Caterina Pesce is a Professor in the Department of Movement, Human and Health Sciences at the Italian University Sport and Movement 'Foro Italico' of Rome, Italy. Her research is focused on exercise and cognition across the lifespan and the rise and fall of motor coordination and enriched physical education in skilled athletes. She is a founding member of the Italian Society of Movement and Sports Sciences. She is on the editorial board of the *Journal of Sport and Exercise Psychology* and an Associate Editor for the *Journal of Aging and Physical Activity*.

Uwe Pühse is a Full Professor and head of sport science at the Department of Sport, Exercise and Health at the University of Basel in Switzerland. In research and teaching he focuses on topics related to psycho-social aspects of physical activity and health. Uwe Pühse has authored and co-authored 199 publications. He is the treasurer of the International Association for Physical Education in Higher Education (AIESEP), member of the board of directors, and a fellow of AIESEP and the National Academy of Kinesiology. As principal investigator he is in charge of numerous research projects, such as the Sport and Social Inclusion (SSINC) study as well as the DASH study (Disease, Activity and Schoolchildren's Health in Marginalized Communities in Port Elizabeth, South Africa), funded by the Swiss National Science Foundation and the National Research Foundation in South Africa.

Nadja Schott is the Chair and Professor of Human Performance at the University of Stuttgart, Germany. She received her PhD in Sport Science from the University of Karlsruhe in 2000, and previously worked at the University of Giessen (Germany), University of Illinois (USA) and Liverpool Hope University (UK). Professor Schott's research and professional interests focus on exercise psychology and psychophysiology, cognitive neuroscience and motor performance across the lifespan. A major focus of her lab's recent research is the understanding of the mechanisms of age-related changes in motor representation in healthy individuals as well as patients with, e.g. developmental coordination disorder or Parkinson disease. She has published seven books, 18 book chapters and 37 articles in peer-reviewed journals. She is a former Associate Editor of *German Journal of Sport Psychology* and is currently a member of two editorial boards. Professor Schott is the Vice-President for Research and International Affairs of the German Society for Sport Psychology, and a fellow of the North American Society for the Psychology of Sport and Physical Activity.

Heidi Syväoja, PhD, is a researcher at LIKES Research Centre for Physical Activity and Health, Finland, with expertise in research on physical activity, cognitive functions and academic achievement. She earned her MS and PhD from the University of Jyväskylä, Finland, and has continued with postdoctoral studies determining the effects of physical activity and fitness on the cognitive prerequisites of learning.

Tuija Tammelin works as a Research Director at LIKES Research Centre for Physical Activity and Health, in Jyväskylä, Finland. Her research interest and expertise are in the epidemiology and physiology of physical activity, fitness and health during the life course. Her current research at LIKES focuses on the enhancement of physical activity: the determinants of physical activity and sedentary behaviours; the effectiveness of physical activity interventions in different populations; and the significance of physical activity on health, well-being and learning outcomes at different phases of life. Dr Tammelin is also responsible for the follow-up research related to the national physical activity programme Finnish Schools on the Move, which aims to make school days more active and pleasant in Finland's comprehensive schools.

Cajsa Tonoli did a joint PhD at the Vrije Universiteit Brussel, Belgium, and at the University of Lille, Nord de France. She currently works as a post-doctoral researcher at the University of Ghent, Belgium. Her research interest is focused on exercise physiology, nutrition, brain function and brain blood flow, especially in the diseased population, such as diabetes mellitus type 1 and 2. In this research, she specifically explores the influences of non-pharmacological interventions (such as exercise and nutritional interventions) on cognitive functions and brain blood flow in populations at risk for cognitive decline. In 2011, she won the Young Investigator Award for the best manuscript in the Dutch journal *Sport en Geneeskunde*. She teaches on exercise physiology and rehabilitation, internal diseases (diabetes type 1 and type 2) and cardiovascular diseases.

Patrizia Tortella is MS of Pedagogy and of Sport Sciences and PhD in Cognitive Sciences and Education. Teacher of disabled children, qualified trainer for several sport specialties, and organizer of physical activities for 0–6-year-old children, she is now post-doc at the Research Center on Child Motor Development of the University of Verona, Italy. Her research interests include interactions between executive functions and basic motor skills and educational strategies to promote physical activities in Italian preschoolers.

Claudia Voelcker-Rehage is Full Professor of Sports Psychology (with focus on Prevention and Rehabilitation) at Chemnitz University of Technology, Germany (since 2015). She graduated in 1998 and received her PhD in 2002 from University of Bielefeld, Germany. After that she was Postdoctoral Fellow at the School of Applied Physiology, Georgia Institute of Technology (Atlanta, GA, USA) and at International University Bremen (Germany). From 2007 she was University Lecturer at the Jacobs Center on Lifelong Learning and Institutional Development of Jacobs University Bremen (Germany), where she was appointed Full Professor of Human Performance in 2010. Claudia is Vice President, Finance and Managing Director of the German Society for Sport Psychology and Editor in Chief (Deputy) of the *German Journal of Exercise and Sport Research*. She is Review Editor at *Frontiers in Movement Science* and on the Editorial Board of the *European Review of Aging and Physical Activity*, the *Journal of Aging and Physical Activity* and

OBM Geriatrics. Her research interests include neurocognition and control of movement, learning and plasticity and the role of physical activity in cognitive development and health. She examines both children and adolescents as well as older adults.

Nadja Walter studied sport science at the Martin Luther University Halle-Wittenberg, Germany, from 2003 to 2008 and received her PhD in 2011, with a thesis entitled 'The Effects of a Specific Exercise Program on Children's Attention Performance in Primary Schools'. After her dissertation, she worked as a personal assistant for the president of the state sports association in Saxony-Anhalt. Since 2015 she has been a research scientist at the Institute for Sport Psychology and Sport Pedagogy (University of Leipzig) and works in the field of sport and exercise psychology. In previous studies she has shown the positive influence of a specific exercise programme on the attention performance of primary schoolchildren compared to regular PE lessons. Beside the focus on the interplay of cognition and motor performances, she is also dealing with psycho-social aspects in lifestyle intervention programmes, particularly in the field of exercise and communication.

Mirko Wegner completed his academic training in sport and exercise science and education at the University of Nebraska, USA, and Humboldt University, Berlin, Germany. He received his PhD in sport and exercise science from the Humboldt-University, Berlin. Mirko Wegner is a certified sport psychologist and his research interests focus on physiological and neurobiological responses to physical and psychological stress, and their affective, health-related and cognitive consequences. He is an expert in motivational processes and their behavioural and physiological associations. Mirko Wegner is currently working as a post-doctoral fellow for the Institute of Sport Science at the University of Bern, Switzerland. His teaching activities include lectures on exercise, health and prevention, sport, exercise and stress relationships as well as motivation and self-regulation in sports.

Introduction

Phillip Tomporowski, Richard Bailey,
Romain Meeusen and Sabine Schaefer

Educational achievement has been a cornerstone of the advances that have been achieved by humans over the past 10,000 years. The capacity for intergenerational transmission of knowledge has allowed each successive generation to build upon the experiences of past generations. With the rise of early cultures across the globe, specialists emerged who had specific skills that were important to the success of communities – builders, farmers, hunters, soldiers, and others. Skilled teachers took on the responsibility of educating the young. With the emergence of schools and universities, educators came to serve as the catalyst for cultural advances and to solve challenges that affected the survival of a culture.

Over the centuries, numerous methods of education have been developed and employed with the intent of preparing the next generation to meet the challenges they will face as adults. Regardless of the method, however, the goal is to have students learn: to acquire knowledge. While the methods of teaching have a very long past, the science of teaching and learning has a relatively short history. Contemporary educational psychologists can trace their philosophical roots to the ancient Greeks. However, the scientific study of learning emerged in the mid 19th century with the first systematic research conducted on processes such as memory, learning, information processing and problem solving. Pioneers in the fields of human development, psychology and physiology contributed seminal theories to explain learning. Jean Piaget hypothesized the emergence of cognition as a stage-like process. Ivan Pavlov explained associative learning in terms of irradiation of neural cortical activation, while Donald Hebb hypothesized the existence of neural networks and how they were modified by experience. Charles Sherrington advanced the view of synaptic communication and the integrative action of the nervous system. Advances in understanding the relation between the mind and body were made during the early to mid decades of the 20th century, although the extent to which these developments have impacted on day-to-day schooling is much less clear.

Technological advances in neuroscience over the past few decades have provided researchers the means to test and validate many of the early theories of learning and mental development. The rate of gain of knowledge of the structures and function of the brain has been astounding. Many of the achievements made by neuroscientists have practical significance for contemporary educators. In some cases, the results obtained by neuroscientists have corroborated long-held psychological and educational methods, whereas findings from brain research reveal the potential benefits of new or modified educational methods.

The contributors of the chapters in this book – *Physical Activity and Educational Achievement: Insights from Exercise Neuroscience* – describe how the neurosciences can enhance the intergenerational transfer of knowledge and support educational achievement. They seek to offer insights into an emerging field of research, with significant practical implications. Recent research has examined a range of processes associated with activity that are of interest and relevance to those working in education, including learning, memory and attention, mood and mental health symptoms. This book aims to build on this existing research, and look to the future. *Where will these lines of enquiry lead researchers and practitioners? What is its scope, and where are its limits? What effects will these developments have on the future practice of education?* So, the book is part *review* and part *preview* of a rapidly emerging and exciting field.

Physical Activity and Educational Achievement: Insights from Exercise Neuroscience begins with three contributions that set the scene for the rest of the book, and explore the possibilities and progress of the field of exercise neuroscience. Erin K. Howie and Russell R. Pate give an overview of the dose–response relationship between physical activity and educational achievement in children from experimental studies, specifically examining the educational effects of both acute exercise bouts and regular physical activity by varying doses of time, intensity and type of activity. Despite the justifiably cautious conclusions drawn by Howie and Pate, it seems clear that this is a key question for researchers to address. Phillip Tomporowski, Daniel M. Pendleton and Bryan A. McCullick set their sights on another fundamental concern for scientists in this area, namely the neurophysiology of learning. Their rich, historical review of contemporary theories of cognitive development and neurological development suggests that researchers should take into consideration evidence that suggests that physical activity may influence some types of learning differently from others. Charles H. Hillman and Darla M. Castelli complete this introductory part by evaluating the state of the science. Their chapter discusses some of the limitations of existing research and provides recommendations for future directions. Hillman and Castelli's thoughtful chapter raises challenging questions about both the science and application of findings from exercise neuroscience in the future.

The second part of the book considers insights and innovations in exercise neuroscience. So, the focus here is on empirical advances and hypotheses. Romain Meeusen, Cajsa Tonoli, Kristel Knaepen and Danusa Dias Soares discuss the several ways in which physical activity stimulates brain processes, and particularly how it can induce a cascade of molecular and cellular processes that support brain plasticity. The topic of Terry McMorris's chapter is the 'catecholamines hypothesis', that short-duration, moderate-intensity acute exercise induces increased concentrations of catecholamines, which aid cognitive performance of many tasks. However, as McMorris argues, matters become more complicated when activity is of a longer duration. Nadja Schott and Thomas Klotzbier discuss an elegant approach to assessing the interdependence of motor and cognitive function that comes from cognitive–motor interference research using dual-task conditions. In addition to reviewing the existing literature on this topic, they present an integrative framework for the interaction of cognition, motor performance and life-course factors, specifically considering the interactions between nature and nurture, embodied cognition and motor behaviour. Eduardo Matta Mello Portugal takes a similarly broad perspective on exercise–cognition interaction, in this case considering how physical activity can improve mental health and academic performance. Portugal argues that improvements in resilience, coping strategies, mood and affective response are positive responses to stress that are generated by molecular and structural neuronal changes. Claudia Voelcker-Rehage, Claudia Niemann and Lena Hübner take a different approach to these themes. Their contribution summarizes effects and associations of different types of physical activity and exercise on and with cognition, motor performance and brain structure and function. Voelcker-Rehage, Niemann and Hübner propose possible mechanisms by which physical activity facilitates cognitive and motor performance by briefly reviewing microscopic structural changes in animal research.

Most of the chapters in *Physical Activity and Educational Achievement* address issues of child and adolescent development. Patrick Müller, Anita Hökelmann and Notger G. Müller demonstrate that the vibrant research in exercise neuroscience also has great relevance for older people. In the context of the demographic change, with its unprecedented increase in absolute and relative numbers of senior citizens, they report accumulating evidence that exercise can induce neuroplasticity in adults and may reduce the risk of dementia. Nadja Walter and Sabine Schaefer return the discussion to children's exercise and cognition. Starting from findings suggesting that acute exercise can improve cognitive performances in children, they explore the conditions that are necessary for optimal performance enhancement. One specific area of recent research into cognitive performance relates to attention deficit-hyperactivity disorder (ADHD). Sebastian Ludyga, Serge Brand, Markus Gerber and Uwe Pühse present neurophysiological evidence of the differences between young people with and without ADHD, and review the impact of exercise interventions on cognitive functioning and ADHD-related behaviour. Henning Budde, Flora Koutsandréou and Mirko Wegner broaden the discussion to review evidence of the link between exercise and cognitive functioning in children and adolescents, considering the effects of different kinds of exercise on cognition. The contribution from R. Davis Moore, Jacob J. Kay and Eric S. Drollette continues this theme by offering an integrative perspective on how health factors, such as physical activity and fitness, translate into changes in academic skills and performance. The second part ends with a reflective and thought-provoking essay by Caterina Pesce, Avery D. Faigenbaum, Marios Goudas and Phillip Tomporowski. Beginning with a review of the evidence on the functional, structural and biological changes in children's brain related to physical activity, they go beyond the standard focus on combatting obesity to propose a vision of activity as a unique form of enrichment that impinges on lifelong brain sculpturing, cognitive flexibility and adaptability of goal-oriented achievement behaviour. Pesce and her colleagues offer a compelling, evidence-based case for a holistic education, grounded in the insights from exercise neuroscience.

The final part of *Physical Activity and Educational Achievement* focuses on practical concerns. Andy Daly-Smith, Jim McKenna, Greta Defeyter and Andrew Manley provide a valuable bridge between research into the impact of bouts of physical activity on cognition and the realities of the school. They review the evidence related to three intervention types: classroom exercise breaks, aerobic exercise outside the classroom, and cognitively engaging physical activity outside the classroom. They conclude that claims for the impact of acute bouts of physical activity on cognition within the school environment are best viewed with cautious optimism. Patrizia Tortella and Guido Fumagalli try to make sense of the sometimes contradictory evidence of the relationship between physical activity and executive functions. They suggest that the development of executive functions in children requires specific conditions, usually brought by movement-based games. Thus, Tortella and Fumagalli reiterate and refine one of the most persuasive general findings of exercise science, namely that the outcomes of physical activity are significantly dependent on the appropriateness of its design and delivery. With this in mind, it is interesting to consider Tuija Tammelin, Heidi Syväoja, Anna Bugge and Karsten Froberg's analysis of the practical application of physical activity research findings. Their case studies from Finland and Denmark highlight the strengths and weaknesses of 'bottom-up' and 'top-down' approaches to school-based programmes. In the final chapter, Richard Bailey sounds a cautionary note on the rise of brain-based ideas in schools. Contrasting the sound scientific research reported in this book with the pseudoscientific ideas and practices about the brain and physical activity that often infiltrate into schools, Bailey offers guidance on spotting bad and ugly science, and preventing it from wasting young people's time, energy and opportunities.

This book is offered as an introduction to, and state-of-the-science review of, a fascinating new area of the sport and exercise sciences. In endorsing this volume, the International Council of Sport Science and Physical Education's (ICSSPE's) Editorial Board was keen to promote a genuinely multidisciplinary and interdisciplinary project of great contemporary importance and urgency. We hope this book meets such a strict expectation. There has been no attempt at compiling these chapters to present a consensus statement for exercise neuroscience, nor of the specific issue of the relationship between physical activity and academic achievement. However, the contributors to this volume do demonstrate a remarkable degree of consistency in their key messages and cautions. That seems encouraging. We sincerely hope that *Physical Activity and Educational Achievement* provokes discussion, stimulates further research and acts as a springboard for new ways of thinking about the relationship between physical activity, cognition and education.

Part I

Progress and possibilities

Chapter 1

Physical activity and educational achievement

Dose–response relationships

Erin K. Howie and Russell R. Pate

Introduction

Mens sana in corpore sano (a sound mind in a sound body). Physical health and fitness have long been thought to benefit thinking and mental health. But how much physical activity do we need for a sound mind? This chapter gives an overview of the dose–response relationship between physical activity and educational achievement. It begins with definitions of key concepts followed by a brief history of the relationship between learning and movement. It then describes the dose–response as it relates to time, intensity and type. The chapter concludes with a summary and practical implications for educators.

Definitions and concepts

Physical activity (the dose)

Physical activity is bodily movement produced by muscle contractions that raise energy expenditure above resting levels (Caspersen, Powell, & Christenson, 1985). For the purposes of this chapter, which examines the effects of physical activity on educational outcomes, two subcategories of physical activity are specified:

1   *acute physical activity* – a single session of physical activity, e.g. 20 minutes of walking on the treadmill or 40 minutes of a physical education class;
2   *regular physical activity (or training)* – physical activity (or training) that is performed multiple times over a period of days, weeks, months or years, e.g. 30 minutes of recess every day for one school year or 8 weeks of an afterschool exercise training programme.

Moderate-to-vigorous physical activity is a specific intensity level of physical activity that is more than three times the amount of energy used while resting. This type of physical activity has been shown to be beneficial for cardiovascular health. Examples of moderate-to-vigorous physical activity include brisk walking (that makes you start to breathe heavily), running, jumping and dancing.

Physical fitness is a set of characteristics related to health or skills, such as aerobic capacity or muscular strength (Caspersen et al., 1985). While physical fitness is likely to be related to educational outcomes it will not be discussed in this chapter, as it is a health characteristic that is influenced but not determined by the behaviour of physical activity.

It is important to describe accurately in detail the dose or exposure when considering the relationship between physical activity and educational outcomes. Often times, a cross-sectional study will show that there is a positive relationship between physical fitness and educational outcomes. The media then interprets it into an article, 'Exercise makes you smart', when in reality there are many factors that contribute to physical fitness (including physiology).

Educational achievement (the outcome)

Educators and researchers have examined a wide variety of educational outcomes. Three different types of educational outcomes are described below and depicted in Figure 1.1.

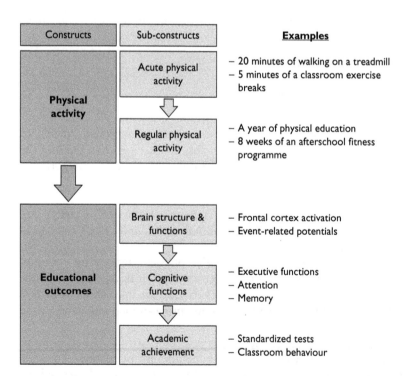

Figure 1.1 Deconstructing the constructs in the relationships between physical activity and educational outcomes.

Brain structure and functions

Physical structures and physiological processes underlie all thought processes. Brain functions can include the anatomy of specific brain structures, such as the size of the hippocampus, or electrical activity measured through electroencephalogram (EEG) to examine the activity of certain areas of the brain (Khan & Hillman, 2014). Many of the tests used to measure brain structure / function may also measure cognitive functions. For example, EEG or functional imaging may be used during the flanker task, which measures executive functions; such combinations are neurocognitive outcomes.

Cognitive functions

Cognitive functions, or mental actions, are the result of the underlying brain functions and consist of several cognitive processes, including attention, memory and problem solving (Aukrust, 2011). One example of a commonly used measure is the d2 test of attention. Many studies have examined executive functions or high-level, complex cognitive processes which control other processes. Executive functions include cognitive flexibility or shifting, working memory and inhibition (Miyake et al., 2000). Executive functions can be assessed through tests such as flanker tasks, the Stroop test (Chan, Shum, Toulopoulou, & Chen, 2008) or batteries such as the Delis-Kaplan Executive Function System.

Academic achievement

The most relevant category of educational outcomes for educators is academic achievement. Measures of academic achievement include standardized batteries, such as the Stanford Achievement test or Wide Range Achievement Test; school grades; or scores on standardized tests such as school- or state-level achievement tests.

It is important to note that brain structure and functions, cognitive functions and academic achievement all interact in multiple ways. For example, improved brain activation in the frontal cortex may lead to improved performance on an executive function cognitive task, which may lead to better maths performance on a standardized test. Similarly, improved inhibition on a cognitive task may relate to improved on-task behaviour in the classroom and ultimately better school grades. In the education literature, it has long been debated if time-on-task directly relates to academic achievement outcomes such as performance on standardized tests (Karweit, 1984).

As well as accurately describing and defining physical activity, it is important to describe the educational outcome of interest. The same cross-sectional study that showed that there was a positive relationship between physical fitness and educational outcomes may have examined electrical activity in the brain during a specific task. The article reports 'Exercise makes you smart'; however, brain activity during a single task does not mean that child had higher intelligence or will do better in school. It is essential to take a critical view when reading and interpreting research studies.

Dose

The dose of physical activity is the amount of physical activity that a child receives. This is composed of the frequency (when considering multiple sessions of regular physical activity), intensity (light or moderate-to-vigorous physical activity), and time (how long is/are the session(s)). A description of the dose can also include the type of activity. In traditional exercise prescription, dose may refer to aerobic activity, muscular strength training or flexibility exercises. The majority of studies about the relationship between physical activity and educational outcomes have examined aerobic physical activity. But within aerobic exercises, the type of activity has varied from skills-based physical education, to walking on a treadmill, to physical activity that is integrated with learning activities also known as active lessons.

Dose–response relationship

This term refers to the varying response in an outcome as the result of varying exposures or treatments. Studies of the dose–response of physical activity on educational outcomes could examine the effect of different durations, differing intensities or different types of physical activity. For example, 10 minutes per day of regular physical activity may result in an increased test score of 10 points on a 100-point scale. However, 20 minutes per day may result in an increased test score of 20 points.

History of physical activity in education

Physical activity has long been considered an important part of overall mental health and intellectual capacity.

In early Greece, excellence in both mind and body were prized (Van Dalen, 1953, p. 35). The Athenians integrated physical education into society as a way to develop the mind through the physical (Van Dalen, 1953, p. 47). Many Greek philosophers supported incorporating physical activity in daily life. One quote that has been attributed to Socrates states:

> For in everything that men do the body is useful. . . Why even in the process of thinking, in which the use of the body seems to be reduced to a minimum, it is a matter of common knowledge that grave mistakes may often be traced to bad health.
>
> (Van Dalen, 1953, p. 61)

The now common phrase of the Roman poet Juvenal, *mens sana in corpore sano*, again emphasized the connection between mental and physical translated into 'a sound mind in a sound body'.

From the early middle ages of the fifth to tenth centuries, when education was controlled by the Church, physical education was included in the curriculum as part of the training to be a functional and valued member of society. Later, in the 14th and 15th centuries, sport and activity were considered critical parts of a humanistic and holistic education (Zeigler, 1967). In the late 17th century, the influential educational philosopher John Locke, who was trained in medicine, opened his work 'Some thoughts concerning education' with the words, 'A sound mind in a sound body, is a short, but full description of a happy state in this world' (Glassford & Redmond, 1967). This shows how educators valued physical health.

Physical activity became more formalized during the 19th century. 'Rational recreation' or the belief that exercise refreshed the mind and body for society and work was promoted by middle- and upper-class Victorians (Rader, 2004). The Greek Olympics was revived in its modern form at the end of the century as a way to promote peaceful competition and national pride (Rader, 2004). John Dewey led educational reforms advocating for formal physical education in schools. Dewey believed in 'education though the physical' (Barney, 1967). By 1967, physical education was a required subject in 72 out of 73 countries studied by the International Council for Health, Physical Education and Recreation (Glassford & Redmond, 1967). The World-wide Survey of School Physical Education of 2013 confirms that 97% of countries have a physical education requirement; however, these policies are often not carried out in practice (United Nations Educational Scientific and Cultural Organization (UNESCO), 2014).

Physical education has thus become a pillar of children's education around the world (Van Dalen, 1953). In addition to traditional physical education, physical activity has been incorporated into the modern school day through other opportunities such as recess, school sports) both extra- and intra-mural), music and dance, and classroom activity breaks. However, with increasing pressure from high-stakes standardized tests, school teachers and administrators are cutting time for physical activities in favour of core subjects (Center on Education Policy, 2011). Decreasing physical activity time may have unintended consequences; emerging research suggests that physical activity promotes learning, as highlighted throughout the chapters in this book. Thus, an understanding of the optimal dose to benefit educational outcomes is needed for educators to incorporate and maintain physical activity in schools.

Review of the evidence on the dose–response of physical activity and academic outcomes

Research on the educational effects of physical activity has been ongoing since the mid 20th century, and the number of studies published each year is increasing exponentially. A key study in France in the 1950s examined the effects of increasing physical education from 8% to 22% of the school day on standardized test performance. After 20 years, schools with increased physical education performed better on French national examinations (Glassford & Redmond, 1967). A review conducted in 2012 located 125 published studies on the topic (Howie & Pate, 2012). While the majority of studies found a positive relationship between physical activity and improved educational outcomes, most of the studies were of low quality and used cross-sectional designs. In addition, studies used varied doses of physical activity exposures and measures of educational outcomes, making comparisons across studies difficult.

This chapter provides a summary of the research to date on the dose–response effect of physical activity on educational outcomes. Because experimental and quasi-experimental research designs provide the best understanding of the causal relationship between physical activity and educational outcomes, this chapter will focus on those types of experimental studies and will not include cross-sectional or longitudinal studies.

For this chapter, a narrative review was conducted. The selection of articles began with the studies identified in the previous review (Howie & Pate, 2012). Thirty additional relevant experimental studies were identified from the literature, in addition to the 66 experimental studies identified in the previous review.

Articles were summarized by three components of dose, as described in an earlier section: time (duration and frequency), intensity and type. Articles were grouped by those looking at the effects of acute physical activity or regular physical activity. Ideally, one could combine the duration, frequency and intensity of physical activity to create a single metric of the exposure dose (i.e. total amount of energy expended). However, due to inconsistencies in reporting it was not possible to compute a single metric.

Time (duration and frequency)

Acute studies

Studies that have examined the effects of a single bout of physical activity on educational outcomes (brain structure and functions, cognitive functions and academic achievement) have varied in duration from 1 minute to 60 minutes of physical activity. Most of the acute studies have examined brain functions, cognitive functions and on-task behaviour. This section will summarize studies that have examined 10 minutes or less of acute physical activity, 11–20 minutes of physical activity, 21–30 minutes of physical activity and greater than 30 minutes of physical activity.

SHORTER BOUTS OF ≤10 MINUTES

Few studies have examined the effects of shorter bouts of acute physical activity on educational outcomes, despite the practicality and feasibility of taking short breaks throughout the school day. Four studies have shown that short bouts of physical activity have improved at least one educational outcome. In a study by Etnier, Labban, Piepmeier, Davis, and Henning (2014), children ($n = 43$, ages 11–12 years) completed the Progressive Aerobic Cardiovascular Endurance test, which took between 2 and 7 minutes to complete. The results showed that children had improved performance during specific trials of the Rey Auditory Verbal Learning Test following the brief physical activity, but did not improve overall performance compared to the control condition. Shorter bouts have also been shown to improve selective attention. A recent study ($n = 88$, ages 9–11 years) of just 4 minutes of high-intensity exercise improved accuracy on the d2 test of attention compared to a control condition (Ma, Le Mare, & Gurd, 2015).

Two small studies have examined the effects of 5 minutes of exercise on maths fluency and behaviour. A small study of 19 second-graders found that a 5-minute walk/run break improved children's maths fluency on a 1-minute maths test (Maeda & Randall, 2003). In a single case study of one 13-year-old boy with hyperactivity, 5 minutes of coached exercise improved observed hyperactivity but not achievement on an arithmetic and reading test (Etscheidt & Ayllon, 1987). However, these were both small studies.

Ten-minute bouts of physical activity have also been shown to improve on-task behaviour (Mahar et al., 2006), attention (Budde, Voelcker-Rehage, Pietrabyk-Kendziorra, Ribeiro, & Tidow, 2008) and executive functions (through performance on the flanker task) (Vazou & Smiley-Oyen, 2014) in three separate studies. In the first study, Mahar et al. (2006) observed on-task behaviour in students ($n = 243$, ages 8–9) following 10 minutes of active lessons and found that behaviour improved following the exercise compared to controls. In the second study, Budde et al. (2008) found that 10 minutes of coordinative exercise ($n = 115$, ages 13–16 years) improved attention on the d2 test of attention. In the third and most recent study, Vazou and Smiley-Oyen (2014) found that 10 minutes of an active lesson improved executive functions ($n = 35$, ages 9–11 years) measured via the flanker task, particularly inhibition, as compared to a control condition.

Summary Short bouts of less than 10 minutes of physical activity may have benefits for educational outcomes, particularly cognitive or on-task behavioural outcomes.

MEDIUM BOUTS OF 11–20 MINUTES

Studies examining 11–20 minutes have found improvements in classroom behaviour (Evans, Evans, Schmid, & Pennypacker, 1985; Jarrett et al., 1998), concentration (Caterino & Polak, 1999), spelling achievement (Duncan & Johnson, 2014) and EEG signals (Hillman, Kamijo, & Scudder, 2011), as well as other cognitive and achievement measures.

Several laboratory studies conducted by the same research group have utilized a 20-minute treadmill walking protocol to study the effects of physical activity on EEG signals, cognitive performance on tasks such as the flanker task and academic achievement. Most of these studies have reported improvements in at least one educational outcome, such as event-related potentials, indicators of executive function or performance on standardized achievement tests (Hillman et al., 2011). For example, in 2009, Hillman et al. found that 20 minutes of treadmill walking ($n = 20$, ages 9–11) resulted in an improvement in brain waves, specifically the P3 wave that indicates attentional allocation as well as response accuracy on a modified flanker task. They also reported improved performance on the reading component of the Wide Range Achievement Test. However, there were no improvements on the spelling or arithmetic components.

Summary   Many studies have examined the acute effects of 11–20 minutes of physical activity and have found positive effects on cognition, behaviour and achievement.

MEDIUM BOUTS OF 20–30 MINUTES

Approximately six studies have used 30-minute acute bouts of exercise and have found improvements in attention (Pellegrini & Davis, 1993; Pellegrini, Huberty, & Jones, 1995), reaction time (Ellemberg & St-Louis-Deschênes, 2010), sustained attention (Palmer, Miller, & Robinson, 2013), time-on-task (Mullender-Wijnsma et al., 2015) and recall (Norris, Shelton, Dunsmuir, Duke-Williams, & Stamatakis, 2015). Pelligrini and colleagues have conducted multiple studies on the effects of manipulating recess scheduling on observed classroom behaviour and found that students are more fidgety and less attentive during prolonged periods without recess (Pellegrini & Davis, 1993; Pellegrini et al., 1995). Children have shown improved on-task behaviour ($n = 81$, ages 7–9) following 30 minutes of a physically active lesson (Mullender-Wijnsma et al., 2015), faster reaction times on a simple computerized reaction test after 30 minutes of cycling on an ergometer ($n = 72$, ages 7–11) (Ellemberg & St-Louis-Deschênes, 2010), and improved sustained attention (but not response inhibition) on the Picture Deletion Task for Preschoolers following a 30-minute movement programme ($n = 16$, ages 3–4) (Palmer et al., 2013). However, Norris et al. (2015) compared a 30-minute active lesson to a non-active lesson ($n = 85$, ages 9–10 years) and found that there were no differences in the content recalled.

Summary Bouts of 30 minutes of acute physical activity have been shown to improve cognitive functions and on-task behaviour, but the evidence is inconclusive.

LONGER BOUTS OF >30 MINUTES

Not many studies have examined the effects of longer bouts of 40, 45, 50 and 55 minutes of physical activity on educational outcomes. After 40 minutes of physical education children showed improved memory recall ($n = 52$, ages 11–12 years) using a free-recall visual memory task (Pesce, Crova, Cereatti, Casella, & Bellucci, 2009).

After 45 minutes of exercise in younger children ($n = 10$, ages 5–6 years) there were no effects of the exercise condition compared to the control condition on the cognitive measures in the Schufried Vienna Test System (Mierau et al., 2014). However, the researchers found differences in EEG monitoring, specifically increased alpha-1 power, following exercise, which indicates reduced arousal in response to visual stimuli and was interpreted as increased inhibition.

After 50 minutes of regular physical education lesson, a cognitive activity or a combined cognitive and physical education class ($n = 113$, ages 8–11), children had equally improved performance on the d2 test of attention (Gallotta et al., 2015).

After 55 minutes of exercise training class ($n = 56$, ages 5–8), children improved maths performance during a timed maths test; however, there was no comparison condition or group (Bala, Adamovic, Madic, & Popovic, 2015).

Summary The limited evidence has found improvements in educational outcomes following longer-duration bouts of physical activity.

COMPARISONS BETWEEN DURATIONS

Due to varying study designs, types of activity and outcome measures, there are many inconsistencies in the findings from these acute studies. Yet, even studies directly comparing durations have had inconsistent results.

Two studies, however, have directly compared short durations of physical activity, with contrasting findings. Molloy (1989) found that children with hyperactivity ($n = 32$, ages 6–11) showed improved attention after a 5-minute session active break but not following the 10-minute session. In contrast, Craft (1983) found no improvements ($n = 62$, ages 7–10) following 1, 5 or 10 minutes of cycling on the Wechsler Intelligence Scale for Children

(WISC) compared to a within-subject no-exercise control. Other studies comparing longer durations in addition to shorter durations of 10 minutes or less will be discussed later.

The majority of studies have found positive effects with longer durations of physical activity. Kubesch et al. (2009) compared a shorter 5-minute bout of exercise to a longer 30-minute physical education class (n = 81, ages 13–14 years) and found that 30 minutes of physical education, but not 5 minutes of exercise, improved inhibition and working memory as measured by the flanker task. In a complex study design, McNaughten and Gabbard (1993) compared 20, 30 and 40 minutes of paced walking on maths performance using a 90-second timed maths test. Children improved maths performance after 30 and 40 minutes of walking compared to 20 minutes, but these differences occurred only during the afternoon, and no improvements in performance occurred during the morning. Gabbard and Barton (1979) compared the effects of 20, 30, 40 and 50 minutes of relay activities on maths performance on a timed maths test in children (n = 108, ages 7–8 years). They found that children performed better only after 50 minutes of physical activity. Similarly, Altenburg, Chinapaw, and Singh (2016) found that one 20-minute bout of video-based dance activities (n = 56, ages 10–13) did not improve selective attention, but two 20-minute bouts (total of 40 minutes with a break in between) did result in improved performance.

However, others have found positive effects with shorter durations of physical activity. Molloy (1989) compared the effects of 5 vs. 10 minutes of exercise and found improved arithmetic performance in the entire class (n = 32) and attention in children with hyperactivity (n = 2) after 5 minutes but not after 10 minutes.

Other studies have suggested that there may be an inverted-U-shaped response, where too short and too long durations do not benefit educational outcomes. Holmes, Pellegrini, and Schmidt (2006) compared the effects of 10, 20 and 30 minutes of recess on observed behaviour in preschool students (n = 27, ages 4–5). They found that attention improved following all durations; however, the highest improvement occurred following 20 minutes. Similarly, Howie, Beets, and Pate (2014) directly compared 5, 10 and 20 minutes of classroom exercise breaks and found that observed classroom behaviour only improved after 10 minutes; however, 10 and 20 minutes of physical activity improved maths fluency during a timed maths test (Howie, Schatz, & Pate, 2015).

Summary   Of these eight studies, five compared 5-minute bouts to longer bouts. Three of the five studies found no improvements in educational outcomes after 5 minutes but did find improvements following longer durations. One of the five studies found no improvements following any duration of exercise, and one found improvements with 5 minutes but not with longer bouts.

Table 1.1 Comparison of duration of physical activity exposure in studies of the acute effects of physical activity on educational outcomes

Study	Physical activity	Outcome	Duration of exposure (minutes)
Craft (1983)	Cycling	WISC	*1 5 10*
Molloy (1989)	Classroom exercise	Arithmetic	**5** *10*
Howie et al. (2015)	Classroom exercise	Maths	*5* **10 20**
Howie et al. (2014)	Classroom exercise	Behaviour	*5* **10** *20*
Kubesch et al. (2009)	Physical education	Flanker	*5* **30**
Holmes et al. (2006)	Recess	Observed behaviour	**10* 20 30***
McNaughten and Gabbard (1993)	Walking	Maths	*20* **30 40**
Altenburg et al. (2016)	Video-based dance	Selective attention	*20* **40**
Gabbard and Barton (1979)	Relay activities	Maths	*20 30 40* **50**

WISC, Wechsler Intelligence Scale for Children.

Bold font indicates an improvement in educational outcomes while *italic* indicates no improvement.

*In Holmes et al. improvements were seen following 10, 20 and 30 minutes; however the strongest effects were seen after 20 minutes.

Four of five studies that examined 30- and 40-minute bouts compared to shorter durations found positive effects in the longer bouts (Table 1.1).

This limited evidence may suggest that longer bouts are more effective in improving educational outcomes. However, these comparative studies are inconclusive. While some have found longer bouts to be effective, others have found shorter bouts. These inconsistencies may be dependent on the study populations (e.g. age, hyperactivity) as well as the educational outcome measures (e.g. WISC, direct observation of behaviour).

Regular physical activity

It is more difficult to summarize the dose of regular physical activity on educational outcomes, as there are many variations in not only the duration of each session, but also the duration of the intervention and the frequency of the sessions. The duration in the interventions tested has varied from five sessions (Klein & Deffenbacher, 1977) to 5 years (Bunketorp Kall, Malmgren, Olsson, Linden, & Nilsson, 2015; Kall, Nilsson, & Linden, 2014), with large variation in durations. Longer interventions seem to have more null findings, but this may be due to more rigorous study designs (i.e. randomized controlled trials) or the choice of measures (i.e. academic achievement or standardized test or report cards vs. cognition).

Almost every study that has examined the effects of regular physical activity has used a different educational outcome measure, as seen in Table 1.2.

Table 1.2 Summary of educational outcome measures used in studies of regular physical activity interventions

Author	Age (years)	Educational outcome measure
Brain structure and function and cognitive measures		
Chasey and Wyrick (1970)	6–12	Winter Haven Perceptual Forms Test
Klein and Deffenbacher (1977)	8–9	Matching Familiar Figures Test, Continuous Performance Task
Sharpe (1979)	4–8	Piagetian tasks
Tuckman and Hinkle (1986)	9–11	Devereaux Elementary School Behavior Rating Scale, Alternate Uses Test, Maze Tracing Speed Test
Bluechardt and Shephard (1995)	8–11	Self-Perception Profile for Learning Disabled Students, Context-based Test of Social Skills
Manjunath and Telles (1999)	12–17	Critical Flicker Fusion Frequency
Davis et al. (2007)	7–11	Cognitive Assessment System
Hill et al. (2010)	8–11	Paced serial addition, size ordering, listening span, digit-span backwards, digit-symbol encoding
Fisher et al. (2011)	5–6	Cambridge Neuropsychological Test Battery, Attention Network Test, Cognitive Assessment System, Conner's Parent Rating Scale
Kamijo et al. (2011)	7–9	Modified Sternberg task, EEG
Chang et al. (2013)	6–7.5	Modified flanker, EEG
Crova et al. (2014)	9–10	Random number generation task
Hillman et al. (2014)	9–11	Modified flanker, color-shape switch task, EEG
de Greeff et al. (2016)	7–8	Golden Stroop, Digit span backward and visual span backward, Wisconsin Card Sorting Test
Reed et al. (2010)	8–9	Standard Progressive Matrices, Palmetto Achievement Challenge Tests (South Carolina, USA)
Davis et al. (2011)	7–11	Cognitive Assessment System, Woodcock-Johnson Tests of Achievement III
Academic achievement		
Corder (1966)	12–17	Wechsler Intelligence Scale for Children
McCormick et al. (1968)	6–7	Lee-Clark Reading Test, Primer
Fretz et al.(1969)	5–11	Wechsler Intelligence Scale for Children
O'Connor (1969)	6–7	Metropolitan Readiness and Metropolitan Achievement Tests
Brown (1976)	12	Stanford-Binet Intelligence Test
Dwyer et al. (1983)	10	Australian Council for Educational Research arithmetic, GAP reading, KAB Child Behaviour Scale

Pollatschek and O'Hagan (1989)	11–13	Gapadol Reading Comprehension test, Staffordshire Test of Computation
Shephard (1996)	6–11	Report cards
Sallis et al. (1999)	10–12	Metropolitan Achievement Tests
Fredericks et al. (2006)	5–7	Aptitude Test for School Beginners, reading and maths age, draw-a-person
Ahamed et al. (2007)	9–11	Canadian Achievement Test (Canada)
Reynolds and Nicolson (2007)	7–11	National Foundation for Educational Research reading test, standardized attainment tests (UK), school reading grades
Uhrich and Swalm (2007)	10–11	Gates-MacGinitie Reading Test 4th Edition
Ericsson (2008)	5–7	Conner' Rating Scales-Teacher, Swedish and maths achievement
Donnelly et al. (2009)	7–11	Wechsler Individual Achievement Test II
Hollar et al. (2010)	6–9	Florida Comprehensive Achievement Test (USA)
Katz et al. (2010)	7–9	Missouri Academic Performance scores (USA), Independence School District progress report
Chaya et al. (2012)	7–9	Malin's Intelligence Scale for Indian Children, Wechsler Intelligence Scale for Children II
Gao et al. (2013)	10–12	Reading and maths scores from Utah Criterion Reference Test (USA)
Ardoy et al. (2014)	12–14	Spanish Overall and Factorial Intelligence Test, school grades in core and other subjects
Kall et al. (2014)	10–11	National standardized tests (Sweden)
Bunketorp Kall et al. (2015)	10–12?	Standardized tests scores (Sweden), MRI
Kirk and Kirk (2016)	4–5	Early literacy skills: picture naming, rhyming and alliteration individual growth and development indicators
Mullender-Wijnsma et al. (2016)	7–8	One-minute reading test, Speed Test-Arithmetic, Child Academic Monitoring System (Netherlands)

EEG, electroencephalogram; KAB, Kaufman Assessment Battery; MRI, magnetic resonance imaging.

Four studies of varying durations of regular physical activity used the WISC as the measure of educational outcomes. Three studies have found improvements on the WISC with regular physical activity. Firstly, exposure of 1 hour of physical education on 5 days per week for 4 weeks found improved full and verbal WISC scores in children with intellectual disabilities ($n = 14$, ages 12–17 years) (Corder, 1966). Secondly, both a 45-minute physical activity condition and yoga condition on 6 days a week for 3 months improved children's performance ($n = 193$, ages 7–9) (Chaya, Nagendra, Selvam, Kurpad, & Srinivasan, 2012). Thirdly, a longer intervention of 10 minutes of physically active lessons nine times per week for three academic years ($n = 203$, ages 7–11 years) found improvements in the composite, reading, maths and spelling scores (Donnelly et al., 2009). Contrastingly, in another study, 8 weeks of physical activity with unreported frequency or duration in a developmental clinic ($n = 84$, ages 5–11 years) resulted in no changes in WISC.

Only two studies of regular physical activity have directly compared duration or frequency. Davis et al. (2007) conducted an after-school programme ($n = 94$, ages 7–11 years) in overweight children. One group received 20 minutes of physical activity on 5 days per week for 15 weeks, while the other group received 40 minutes for the same period. Before and after the intervention, children completed four subscales of cognitive functions: Planning, Attention, Simultaneous and Successive. Only the group which received 40 minutes of physical activity per session improved on the Planning subscale of the Cognitive Assessment System, which is a measure of executive functions.

In the second comparative study, Ardoy et al. (2014) compared performance ($n = 67$, ages 12–14 years) on the Spanish Overall and Factorial Intelligence Test in classes that had received 55 minutes of physical education twice a week and classes that had four classes per week. There were no differences in cognitive performance between the groups; however, a third group that received four sessions of high-intensity physical education did improve performance, suggesting that intensity of physical activity may be important.

Summary

The optimal duration and frequency of regular physical activity are unknown.

Intensity

In addition to the time of physical activity, the intensity of physical activity contributes to the dose. A child who participates in high-intensity activity would receive a higher dose of physical activity compared to another child participating in the same duration of light activity. The majority of studies, on both acute and regular physical activity, have examined moderate-to-vigorous intensity. The most common measure of intensity reported is heart rate. Other studies have not measured, not reported or used mixed intensities such as in a physical education class. As the studies on moderate-to-vigorous activity are numerous and have been described in the previous section on time, the following examines the potential differential effects of light- and high-intensity activity.

Light-intensity activity

Three studies have examined the acute effects of light physical activity on educational outcomes. Both Krebs, Eickelberg, Krobath, and Baruch (1989) and Eickelburg and Less (1975) examined the effects of 6 minutes of passive exercise on children with physical disabilities and found improved figural and associative learning respectively. Norlander, Moås, and Archer (2005) also found improvements, but in concentration, following 5–10 minutes of stretching and relaxation.

Slightly more studies have examined regular light activity on educational outcomes. The light activity has ranged from yoga (Chaya et al., 2012; Manjunath & Telles, 1999) to active lessons (Valle et al., 1986) and the majority of studies found improvements in various cognitive tasks.

High-intensity activity

Few studies have examined the effects of high-intensity activity. In one study using only high-intensity activities, Ma et al. (2015) examined the effects of 4 minutes of high-intensity acute physical activity. The researchers found improved accuracy on the d2 test of attention following the high-intensity activity compared to no activity.

Four studies have directly compared varying intensities. Three out of the four studies directly comparing intensities found no differences in educational outcomes between intensities for equivalent durations of activity. Ardoy et al. (2014) compared 55 minutes of high (heart rate above 120 beats per minute) versus moderate intensity of a traditional physical education class activity over 4 weeks. Only the high-intensity group improved cognition on the Spanish Overall and Factorial Intelligence Test and academic performance assessed by student grades.

The remainder of the studies, however, have found no differences in the effects between intensities. Chang, Tsai, Chen, and Hung (2013) compared 35 minutes of low (40–50% maximum heart rate) versus moderate intensity (60–70% of maximum heart rate) for two sessions per week for 8 weeks and found that both groups improved on the flanker task and EEG equally. Chaya et al. (2012) compared 45 minutes of light-intensity yoga 6 days per week for 3 months to moderate physical activity sessions and found no differences as both groups improved on the WISC equally. Finally, Duncan and Johnson (2014) compared moderate activity (50% of heart rate reserve) to high-intensity activity (75% of heart rate reserve) on a cycle ergometer and found that both conditions equally improved spelling performance.

SUMMARY

With such limited evidence examining varying intensities of physical activity, it is difficult to make conclusions about the ideal intensity of physical activity either acutely or regularly to improve educational outcomes.

Type of activities

The types of activities used in these research studies have varied greatly from monitored physical activity on a cycle ergometer, to game and skill-based physical activity during physical education, to physical activity that is combined with educational activities. Often, the exact type of activity is not described.

Several studies on the acute effects of physical activity have used brief classroom exercise breaks integrated with academic content (i.e. jumping while counting) (Mahar et al., 2006) to longer active lessons such as an active lesson about the London Olympics (Norris et al., 2015). These active lessons are ideal for teachers with limited time as they efficiently integrate both learning and physical activities. Active lessons of varying durations have been found to improve observed on-task behaviour (Mahar et al., 2006; Mullender-Wijnsma et al., 2015) or prevent a decline in behaviour (Grieco, Jowers, & Bartholomew, 2009), but findings have been controversial about other cognitive outcomes such as recall (Norris et al., 2015; Valle et al., 1986).

Studies on the effects of regular physical activity have ranged from brief classroom exercise breaks (Donnelly et al., 2009) to physical activity incorporated into a healthy lifestyle, nutrition and physical activity curriculum (de Greeff et al., 2016). Donnelly et al. (2009) found the classroom exercise breaks improved children's ($n = 167$, ages 7–12) performance on the Wechsler Individual Achievement Test – 2nd edition, while de Greeff et al. (2016) found improvements in speed coordination ($n = 499$, ages 7–8) but no changes in executive functions. Most of these studies have examined academic achievement outcomes such as state-standardized tests and have either improved achievement or found no differences compared to controls.

Two studies have directly compared types of physical activity on educational outcomes using the d2 test of attention. Gallotta et al. (2015) directly compared performance on the d2 test of attention between three types of activities: coordinated exercises with movement-based problem solving, traditional physical education and a sedentary cognitive challenge. They found that the group which combined cognitive and physical exertion had less improvement in attention than the other two groups. The authors concluded the dual task may have exceeded resources and led to decreased improvements.

Budde et al. (2008) also examined the effects of different types of physical activity on performance on the d2 test of attention. They compared bilateral coordinative exercise to a normal sport lesson. Both groups had the same duration and intensity; however the coordinative exercise group performed better on the tests of concentration and attention.

Summary

Active lessons combining learning with acute physical activity have either shown improvements in educational outcomes or no benefit. The two studies on regular active lessons had opposing findings. Thus, more research is needed directly comparing the effects of different types of physical activity on educational outcomes.

Offset box 1

Note on special populations: while the majority of studies have examined the effects of physical activity on typically developing or a heterogeneous sample of children in the classroom, some studies have examined special populations (Corder, 1966; Craft, 1983; Etscheidt & Ayllon, 1987; Molloy, 1989; Pontifex, Saliba, Raine, Picchietti, & Hillman, 2013). It is possible that physical activity may have a differential dose–response effect in varying populations, but thus far the research is limited comparing the response between populations.

Overall summary: how much activity do we need?

There are many types of educational outcomes that have been shown to be influenced by both acute and regular physical activity. Physical activity has been an important part of education throughout history. There is likely to be a dose–response relationship, as evidenced by the few studies that have directly compared time, intensities and types of physical activity, but the exact nature of the response is still unknown.

Based on current evidence, it is not possible at this time to specify the ideal dose of physical activity needed to improve educational outcomes. Studies need to quantify better the dose of physical activity to compare to other studies (report frequency, intensity, time and type). More studies are needed that directly compare doses of physical activity by time frequency, intensity, time (duration) and type. Effects may be context-dependent: what works best for one teacher and classroom may not work best for another classroom. Educators and stakeholders should be encouraged to implement any dose of physical activity. Importantly, there are limited instances where any dose of physical activity has harmed educational outcomes compared to sedentary classroom time.

Considerations for educators

How much physical activity should I incorporate into my classroom each day?

Some is better than none and more is likely to be better. Teachers who are currently not implementing any physical activity into the school day should start with smaller amounts and increase over time. Physical activity should be included on most days, preferably every day, of the week, and throughout the entire school year. Changing the types of activities may help to keep students and teachers motivated for longer periods of time.

What intensity activity should I aim for?

It is likely that different intensities have different benefits for children, thus teachers should incorporate a variety of intensity activity throughout the day. Teachers should aim for quality physical activity. Similarly to quality physical education (United Nations Educational Scientific and Cultural Organization (UNESCO), 2015), quality physical activity should be intentional, give children adequate opportunity to be active for the intended dose and provide them with a positive experience to want to continue engaging in physical activity through their lives. This could include yoga or stretching in the morning, a 30-minute break with teacher-led moderate-to-vigorous physical activity, 30-minute recess for free play (with teacher-encouraged physical activity) and brief bursts of high-intensity activity throughout the classroom day.

What type of activity should I use?

The evidence is not conclusive about which type is best. Some lessons may be enhanced through physical activity while others may not benefit, or be harmed, by incorporating physical activity. If curriculum activities can be designed and incorporated into daily classroom lessons, they should be encouraged. Physical activity without an academic component is also important for children's development. As different types of activities may have different purposes, teachers should implement multiple types, similar to varying intensities, of activity throughout the school day.

References

Altenburg, T. M., Chinapaw, M. J., & Singh, A. S. (2016). Effects of one versus two bouts of moderate intensity physical activity on selective attention during a school morning in Dutch primary schoolchildren: A randomized controlled trial. *J Sci Med Sport, 19*(10), 820–824. doi: 10.1016/j.jsams.2015.12.003.

Ardoy, D. N., Fernandez-Rodriguez, J. M., Jimenez-Pavon, D., Castillo, R., Ruiz, J. R., & Ortega, F. B. (2014). A physical education trial improves adolescents' cognitive performance and academic achievement: the EDUFIT study. *Scand J Med Sci Sports, 24*(1), e52–61. doi: 10.1111/sms.12093.

Aukrust, V. G. (2011). *Learning and cognition.* Oxford: Elsevier.

Bala, G., Adamovic, T., Madic, D., & Popovic, B. (2015). Effects of acute physical exercise on mathematical computation depending on the parts of the training in young children. *Coll Antropol, 39*(Suppl 1), 29–34.

Barney, R. K. (1967). Physical education and sport in North America. In E. F. Zeigler (Ed.), *History of physical education and sport* (Vol. 67, pp. 171–227). Englewood Cliffs, NJ: Prentice-Hall.

Bluechardt, M. H., & Shephard, R. J. (1995). Using an extracurricular physical activity program to enhance social skills. *J Learn Disabil, 28*(3), 160–169.

Brown, B. (1976). The effect of an isometric strength program on the intellectual and social development of trainable retarded males. *Am Correct Ther J, 31*(2), 44–48.

Budde, H., Voelcker-Rehage, C., Pietrabyk-Kendziorra, S., Ribeiro, P., & Tidow, G. (2008). Acute coordinative exercise improves attentional performance in adolescents. *Neurosci Lett, 441*(2), 219–223. doi: 10.1016/j.neulet.2008.06.024.

Bunketorp Kall, L., Malmgren, H., Olsson, E., Linden, T., & Nilsson, M. (2015). Effects of a curricular physical activity intervention on children's school performance, wellness, and brain development. *J Sch Health, 85*(10), 704–713. doi: 10.1111/josh.12303.

Caspersen, C. J., Powell, K. E., & Christenson, G. M. (1985). Physical activity, exercise, and physical fitness: definitions and distinctions for health-related research. *Public Health Rep, 100*(2), 126–131.

Caterino, M. C., & Polak, E. D. (1999). Effects of two types of activity on the performance of second-, third-, and fourth-grade students on a test of concentration. *Percept Mot Skills, 89*(1), 245–248. doi: 10.2466/pms.1999.89.1.245.

Center on Education Policy. (2011). Strained schools face bleak future: Districts foresee budget cuts, teacher layoffs, and a slowing of education reform efforts. Retrieved from www.cep-dc.org/cfcontent_file.cfm?Attachment=KoberRentner_Report_StrainedSchools_063011.pdf.

Chan, R. C. K., Shum, D., Toulopoulou, T., & Chen, E. Y. H. (2008). Assessment of executive functions: Review of instruments and identification of critical issues. *Arch Clin Neuropsychol, 23*(2), 201–216. doi: http://dx.doi.org/10.1016/j. acn.2007.08.010.

Chang, Y. K., Tsai, Y. J., Chen, T. T., & Hung, T. M. (2013). The impacts of coordinative exercise on executive function in kindergarten children: An ERP study. *Exp Brain Res, 225*(2), 187–196. doi: 10.1007/s00221-012-3360-9.

Chasey, W. C., & Wyrick, W, (1970). Effect of a gross motor developmental program on form perception skills of educable mentally retarded children. *Res Q. Am Assoc Hlth Phys Ed Recr, 41*(3), 345–352.

Chaya, M. S., Nagendra, H., Selvam, S., Kurpad, A., & Srinivasan, K. (2012). Effect of yoga on cognitive abilities in schoolchildren from a socioeconomically disadvantaged background: A randomized controlled study. *J Altern Complement Med, 18*(12), 1161–1167. doi: 10.1089/acm.2011.0579.

Corder, W. O. (1966). Effects of physical education on the intellectual, physical, and social development of educable mentally retarded boys. *Except Child, 32*, 357–364.

Craft, D. H. (1983). Effect of prior exercise on cognitive performance tasks by hyperactive and normal young boys. *Percept Mot Skills, 56*(3), 979–982. doi: 10.2466/pms.1983.56.3.979.

Crova, C., Struzzolino, I., Marchetti, R., Masci, I., Vannozzi, G., Forte, R., & Pesce, C. (2014). Cognitively challenging physical activity benefits executive function in overweight children. *J Sports Sci, 32*(3), 201–211.

Davis, C. L., Tomporowski, P. D., Boyle, C. A., Waller, J. L., Miller, P. H., Naglieri, J. A., & Gregoski, M. (2007). Effects of aerobic exercise on overweight children's cognitive functioning: A randomized controlled trial. *Res Q Exerc Sport, 78*(5), 510–519. doi: 10.1080/02701367.2007.10599450.

Davis, C. L., Tomporowski, P. D., McDowell, J. E., Austin, B. P., Miller, P. H., Yanasak, N. E., Allison, J. D., & Naglieri, J. A. (2011). Exercise improves executive function and achievement and alters brain activation in overweight children: A randomized, controlled trial. *Hlth Psychol, 30*(1), 91.

de Greeff, J. W., Hartman, E., Mullender-Wijnsma, M. J., Bosker, R. J., Doolaard, S., & Visscher, C. (2016). Long-term effects of physically active academic lessons on physical fitness and executive functions in primary school children. *Health Educ Res, 31*(2), 185–194. doi: 10.1093/her/cyv102.

Donnelly, J. E., Greene, J. L., Gibson, C. A., Smith, B. K., Washburn, R. A., Sullivan, D. K., . . . Ryan, J. J. (2009). Physical Activity Across the Curriculum (PAAC): A randomized controlled trial to promote physical activity and diminish overweight and obesity in elementary school children. *Prev Med, 49*(4), 336–341.

Duncan, M., & Johnson, A. (2014). The effect of differing intensities of acute cycling on preadolescent academic achievement. *Eur J Sport Sci, 14*(3), 279–286. doi: 10.1080/17461391.2013.802372.

Dwyer, T., Coonan, W. E., Leitch, D. R., Hetzel, B. S., & Baghurst, R. (1983). An investigation of the effects of daily physical activity on the health of primary school students in South Australia. *Int J Epidemiol, 12*(3), 308–313.

Eickelberg, W., & Less, M. (1975). The effects of passive exercise of skeletal muscles on cardiac cost, respiratory function and associative learning in severe myopathic children. *J Hum Ergol, 3*, 157–162.

Ellemberg, D., & St-Louis-Deschênes, M. (2010). The effect of acute physical exercise on cognitive function during development. *Psychol Sport Exerc, 11*(2), 122–126.

Etnier, J., Labban, J. D., Piepmeier, A., Davis, M. E., & Henning, D. A. (2014). Effects of an acute bout of exercise on memory in 6th grade children. *Pediatr Exerc Sci, 26*(3), 250–258. doi: 10.1123/pes.2013-0141.

Etscheidt, M. A., & Ayllon, T. (1987). Contingent exercise to decrease hyperactivity. *J Child Adolesc Psychother, 4*, 192–198.

Evans, W. H., Evans, S. S., Schmid, R. E., & Pennypacker, H. (1985). The effects of exercise on selected classroom behaviors of behaviorally disordered adolescents. *Behav Disord*, 42–51.

Fisher, A., Boyle, J. M., Paton, J. Y., Tomporowski, P., Watson, C., McColl, J. H., & Reilly, J. J. (2011). Effects of a physical education intervention on cognitive function in young children: Randomized controlled pilot study. *BMC Pediatrics, 11*(1), 1.

Fretz, B. R., Johnson, W. R., & Johnson, J. A. (1969). Intellectual and perceptual motor development as a function of therapeutic play. *Res Q. Am Assoc Hlth, Phys Ed Recr, 40*(4), 687–691.

Gabbard, C., & Barton, J. (1979). Effects of physical activity on mathematical computation among young children. *J Psychol, 103*(2), 287.

Gallotta, M. C., Emerenziani, G. P., Franciosi, E., Meucci, M., Guidetti, L., & Baldari, C. (2015). Acute physical activity and delayed attention in primary school students. *Scand J Med Sci Sports, 25*(3), e331–338. doi: 10.1111/sms.12310.

Glassford, R. G., & Redmond, G. (1967). Physical education and sport in modern time. In E. F. Zeigler (Ed.), *History of physical education and sport* (Vol. 67, pp. 103–170). Englewood Cliffs, NJ: Prentice Hall.

Grieco, L. A., Jowers, E. M., & Bartholomew, J. B. (2009). Physically active academic lessons and time on task: The moderating effect of body mass index. *Med Sci Sports Exerc, 41*(10), 1921–1926.

Hill, L., Williams, J. H., Aucott, L., Milne, J., Thomson, J., Greig, J., Munro, V., & Mon-Williams, M. (2010). Exercising attention within the classroom. *Dev Med Child Neurol, 52*(10), 929–934.

Hillman, C. H., Kamijo, K., & Scudder, M. (2011). A review of chronic and acute physical activity participation on neuroelectric measures of brain health and cognition during childhood. *Prev Med, 52*(Suppl 1), S21–S28. doi: 10.1016/j.ypmed.2011.01.024.

Hillman, C. H., Pontifex, M. B., Castelli, D. M., Khan, N. A., Raine, L. B., Scudder, M. R., Drollette, E. S., Moore, R. D., Wu, C. T., & Kamijo, K. (2014). Effects of the FITKids randomized controlled trial on executive control and brain function. *Pediatrics, 134*(4), e1063–e1071.

Hillman, C. H., Pontifex, M. B., Raine, L. B., Castelli, D. M., Hall, E. E., & Kramer, A. F. (2009). The effect of acute treadmill walking on cognitive control and academic achievement in preadolescent children. *Neuroscience, 159*(3), 1044–1054.

Holmes, R. M., Pellegrini, A. D., & Schmidt, S. L. (2006). The effects of different recess timing regimens on preschoolers' classroom attention. *Early Child Devel Care, 176*(7), 735–743.

Howie, E. K., Beets, M. W., & Pate, R. R. (2014). Acute classroom exercise breaks improve on-task behavior in 4th and 5th grade students: A dose–response. *Ment Health Phys Act, 7*(2), 65–71. doi: http://dx.doi.org/10.1016/j.mhpa.2014.05.002.

Howie, E. K., & Pate, R. R. (2012). Physical activity and academic achievement in children: A historical perspective. *J Sport Health Sci, 1*(3), 160–169. doi: http://dx.doi.org/10.1016/j.jshs.2012.09.003.

Howie, E. K., Schatz, J., & Pate, R. R. (2015). Acute effects of classroom exercise breaks on executive function and math performance: a dose–response study. *Res Q Exerc Sport, 86*(3), 217–224. doi: 10.1080/02701367.2015.1039892.

Jarrett, O. S., Maxwell, D. M., Dickerson, C., Hoge, P., Davies, G., & Yetley, A. (1998). Impact of recess on classroom behavior: Group effects and individual differences. *J Educ Res, 92*(2), 121–126.

Kall, L. B., Nilsson, M., & Linden, T. (2014). The impact of a physical activity intervention program on academic achievement in a Swedish elementary school setting. *J Sch Health, 84*(8), 473–480. doi: 10.1111/josh.12179.

Kamijo, K., Pontifex, M. B., O'Leary, K. C., Scudder, M. R., Wu, C. T., Castelli, D. M., & Hillman, C. H. (2011). The effects of an afterschool physical activity program on working memory in preadolescent children. *Dev Sci, 14*(5), 1046–1058.

Karweit, N. (1984). Time-on-task reconsidered: Synthesis of research on time and learning. *Educ Leader, 41*(8), 32–35.

Khan, N. A., & Hillman, C. H. (2014). The relation of childhood physical activity and aerobic fitness to brain function and cognition: A review. *Pediatr Exerc Sci, 26*(2), 138–146. doi: 10.1123/pes.2013-0125.

Klein, S. A., & Deffenbacher, J. L. (1977). Relaxation and exercise for hyperactive impulsive children. *Percept Mot Skills, 45*(3f), 1159–1162.

Krebs, P., Eickelberg, W., Krobath, H., & Baruch, I. (1989). Effects of physical exercise on peripheral vision and learning in children with spina bifida manifesta. *Percept Mot Skills, 68*(1), 167–174.

Kubesch, S., Walk, L., Spitzer, M., Kammer, T., Lainburg, A., Heim, R., & Hille, K. (2009). A 30-minute physical education program improves students' executive attention. *Mind, Brain, Educ, 3*(4), 235–242.

Ma, J. K., Le Mare, L., & Gurd, B. J. (2015). Four minutes of in-class high-intensity interval activity improves selective attention in 9- to 11-year olds. *Appl Physiol Nutr Metab, 40*(3), 238–244. doi: 10.1139/apnm-2014-0309.

Maeda, J. K., & Randall, L. M. (2003). Can academic success come from five minutes of physical activity? *Brock Educ J, 13*(1).

Mahar, M. T., Murphy, S. K., Rowe, D. A., Golden, J., Shields, A. T., & Raedeke, T. D. (2006). Effects of a classroom-based program on physical activity and on-task behavior. *Med Sci Sports Exerc, 38*(12), 2086–2094. doi: 10.1249/01.mss.0000235359.16685.a3.

Manjunath, N., & Telles, S. (1999). Improvement in visual perceptual sensitivity in children following yoga training. *J Ind Psychol, 17*(2), 41–45.

McCormick, C. C., Schnobrich, J. N., Footlik, S. W., & Poetker, B. (1968). Improvement in reading achievement through perceptual-motor training. *Res Q. Am Assoc Hlth, Phys Ed Recr, 39*(3), 627–633.

McNaughten, D., & Gabbard, C. (1993). Physical exertion and immediate mental performance of sixth-grade children. *Percept Mot Skills, 77*(3 Pt 2), 1155–1159. doi: 10.2466/pms.1993.77.3f.1155.

Mierau, A., Hulsdunker, T., Mierau, J., Hense, A., Hense, J., & Struder, H. K. (2014). Acute exercise induces cortical inhibition and reduces arousal in response to visual stimulation in young children. *Int J Dev Neurosci, 34*, 1–8. doi: 10.1016/j.ijdevneu.2013.12.009.

Miyake, A., Friedman, N. P., Emerson, M. J., Witzki, A. H., Howerter, A., & Wager, T. D. (2000). The unity and diversity of executive functions and their contributions to complex 'frontal lobe' tasks: A latent variable analysis. *Cogn Psychol, 41*(1), 49–100.

Molloy, G. N. (1989). Chemicals, exercise and hyperactivity: A short report. *Int J Disabil Devel Educ, 36*(1), 57–61.

Mullender-Wijnsma, M. J., Hartman, E., de Greeff, J. W., Bosker, R. J., Doolaard, S., & Visscher, C. (2015). Moderate-to-vigorous physically active academic lessons and academic engagement in children with and without a social disadvantage: A within subject experimental design. *BMC Publ Hlth, 15*, 404. doi: 10.1186/s12889-015-1745-y.

Norlander, T., Moås, L., & Archer, T. (2005). Noise and stress in primary and secondary school children: Noise reduction and increased concentration ability through a short but regular exercise and relaxation program. *School Effective School Improve, 16*(1), 91–99.

Norris, E., Shelton, N., Dunsmuir, S., Duke-Williams, O., & Stamatakis, E. (2015). Virtual field trips as physically active lessons for children: A pilot study. *BMC Publ Hlth, 15*, 366. doi: 10.1186/s12889-015-1706-5.

O'Connor, C. (1969). Effects of selected physical activities upon motor performance, perceptual performance and academic achievement of first graders. *Percept Motor, 3*, 703–709.

Palmer, K. K., Miller, M. W., & Robinson, L. E. (2013). Acute exercise enhances preschoolers' ability to sustain attention. *J Sport Exerc Psychol, 35*(4), 433–437.

Pellegrini, A. D., & Davis, P. D. (1993). Relations between children's playground and classroom behaviour. *Br J Educ Psychol, 63*(1), 88–95.

Pellegrini, A. D., Huberty, P. D., & Jones, I. (1995). The effects of recess timing on children's playground and classroom behaviors. *Am Educ Res J, 32*(4), 845–864.

Pesce, C., Crova, C., Cereatti, L., Casella, R., & Bellucci, M. (2009). Physical activity and mental performance in preadolescents: Effects of acute exercise on free-recall memory. *Ment Health Phys Act, 2*(1), 16–22.

Pontifex, M. B., Saliba, B. J., Raine, L. B., Picchietti, D. L., & Hillman, C. H. (2013). Exercise improves behavioral, neurocognitive, and scholastic performance in children with attention-deficit/hyperactivity disorder. *J Pediatr, 162*(3), 543–551. doi: 10.1016/j.jpeds.2012.08.036.

Rader, B. G. (2004). *American sports: From the age of folk games to the age of televised sports* (5th ed.). Upper Saddle River, NJ: Pearson College Division.

Reed, J. A., Einstein, G., Hahn, E., Hooker, S. P., Gross, V. P., & Kravitz, J. (2010). Examining the impact of integrating physical activity on fluid intelligence and academic performance in an elementary school setting: A preliminary investigation. *Journal of Physical Activity and Health, 7*(3), 343.

Sharpe, P. (1979). The contribution of aspects of movement education to the cognitive development of infant school children. *J Hum Move Stud, 5*, 125–140.

Tuckman, B. W., & Hinkle, J. S. (1986). An experimental study of the physical and psychological effects of aerobic exercise on schoolchildren. *Hlth Psychol, 5*(3), 197.

United Nations Educational Scientific and Cultural Organization (UNESCO). (2014). *World-wide survey of school physical education*. Retrieved from: http://unesdoc.unesco.org/images/0022/002293/229335e.pdf.

United Nations Educational Scientific and Cultural Organization (UNESCO). (2015). *Quality physical education (QPE): Guidelines for policy-makers*. Retrieved from: http://unesdoc.unesco.org/images/0023/002311/231101E.pdf.

Valle, J. D., Dunn, K., Dunn, R., Geisert, G., Sinatra, R., & Zenhausern, R. (1986). The effects of matching and mismatching students' mobility preferences on recognition and memory tasks. *J Educ Res, 79*(5), 267–272.

Van Dalen, D. B. (1953). *A world history of physical education: Cultural, philosophical, comparative*. New York: Prentice-Hall.

Vazou, S., & Smiley-Oyen, A. (2014). Moving and academic learning are not antagonists: Acute effects on executive function and enjoyment. *J Sport Exerc Psychol, 36*(5), 474–485. doi: 10.1123/jsep.2014-0035.

Zeigler, E. F. (1967). Physical education and sport in the middle ages. In E. F. Zeigler (Ed.), *History of physical education and sport* (Vol. 67, pp. 57–102). Englewood Cliffs, NJ: Prentice-Hall.

Chapter 2

Varieties of learning and developmental theories of memory

Neurophysiological evidence and its relevance for researchers and educators

Phillip Tomporowski, Daniel M. Pendleton and Bryan A. McCullick

Introduction

Learning has been defined as a set of internal processes associated with practice or experience that lead to relatively permanent changes in the potential to behave (Schmidt & Wrisberg, 2008). Several assumptions are central to this definition; learning is: (1) an internal process that cannot be seen directly but is inferred from observations of behaviour; (2) related to experience and is not a function of maturation or development; (3) relatively permanent and expressed in behaviours performed following delays in time or in multiple contexts; and (4) sometimes obscured by environmental conditions, such as fatigue or motivation.

Does physical activity affect children's learning? Over the past decade, there has been a substantial increase in the number of studies that focus on physical activity's impact on children's cognitive performance, particularly on tasks that emphasize response speed and accuracy (Donnelly et al., 2016). Far fewer controlled experiments have focused on children's memory and learning. The present chapter draws upon neurophysiological evidence, research conducted with adults and theories of child development to determine the plausibility that acute bouts of physical activity or chronic exercise training will influence children's memory and learning. The chapter has five sections. The first provides a historical overview of the constructs of memory and learning and experimental approaches that have been used to study the phenomena. The second introduces neurobiology of learning, theories of memory consolidation and plasticity. The third examines the neurological underpinnings of four types of learning. The fourth links the four types of learning to contemporary theories of children's cognitive development. The final section concludes with recommendations concerning physical activity interventions and children's academic achievement.

The study of learning

The earliest written account of memory stretches back roughly 2.4 millennia to the time of ancient Greeks. Initial investigations by philosophers such as Plato (428–348 BCE), Aristotle (384–322 BCE) and Erasistratus (304–250 BCE) provide examples of qualitative approaches to understanding human memories. The beginning of the scientific study of memory is credited to Herman Ebbinghaus (1850–1909) and Georg Elias Müller (1850–1934) who developed quantitative methods to assess memory storage (Hergenhahn, 2001). Ebbinghaus developed a number of laboratory-based methods to measure memory. He created a pool of about 2,300 trigrams, 'nonsense' three-letter words that were used to reduce individual differences in reading experiences. Trigrams enabled him to create lists that could be varied in length and item difficulty, providing him insight into the effects of various practice conditions on word learning (e.g. presentation duration, inter-item interval) and enabling him to generate empirical word-recall curves that reflected the processes of learning. He also varied the duration between word-list encoding and recall, which provided quantitative indices of forgetting.

Ebbinghaus' work (1885/1913) provided the initial quantitative methods to describe memory storage. The practice-test methods he developed revealed that memories of words decayed rapidly unless some form of intentional rehearsal strategy was employed. With repeated practice, however, words could be retained for longer periods of time. These observations led memory researchers to propose that information was retained in either short-term or long-term memory. The characteristics of memory stores and how they develop have been central to many theories of memory and the emergence of alternative conceptualizations of memory storage (Baddeley, 2000; Baddeley & Hitch, 1974).

Regardless of theoretical orientation, however, the methods used by contemporary researchers are fundamentally akin to those developed by Ebbinghaus. In memory experiments, a participant is provided time to practise (encode) information. Then, following a specified delay interval, he or she is asked either to recall or recognize the studied material. The participant's performance is taken to infer the degree to which the material was learned. Attempts to explain these direct observations have led to numerous theories of memory and cognition (Puff, 1982); many are based on changes that are hypothesized to occur within the central nervous system.

Emergence of the neurobiology of learning, theories of memory consolidation and brain plasticity

Memories reflect neurological changes that occur during and following our experiences; memories are the linchpins for the changes in behaviours that allow one to infer that learning has occurred. Methodological advances in neuroscience made over the past few decades provide researchers the means to explore how experiences affect the brain at multiple levels; i.e. the whole brain, brain networks, individual brain cells and the processes that occur within neurons. The observations of neuroscientists have supported predictions made by early experimental researchers concerning how learning occurs. At the beginning of the 20th century, based on his pioneering research in animal learning, Ivan Pavlov suggested that repeated experiences (e.g. between an auditory tone and food presentation) led to alterations of neural tracks in the cortex of the brain that result in the formation of increasingly stronger memory traces that reinforce learned associations between events (Pavlov, 1963). In the mid 20th century, Donald Hebb suggested a similar, but more precise, neurological hypothesis to explain associative learning in animals (Hebb, 1949). Observations that neurons communicate via chemical and electrical events that occur at the level of the synapse, or space, between neurons led Hebb to propose that stimuli came to control behaviours via changes within neurons, which resulted in a strengthening of the impact of what was initially a weak neural signal. What came to be known as Hebb's Rule provided researchers with several testable hypotheses that were supported decades later with the emergence of advanced methods of assessing neurological processes. The study of hippocampal neurons using single-unit recording revealed mechanisms that underlie long-term potentiation and how molecular events occurring within a specific time range on the neuronal dendrites lead to synaptic plasticity (Carlson, 2013, pp. 443–448).

Memory consolidation

The transfer of memory short-term, long-term storage has been explained in terms of a process referred to as memory consolidation and how the strength of a memory of an event depends on the passage of time. Teachers and researchers have long known that students retain information better when study time is distributed over several sessions, as opposed to a single night of 'cramming' before a test. Over the past four decades, researchers have focused considerable attention on the neurobiology of memory consolidation. Much of what is known of the neurobiology of memory consolidation is reflected in work conducted by James McGaugh and his students and colleagues, who set about answering a question posed by William James over a century ago – why are some experiences 'so exciting emotionally as almost to leave a scar on the cerebral tissues' (James, 1981/1890, p. 670) and yet experiences have less of an effect on memory (McGaugh, 2015)?

Laboratory research conducted with animals undergoing learning training involving aversive stimuli (e.g. shock) led to insights on the biological consequences of physical stress on memory consolidation. Animals involved in classically conditioned escape behaviour training showed rapidly learned associations between environmental conditions and the onset of aversive events (Gold, 2001). The rapid and long-lasting memories of the animals' experiences were explained in terms of the biological stress response elicited during training. When an animal becomes emotionally aroused, a cascade of neurohormonal changes occurs. The release of adrenal stress hormones results in widespread changes throughout the peripheral and central nervous system. In particular, the stress hormones adrenaline (epinephrine) and cortisol were implicated in memory consolidation.

In a seminal study (Gold & van Buskirk, 1975), rats experienced a single foot shock and then received administrations of adrenaline at several time points of up to 2 hours following the shock. Memory consolidation was time-dependent; the greatest enhancements were observed when adrenaline was given immediately following training. Reductions in memory recall occurred with the temporal delays between training and adrenaline administration.

A similar demonstration of the effects of adrenaline on memory consolidation was observed following training that did not involve aversive experiences. Dornelles and his colleagues (2007) reported that adrenaline administered to rats immediately after an opportunity to explore a novel environment enhanced memory for objects when the animals were tested 4 days later.

A substantial body of research has shown that corticosterone (in animals) has effects on memory consolidation that are similar to those of adrenaline. The activation of glucocorticoid receptors influences the strength of memories to both aversive events (Roozendaal, 2000) and novel environmental experiences (Roozendaal, Okuda, Van der Zee, & McGaugh, 2006).

The observation that animals' memories of their experiences in novel environments are enhanced by the administration of adrenaline and corticosterone has implications for predictions concerning children's physical activity and learning. Animals placed in new environments evidence a stress-like arousal response during which adrenal glands release endogenous adrenaline. As animals habituate to new learning conditions, the level of adrenaline release declines. Roozendaal et al. (2006) observed that glucocorticoid activation enhanced the consolidation of animals' memory, but only when they were first placed in the learning situation. If allowed to habituate to the learning environment, memory consolidation was not enhanced by corticosterone administration. Thus, under laboratory conditions, rodent memory consolidation depends on the presence of arousal. Should these finding generalize to human children, it would predict that bouts of physical activity that elicit the physiological stress response may moderate learning.

In summary, the results of a large body of animal studies converge on the perspective that physically arousing experiences lead to the release of hormones that moderate memory consolidation and learning. Such observations reflect the adaptive nature of learning in animals and humans. The capacity to recall emotional events and the context in which they occur has tremendous survival value for the individual as well as the evolution of the species (Kempermann et al., 2010). Several anthropologists and neuroscientists have highlighted the importance of the evolution of memory systems for the successful survival of *Homo sapiens* (Mithen, 1996). Our ancient ancestors experienced many life-or-death experiences on a regular basis. Retaining the memories of escape from predators or remembering the location of water or food would provide a substantial survival benefit. The evidence amassed on the neurobiology of emotional memory consolidation supports hypotheses generated in the field of evolutionary psychology. Our ancient ancestors may have had limited language or capacity to store general knowledge, but they certainly possessed memories of 'fight or flight' situations that aided survival. The various forms of learning that are described later in this chapter are grounded in the evolution of the human brain. Some forms of learning occur with no conscious awareness of mental effort and reflect the memory systems of our ancient foreparents, whereas other forms of learning are linked to brain structures involved in effortful mental engagement.

Brain structures involved in memory and learning

Experimental psychologists who have studied human memory using behavioural tests suggest that there are a number of different types of memory (Squire, 2004). Likewise, neuroscientists who conduct laboratory studies of animals and clinicians who observe the effects of brain injury or disease on human performance provide evidence for multiple brain structures and networks that are involved in memory and learning (Morris, 2013). A key observation made by both behaviourally oriented and biologically based researchers is that, while memory systems can function relatively independently, they demonstrate unitary function (Schneider, 2015). For example, visual, auditory, proprioceptive and olfactory experiences are encoded in various modality-specific areas of the brain. When individuals are asked to 'bring to mind' a person they know well, memories are retrieved simultaneously from many different areas. An image of one's mother, for example, may include a memory of her appearance, memory of a location, memory of the smells associated with her. The study of emotional memories provides insights into the interrelations that exist among brain structures that underlie specific types of learning. Convergent research evidence gathered over the past four decades led McGaugh (2004) to highlight the role of the amygdaloid complex in the consolidation of emotional memories. Experiences provide multiple inputs into the central nervous system; the likelihood that the experience will be remembered is modulated by the amygdala, particularly the basolateral area. The modulating impact of the basolateral area is, in turn, influenced by the presence of the hormones released by the adrenal gland, specifically adrenaline and cortisol. These hormones may also influence other brain structures involved in memory consolidation.

Thus, for memories that are developed during conditions of physiological arousal, the amygdaloid complex is not the place where memories are stored; rather, it plays a role in the neurological changes that occur as experiences alter the brain networks.

Brain plasticity

Until the last decade of the 20th century, the general consensus of neuroscience researchers was that the human brain developed following a genetically determined sequence; further, the neurological circuitry of the brain was relatively fixed with the onset of adulthood and remained so across the lifespan. These views were changed radically following studies showing specific areas of the brain could be altered as a function of experience and learning (Voss, Vivar, Kramer, & Van Praag, 2013). Several classic studies provided the impetus for acceptance of brain plasticity and how experiences alter brain structure and function.

The London taxi study was a naturalistic experiment that provided some of the first solid evidence of brain plasticity in humans (Maguire et al., 2000). London taxi drivers undergo extensive training in order to pass a test required for licensure; it typically requires 2 years of study and navigation of the complex London streets. Functional magnetic resonance imaging (fMRI) techniques were used to scan the drivers' brains, focusing on hippocampal structures. The images were compared to those of non-taxi drivers. The posterior hippocampi of taxi drivers were significantly larger than those of controls; further, the hippocampal volume was related to the number of years spent as a taxi driver. These findings were taken to suggest that training altered brain areas involved in the storage of spatial representations and the development of navigational skills.

Similar results were obtained from an early animal study that assessed the effects of different types of physical movement on brain plasticity (Black, Isaacs, Anderson, Alcantara, & Greenough, 1990). Groups of rats received 30 days of aerobic running exercise training or acrobatic training requiring the animals to maximize the use of their paws by climbing ropes. Compared to animals that did not exercise, animals that trained acrobatically generated significantly more new cerebellar synapses than animals that exercised aerobically or were inactive. Animals that exercised aerobically had greater density of cerebellar blood vessels than animals that exercised acrobatically or were inactive. These results demonstrate not only that physical activity modifies brain structure, but that the types of changes that take place in the brain are driven by specific types of movements. In the case of the Black et al. (1990) study, complex movements resulted in synaptogenesis and continuous aerobic training resulted in angiogenesis.

These early experiments led to a sharp rise in the number of studies that examined the effects of exercise on brain plasticity. Early reviews of these studies that focused on brain adaptations to exercise highlighted four ways that exercise training affects the brain (Churchill et al., 2002): (1) synaptogenesis, which is the alteration of the pre- and post-synaptic membrane of neurons; (2) neurogenesis, which is the proliferation of new neurons; (3) glial plasticity, which involves changes in astrocyte processes; and (4) angiogenesis, which is a growth in vascular density.

Of particular interest has been the hippocampus, a structure long been thought to play a role in the storage of episodic memory. A unique characteristic of the hippocampus is that new neurons are created across the lifespan. The proliferation of these neurons has been linked to both physical activity and environmental enrichment. Fabel et al. (2009) examined how physical activity, environmental enrichment and a combination of the two conditions affect the generation of new neurons in rodent hippocampi. They observed that both conditions led to increased generation of hippocampal neurons and that there was an additive effect when combined. These observations led them to hypothesize that exercise and enrichment worked via different mechanisms: Physical activity primes the hippocampus to increase precursor neuron production; environmental enrichment provides a survival-promoting effect.

The importance of the combined effects of physical activity and environmental enrichment on neuronal survival was stressed in a review of the exercise cognition literature that focused on how quickly exercise results in brain plasticity and the durability of those changes. A review of the literature by Thomas and colleagues (Thomas, Dennis, Bandettini, & Johansen-Berg, 2012) highlighted the unique temporal profile of brain changes that occur with exercise training. Animal studies show rapid increases in capillary density within 3 days of aerobic training; further, the creation of new neurons mirrors angiogenesis. Importantly, new neurons are retained only if animals are provided with learning opportunities or novel experiences. Without the added influence of learning experiences, neurogenic growth returns to pre-exercise levels (van Pragg, Christie, Sejnowski, & Gage, 1999).

Kempermann (Kempermann, 2008; Kempermann et al., 2010) highlighted the importance of physical activity during youth and early adulthood. He proposed that physical activity such as locomotion that takes place in complex challenging environments signals the hippocampus to alter the characteristics of emerging neurons and to create a neurogenic reserve. While neurogenesis takes place in the hippocampus across the lifespan, evidence suggests that the bulk of neurogenic reserve development occurs during youth and young adulthood. As such, increases in neurogenesis derived from physical activity or enriched environments would be particularly important for older individuals, whose production of new hippocampal neurons is sparse. Kempermann (2008) proposed that 'Broad ranges of physical activity early in life would not only help to build a highly optimized hippocampal network adapted to a complex life. . .[but] would also contribute to a neurogenic reserve by keeping precursor cells in cycle' (p. 167). From this perspective, physical activity during childhood could potentially influence an individual's capacity to respond adaptively to challenges that are encountered across the lifespan.

A recent review of neuroimaging studies provides evidence for exercise-related increases in hippocampal size and density (Prakash, Voss, Erickson, & Kramer, 2015). The majority of available studies reviewed focused on older adults' brain structure. A randomized controlled experiment provided clear evidence for the effects of a 12-month aerobic exercise programme on hippocampal volume, with increased volume associated with spatial memory performance (Erickson et al., 2011).

Although fewer neuroimaging studies have been conducted with children, the available evidence indicates that brain volume is associated with children's physical fitness. Chaddock et al. (2010) employed fMRI to measure hippocampal volume in children between 9 and 10 years of age who differed in aerobic fitness. Similar to research conducted with older adults, the more aerobically fit children's hippocampi had greater volume than those of less-fit children. These children also performed a simple memory test that involved recognizing specific items or a complex relational memory test that required the association of items. The more aerobically fit children performed better on the complex relational memory test than did less aerobically fit children. In addition, hippocampal volume was significantly correlated with accuracy on the complex memory task but not the simple memory test, suggesting that fitness levels may be particularly important when challenged with a complex learning condition.

These findings were extended by Chaddock, Hillman, Buck, and Cohen (2011) in a cross-sectional study that examined the roles of fitness levels on 9–10-year-old children's executive function and memory. As in their previous study, children with higher aerobic fitness showed greater accuracy on a cognitively demanding relational memory test than less aerobically fit children. The level of children's aerobic fitness did not influence performance on a simple item-recognition memory test. These results were interpreted as evidence of the benefits of aerobic fitness on prefrontal and hippocampal systems and on memory encoding and retrieval.

In summary, a growing literature provides evidence for the plasticity of the human brain and that specific types of environmental experiences affect neurological changes that have long-term effects on learned behaviour. While very little research has been conducted with children to assess the impact of exercise on brain structures that are involved in memory and learning, there is sufficient evidence from animal research and research conducted with mature and older adult humans to support the view that exercise, performed under specific conditions and times, may benefit children's learning. Of particular import are recent studies that consider the interplay between the emerging control of executive functions and long-term memory, and how exercise may play a role not only in the storage of information gained from experience but also in how prefrontal executive processes control and utilize memory (Chaddock et al., 2011).

As discussed previously, there are several different types of learning, each involving specific brain systems. The varieties of learning pose challenges for researchers who are intent on determining whether children's learning benefits from exercise. In the next section, four types of learning are described, each with specific brain systems.

Taxonomies of learning

Laboratory findings, typically from animal studies, in conjunction with observations made by clinical neuroscientists of humans with brain injury or disease, support the view that there are several different types of memory, each defined by specific brain circuitry (Morris, 2013; Schneider, 2015). Contemporary research provides a wealth of information concerning the neurological basis of learning. Taxonomies have been proposed that categorize memory and learning in terms of specific brain circuitry. The terms 'memory' and 'learning' are often used interchangeably as they represent the two sides of a coin. Memory reflects the experiences that individuals 'capture' and lead to alterations in neuronal networks that are called upon when asked to remember past experiences. Carlson (2013), for example, highlights four types of memory and brain areas presumed to be involved in learning: (1) perceptual learning, which is due to changes in neural circuitry involved in stimulus detection; (2) associative learning, brought about by changes in neural circuitry involved in classical condition or instrumental conditioning; (3) motor learning, which reflects changes in neural circuits that control movements; and (4) relational learning, which is based on the organization of multiple sensory inputs and the ability to recognize the spatial location of objects in the environment and to remember the temporal sequence in which events occur. Carlson's method of classifying memory types was selected for the present review as it helps systematically answer questions concerning the impact of physical activity on children's learning.

Perceptual learning

Central to perceptual learning is the capacity to capture and recognize events as they occur. At a fundamental level, humans learn about the world they live in based on the experiences they derived from the stimulation of the sensory systems. Consider, for instance, how one can pick out the face of a friend in a crowded room. As the features of every person's face are unique, they reflect a specific array of light waves that enter the eyes and stimulate photoreceptors on the retina that, in turn, send neural transmissions through the lateral geniculate of the thalamus and on to the striate cortex and the primary visual cortex. There the attributes of the incoming information flow are analysed in terms of form, colour and movement. Information then separates into two streams: the ventral stream flows towards the inferior temporal lobe and is used to recognize the visual experience; the dorsal stream flows toward the posterior parietal cortex and provides information concerning the location of what is seen. Together, the two streams provide the basis for our ability to recognize objects and their locations.

Importantly, these neurological processes result in the formation of unconscious memories of what was experienced. Recognition prompts neural circuits that remain active for a short period of time and allows one to consider how to respond. Perceptual short-term memory has been linked to activity in the sensory association cortex, parahippocampal area and the prefrontal cortex, implicating the role of working memory (Miyashita, 2004). The encoding of the information enables one to remember a friend's face and her location even if one loses sight of her as one navigates toward her through the crowd.

Associative learning

The notion that memories are solidified via the connection or 'associations' between events or experiences has been postulated since the times of the ancient Greek philosophers. Writings by Aristotle, in the third century BC, clearly articulated the phenomenon of memory and the conditions under which memories either gain strength or fade. Indeed, memory aids referred to as mnemonics were used by ancient orators and story tellers to assist in recalling verse. The 'method of loci', which continues to be used today by orators, involves the connection of thoughts or lines to be spoken at specific landmarks on stage. While these methods have been used for thousands of years, the neurobiological mechanism by which associative learning occurs has been revealed only recently.

Two forms of associative learning have been identified, each with its own underlying neurobiological networks. Classical conditioning is a learning method that focuses on the temporal pairing of events; for example, a tone that precedes the presentation of food. As described previously, the pioneering research conducted by Ivan Pavlov with dogs provided quantitative measures of an animal's unconditional response (UCR; e.g. salivation) to an unconditional stimulus (UCS; e.g. food). Pavlov explored how a seemingly benign stimulus, such as a tone, paired closely in time with an UCS, could begin to take on the eliciting characteristics of the UCS. The temporal association between the CS and the UCS strengthened the capacity of the tone to elicit salivation.

The neurobiology that underlies classical conditioning implicates the structures involved in emotional learning described in the previous section of this chapter. Aversive events unconditionally elicit an array of behavioural, autonomic and hormonal responses. The lateral nucleus of the amygdala receives converging input from both the auditory sensory system and the somatosensory systems; as the weak (tone) stimulus precedes the strong (shock), changes at the level of the synapses modify the sensitivity of the dendrites of neurons to the weak stimulus and lead to long-term potentiation.

Instrumental conditioning, sometimes referred to as operant learning, focuses on the association between behaviours and the results of those actions on the environment. Unlike classical conditioning, in which behaviours are reflexively elicited, instrumental conditioning prompts behaviours that are emitted. Behavioural actions in operant learning 'operate' on the environment; the consequences of actions reinforce, or strengthen, the likelihood that the frequency of behaviours will occur. Instrumental conditioning involves the recognition of an environmental condition that provides a signal for behaviour which, if performed, leads to a reinforcer. B. F. Skinner and his colleagues conducted many studies with rats and pigeons under controlled laboratory conditions demonstrating that environmental cues (e.g. a light) which signalled to an animal that a response, such as a lever press, would lead to food reward came to control lever-pressing behaviours (Skinner, 1938, 1990). Similarly, the sight of a red light at a traffic intersection sets the conditions for a driver to remove her foot from the gas pedal and place it on the brake pedal; not reflexively, but because of possible negative consequences of failing to stop at the intersection.

The neurobiology of operant learning has been studied extensively. There are specific neural pathways that are involved in the recognition of environmental cues and the initiation of motor movements. Important for the present discussion are the neural pathways that are engaged as the reinforcing consequences of actions are experienced. Animal research conducted in the mid-1950s (Olds & Milner, 1954) revealed the 'reward centres' of the brain; that is, structures that are involved in establishing memories of actions that lead to reward or to punishers. The medial forebrain bundle is a network of axons, primarily dopaminergic in nature, that extend between the midbrain and the rostral basal forebrain. Various tracts project to the prefrontal cortex, limbic cortex, nucleus accumbens and the hippocampus and all play roles in reinforcement circuitry.

Similarly to studies of classically conditioned emotional memory, which showed that animals learned more when placed in a novel environment than in a familiar environment, operant learning studies conducted with animals and humans have shown that the learning that takes place where a reward is presented depends on the novelty or predictability of the learning context. For example, Mirenowicz and Schultz (1994) observed that the dopaminergic activity in the ventral tegmentum area of the brain increased as primates learned a task that was rewarded by a sweet drink. However, as the task was repeated and became well learned, dopaminergic activity decreased when the reward was delivered. Similarly, an MRI study of young adult humans showed that word learning (declarative memory) improved more when words were presented in a novel setting than when presented in a familiar setting (Schott et al., 2004). These data have been interpreted as evidence for bias toward remembering novel events and information associated with them. Unique events activate the brain's systems and prepare it to encode or remember the event; expected and routine events signal the brain to prepare for redundant information, which need not be remembered.

Motor learning

Fundamentally, everything the brain and spinal cord does involves the control of movements. The capacity of individuals to survive and thrive in a complex world depends on how muscular contractions are controlled. The vast majority of the movements executed are reflexive and occur without, or with limited, conscious awareness; however, other movements are acquired though conscious, deliberate practice (Song, 2009). Skills that are learned provide an individual with the capacity to engage with and adapt to changing environmental conditions and challenges. The acquisition of skill and the quality of movement production are highly valued in human society, with much attention focused on experts in the arts and sports.

Reflex pathways involve connections between the sensory association cortex and the motor association cortex. The motor control involved in even the simplest reflexive behaviour, such as maintaining balance while standing, is exceedingly complex (Baudry, 2016). Skilled movements are thought to emerge from the neurobiological processes involved in motor control (Willingham, 1999). Motor skills are learned gradually and only with practice. Evidence from studies evaluating neurological systems that control movement suggests that transcortical connections, aided by input from the hippocampus, dominate the early stages of skill learning. With each attempt, the learner develops a memory of conditions that existed during previous attempts (recall memory) and a memory of the action itself (recognition memory) (Schmidt, 1975). As a skill is developed, the control of movements is influenced by neural pathways that include the basal ganglia and thalamus (Kerick, Douglas, & Hatfield, 2004). The activation of these structures is hypothesized to underlie the increased automatization of movement sequences observed with extensive practice. Skilled individuals exhibit the ability to control long sequences of complex actions without having to think or attend to their movements.

Relational learning

Taxonomies of memory typically differentiate between two types of long-term memory: implicit and explicit (e.g. Morris, 2013). Implicit memories are those that are acquired without the need for conscious awareness.

The types of learning discussed thus far – perceptual, associative and motor – reflect knowledge that can be acquired based on neural circuits, both those involved in stimulus detection and those involved in the responses that are made to those stimuli. Language or other types of symbolic processing are not necessary for these 'simple' types of learning. Explicit memory, also referred to as declarative memory, differs from implicit memory in three ways. Information is encoded and stored in terms of: (1) semantic memory, which is the factual information gained from learning experiences; (2) spatial memory, which provides information about the location of objects in the environment; and (3) episodic memory, which is a catalogue of an individual's experiences. One might remember a trip to go to the library (an episode of one's life), reading a book about mathematics (semantic information) and remembering the location on the page where a particular mathematical equation was printed (spatial memory). These three forms of memory storage and their interrelationship are central to understanding 'higher' types of learning, referred to a relational learning.

Unique to relational memory is the integration of multiple data inputs; for example, 'what, where, and when'. The neural systems that have been implicated in the encoding, storage, consolidation and recall of declarative memories include the hippocampal formation and the neocortex. While the exact mechanisms for the establishment of long-term declarative memories are debated, there is a general consensus that changes or alterations of synaptic synapses (plasticity) and changes in neural networks throughout the neocortex provide the basis for stored knowledge (Morris, 2013; Squire, 2004). The notion that relational learning reflects a 'higher-order' form of learning that involves the integration of information that is available in multiple networks distributed throughout the neocortex, which can impact 'lower-order' learning, has led to 'top-down, bottom-up' explanations of how the brain functions.

Two early theoretical approaches to memory and learning are informative. The 'top-down' view of perception posits that one's past experiences aid in the construction of perceptions (e.g. Gregory, 1970). From this perspective, when a person experiences an event, stored memories of past events are drawn upon to shape perceptions. In a sense, the knowledge acquired from past experiences prepares the individual's perception of the new event. The 'bottom-up' view of perception considers that raw sensory information is gathered and analysed without the need for stored past memories (e.g. Gibson, 1969).

Contemporary neurobiological theories of memory and learning continue to promote the notion of 'top-down' and 'bottom-up' processing (Schneider, 2015). Attempts have been made by neuroscientists to map neural networks in the brain. For example, Miyashita (2004) proposed a cognitive memory system that describes the interrelations among three brain subdivisions: (1) the medial temporal cortex, which includes the hippocampus and its related structures; (2) the temporal cortex, which is critical in reactivating neural nodes that lead to the representation of memories; and (3) the pre-frontal cortex, which monitors and organizes the flow of reactivated memories in ways that lead to the initiation of movement plans and actions.

In summary, questions concerning the effects of physical activity on learning should take into consideration the various types of learning. Mounting neurobiological evidence suggests that physical activity or the type of physical activity may influence some types of learning more than others. An additional challenge facing researchers with interests in assessing how physical activity may affect children's cognitive development is to understand and account for the rapid brain development that takes place during the first two decades of life. It is well established that specific types of cognitive processing emerge as the central nervous system develops (Casey, Galvan, & Hare, 2005), suggesting that the impacts of specific type of physical activity experiences may differ as a function of the timing of an intervention. To illuminate the role of cognitive development in understanding the exercise–learning relation, overviews of contemporary theories of children's cognitive development are presented in the next section.

Developmental theory

Brain development

The adult human brain consists of at least 100 billion neurons, and the structures of the central nervous system interact in an extremely complex fashion (Chaddock-Heyman, Hillman, Cohen, & Kramer, 2014). The study of normal brain and spinal cord development from the point of conception to adulthood provides insight into how environmental factors such as physical activity may modify structures and functions of the central nervous system. As shown in Figure 2.1 (Thompson & Nelson, 2001), networks of cells continue to form and emerge at different times throughout childhood, adolescence and adulthood. The prefrontal cortex, which has been associated with basic information processing (e.g. working memory, short-term memory and long-term memory) and intellectual functioning (e.g. problem solving, reasoning and planning), develops in a non-linear fashion from infancy through young adulthood (Bunge & Wright, 2007; Casey, Giedd, & Thomas, 2000; Diamond, 2000, 2002; Diamond & Goldman-Rakic, 1989; Luciana, 2003). In general, frontal-lobe processes develop rapidly through the elementary-school years and then at a slower pace during adolescence (Brocki & Bohlin, 2004; Huizinga, Dolan, & van der Molen, 2006). The emergence and development of processes that underlie cognition continue throughout childhood and adolescence and even into young adulthood (Casey, Amso, & Davidson, 2006; Posner & Rothbart, 2007).

While neuroimaging studies of the development of executive functions in children are rare, studies conducted with older children suggest that the

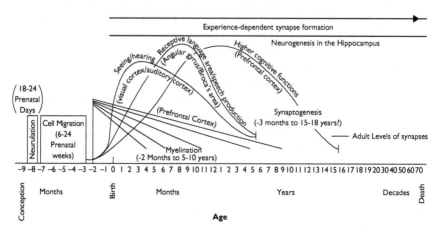

Figure 2.1 The course of human brain development.

Note. This graph illustrates the importance of prenatal events, such as the formation of the neural tube (neurulation) and cell migration; critical aspects of synapse formation and myelination beyond age three; and the formation of synapses based on experience, as well as neurogenesis in a key region of the hippocampus (the dentate gyrus), throughout much of life.

networks involved in their spatial working memory are similar to those of adults. Using fMRI methods, Nelson and his colleagues (2000) observed that the structures activated during non-verbal working-memory tasks were similar to those seen in of adults; i.e. activation of the posterior parietal regions and dorsal regions of the prefrontal cortex. Similarly, Scherf and his colleagues (Scherf, Sweeney, & Liuna, 2006) focused on changes in the integration of the brain regions that are purported to underlie visuospatial working memory. Compared to adolescents and adults, children evidenced less functional connectivity among the dorsolateral prefrontal cortex (considered responsible for maintenance of spatial representations), the premotor regions (responsible for actions) and the parietal regions. Age-related improvements in children's working-memory abilities were hypothesized to depend on the integration of these regions. Based on neurophysiological evidence available at the time, Nelson (2000) concluded that children's early experiences could fundamentally impact memory systems, both detrimentally and positively. The determining factor suggested by Nelson is need for continual challenge to memory/learning systems. Similar arguments have been proposed more recently by Pesce et al. (2013) and Diamond and Ling (2016) and several authors providing chapters in this text..

Cognitive development

The manner in which infants, children and adolescents behave and verbally describe how they solve problems often parallels the rapid changes that occur during brain development (Amso & Casey, 2006). Systematic observations of children's behaviours have led several researchers to posit general theories of cognitive development. One of the earliest and most influential theories was developed by Jean Piaget (1896–1980), who proposed that children's mental development, like physical development, is characterized by an invariant progression through distinct stages (Piaget, 1963). Piaget posited that children's experiences and personal interaction with their environments drive their cognitive development; he also proposed that children are forced to reorganize their thoughts or schemas when challenged by new problems.

Since Piaget's seminal early conceptualizations, numerous theories have been developed to explain cognitive development. Contemporary theories tend to reflect specific aspects of mental development; for example, spatial processing, information processing, executive processing, metacognition, memory, language and others (Bjorklund, 2005; Schneider, 2015). Using the neurological taxonomy introduced in the previous section, we have selected four theory-based approaches to explain cognitive development in an attempt to shed light on the role of physical activity in children's learning.

Development and perceptual learning

Proponents of theories of embodied learning propose that dynamic interactions occur among children's body movements, the sensory experiences obtained from the movements and the context of the movements (Campos et al., 2000; Kontra, Goldin-Meadow, & Beilock, 2012; Moreau, Morrison, & Conway, 2015; Thelen, 1996). As infants and young children learn to control their movements, they begin to understand implicitly how actions provide the means to achieve goals. From this perspective, learning depends on sensory and motor experiences. However, while children are thought to come to understand their surrounding environment through movement, the world they live in limits or constrains what they learn. An unchanging, repetitive world provides few opportunities for children to learn from their movements, but complex, changing and unpredictable environments are assumed to broaden potential learning opportunities. These very early learning experiences have been hypothesized to benefit mental imagery (Adolph, 2008; Sommerville & Decety, 2006), reasoning and problem solving (Gallese & Metzinger, 2003; Jackson & Decety, 2004) and operations necessary for children and adults to solve mathematical and science problems (Kontra, Lyons, Fischer, & Beilock, 2015; Newcombe & Frick, 2010). The central viewpoint of embodied cognition holds that cognitive processes are deeply rooted in the body's interactions with the world (Koziol, Budding, & Chidekel, 2011; Koziol & Lutz, 2013; Wilson, 2002). Taken together, these findings suggest that the manner in which infants and children learn about their environments is through physical activity and movement.

Development and associative learning

Considerable research was conducted during the first half of the 20th century that reflected the long-held view that memories are based upon the strength of the connections between events that occur in close temporal proximity, or connections between responses and their immediate consequences (Hull, 1952; Thorndike, 1914; Woodworth & Schlosberg, 1954). The results of experiments conducted by a generation of researchers who focused on verbal learning had a profound impact on theories of learning and subsequent methods of instruction and education (Hintzman, 1978). Verbal-learning researchers have been particularly interested in factors that influenced the strength of associations between lists of items to be remembered. One factor that garnered considerable interest was physiological arousal. Indeed, the Yerkes–Dodson Law (1908), which explained changes in performance in terms of an inverted-U relation, continues to influence contemporary exercise researchers. For example, the research conducted over the past decades by Terry McMorris, Michel Audiffren, and their colleagues has explored the effects of acute bouts of exercise on tests of attention, information processing and decision making. Exercise-related improvements on information-processing tests have been explained in terms of the activation of brain neuromodulators (e.g. noradrenergic and dopaminergic networks) that modify brain structures involved in attention and speeded mental processing (Audiffren, 2009; Dietrich & Audiffren, 2011; McMorris, Collard, Corbett, Dicks, & Swain, 2008; McMorris & Graydon, 2000; McMorris & Hale, 2015; McMorris, Hale, Corbett, Robertson, & Hodgson, 2015). While the majority of research that assessed the effects of acute bouts of exercise on information processing has been conducted with young adults (Chang, Labban, Gapin, & Etnier, 2012; Lambourne & Tomporowski, 2010; McMorris & Graydon, 2000; Tomporowski, 2003b), there is sufficient evidence that similarly beneficial effects are observed in children (Sibley & Etnier, 2003; Tomporowski, 2003a). Physiological arousal also appears to enhance memory encoding of declarative information in older adults (Stones & Dawe, 1993), young adults (Labban & Etnier, 2011) and children (Etnier, Labban, Piepmeier, Davis, & Henning, 2014; Pesce, Crova, Cereatti, Casella, & Bellucci, 2009). The neurological mechanisms that underlie emotional memories include structures of the limbic system and, predominantly, the amygdala and hippocampus. Emotional experiences and their widespread physiological impact via the autonomic nervous system are often explained in term of classically conditioned learning. Thus, it is plausible that physical activity performed in close proximity to information to be learned may enhance learning in at least two different ways: first, via the short-term changes in neuromodulators that enhance attention to task, and second, via changes in the long-term potentiation of hippocampal neurons that enhance encoding and recall (Roig, Nordbrant, Geertsen, & Nielsen, 2013; Roig et al., 2016).

Development and motor learning

There is a general consensus concerning the development of movement control in early childhood (18 months to about 6 years) and later childhood (6–12 years) (Gabbard, 2004). During early childhood, fundamental movement skills emerge; these include movement patterns required for locomotion (walking and running), non-locomotor actions (bending, twisting and balancing) and manipulative actions (finger dexterity). These movement patterns typically become more refined in later childhood as children become involved in games and sport. Theories of skill acquisition propose that skills are learned in a series of stages: cognitive, associative and automaticity (Fitts & Posner, 1967; Proctor, Reeve, & Weeks, 1990). The initial cognitive stage of learning is characterized by attention and mental effort, which is required to help the learner understand how a movement 'problem' is to be solved and how muscles will be selected, sequenced and timed. Neurophysiological measures of neural activity during skill development provide ample evidence of the triggering of cortical and cerebellar structures during this period of skill learning (Hatfield, Haufler, Hung, & Spalding, 2004). With practice, both motor and cognitive skills improve in terms of their effectiveness (e.g. increased accuracy) and efficiency (e.g. decreased physical and mental effort).

Paralleling the improvement in skills during the associative stage are shifts in activations of brain areas that come to control motor movements; for example, subcortical structures such as the basal ganglia and its connections to the cerebellum result in the construction of the motor programs that provide the basis for skilled movements. Historically, the primary role of the cerebellum was thought to relate to the control of rapid programmed movements (Diamond, 2000). For example, when skilled actions are required, higher-level systems such as those in the prefrontal cortex plan the execution of motor movements; lower-level systems such as the cerebellum alter the general motor program in terms of the timing and force of muscle contractions.

Recent research suggests that the cerebellum plays a considerably greater role than previously thought. Diamond (2000) and Pesce et al. (2016) suggest that skill acquisition involves an interplay between executive processes and cerebellar processes. Both forms of processing come online when an individual is faced with a task that is complex; i.e. one that is novel, unpractised, variable, challenging and requires a quick response. The results obtained from several studies conducted with children (Best, 2013; Lakes et al., 2013; Lakes & Hoyt, 2004) provide support for the task complexity hypothesis (see reviews by Best, 2010; Diamond, 2012, 2015; Diamond & Lee, 2011; van der Fels et al., 2015). Additional support for the role of task complexity on psychomotor skill learning is provided by neurorehabilitation researchers (Mang, Campbell, Ross, & Boyd, 2013; Petzinger et al., 2013; Stoykov & Madhavan, 2015).

Of particular interest in many of these studies is the effect of contextual interference on psychomotor learning. The contextual interference effect is observed when learning is more robust when training occurs under conditions that vary from trial to trial than when conditions are fixed and predictable. First observed in verbal-learning studies (Battig, 1956), several contemporary researchers who focus on psychomotor skills found that individuals who practise skills under varied training conditions (i.e. actions are varied across practice trials) learned more than those who practised skills under constant training conditions (i.e. actions remain constant across practice trials). Explanations for the facilitating effects of varied practice on learning have focused on the amount of mental involvement required of the individual during practice (Guadagnoli & Lee, 2004; Tomporowski, McCullick, & Horvat, 2010). Of particular interest are studies conducted by Curlik and his colleagues (Curlik & Shors, 2012; Shors, Anderson, Curlik, & Nokia, 2012), which explicitly hypothesize that mentally challenging physical activities promote greater learning than just physical activity alone and explain the improvements in terms of hippocampal plasticity. Their data suggest that the survival of newly formed hippocampal cells in rodents depends on the motor training experiences that occur along with physical activity. Hippocampal neurons fail to survive without challenging training.

The importance of physical activity for psychomotor skill learning is unquestioned; physical practice is the main factor in determining the rate and level of skill acquisition (Kantak & Winstein, 2011; Newell & Rosenbloom, 1981). Of interest to the present chapter is evidence showing that bouts of physical activity that are mentally challenging may be critical for long-term changes in children's cognition and memory.

Development and relational learning

Relational memory reflects experiences that are remembered on the basis of factual (semantic) information, spatial information about the location of objects and episodic information that catalogues an individual's experiences. Relational memory is central to understanding 'higher' types of learning. As such, relational learning is of particular importance for those who are interested in linkages between physical activity and children's academic achievement. The goal standards for academic progress, such as grades or scores on standardized tests of academic achievement, reflect how well children encode and store information in long-term memory, and then access and retrieve declarative information when faced with test items.

A significant number of theory-based research studies have been conducted over the past four decades to assess infants' and children's memory development (Schneider, 2015). As described previously, the focus of some researchers has been on 'bottom-up' processing that is reflected in theories of information processing while other researchers have focused on 'top-down' processing reflected in theories of strategy utilization and metamemory.

Information-processing theories draw heavily on the computer models of human cognition and propose that learning involves the encoding of sensory experience into short-term memory and then transferring it into long-term stores (Atkinson & Shiffrin, 1971). Short-term systems are characterized by their limited storage capacities and rapid loss of information (e.g. forgetting). Memory span tests reveal clear evidence that there are age-related differences in memory storage capacity (Dempster, 1981). Short-term memory differs from working memory, which involves not only the storage of information but the additional organization and transformation of that information (Schneider, 2015). While the two systems are related, imaging data suggest that working memory relies on the dorsolateral prefrontal cortex, while short-term memory does not (Diamond, 2013). Working memory, also referred to as information updating, is considered to be a component of executive functions and interacts with or is modulated by inhibition and switching components (Miyake et al., 2000).

The executive function hypothesis introduced by Kramer and his colleagues (Kramer et al., 2002) served as the basis for the majority of studies over the past two decades of the effects of acute bouts of exercise and chronic exercise training on cognition. Numerous systematic and narrative reviews have been conducted and those that have focused on children's performance suggest that, in general, acute bouts of exercise have small but significant effects on the components of executive function (Donnelly et al., 2016). While assumptions have been made concerning the relation between children's executive functions and academic achievement (Howie & Pate, 2012; Tomporowski, McCullick, Pendleton, & Pesce, 2015), there is insufficient evidence to support the contention that chronic exercise interventions improve children's performance on the global indices of academic performance (e.g. grades, standardized tests of academic achievement).

Theories of children's cognitive development also focus on 'top-down' processes such as strategy utilization and metamemory. Children's memory performance is known to be influenced by the emergence of several strategic variables. These include the ability to rehearse information in working memory (Belmont & Butterfield, 1977; Flavell, Beach, & Chinsky, 1966; Hagen & Stanovich, 1977), to group and regroup information to be retained (Dempster, 1981) and to chunk information to be remembered on the basis of recoded information (Chi, 1977). Given the importance of these strategic processes on memory, numerous attempts have been made to enhance them via cognitive training programmes. A recent review of the success of computer-based working-memory training programmes on children between 5 and 12 years of age suggests that training did improve children's working-memory performance, but the effects were temporary and did not appear to affect children's performance on global indices of academic performance (Randall & Tyldesley, 2016).

Metamemory refers to knowledge about one's memory processes (Flavell, 1971). The term metacognition is used by contemporary developmental researchers to include not only metamemory but also comprehension, communication and problem-solving skills (Flavell, 2000). Further, the construct is delineated as procedural metamemory, which is awareness that a particular well-learned and automatized movement or complex action requires some form of preplanning prior to execution, and declarative metamemory, which is the awareness of explicit factual knowledge that requires selection and proper utilization (Schneider, 2015).

Metacognition differs from executive functioning in terms of the depth of monitoring involved. Unlike executive functions, which are important for making decisions in the 'here and now', metacognition involves continuous bottom-up and top-down feedback loops that are critical when considering future actions to be taken. 'Mulling over' the solution to a problem allows time to consider the costs and benefits of actions and brings into play such factors as emotional states, social demands and personality factors, which may have minimal influence on rapid decision making that is characteristic of most methods of assessing executive functions (Roebers, in press; Tomporowski et al., 2015). Theories that focus on strategic processing and metacognition have led to large literatures and methods that can be used to measure the constructs. At this time, studies examining the effects of physical activity on children's use of strategic memory aids or metacognition have not been systematically conducted.

In summary, hypotheses generated from the various theories of cognitive development are well suited for research that includes physical activity interventions. However, as discussed by Etnier and Chang (2009), exercise researchers have tended to employ a limited number of tests developed to assess adults' executive function; as a result, relatively little progress has been made in understanding how physical activity might affect variables that impact children's memory and learning. Advances in understanding the human brain have accelerated over the past decade; however, few researchers have taken into consideration quantitative and qualitative age-related differences in cognitive processing. Exercise researchers will benefit by incorporating contemporary theories of children's cognitive development and selecting tests that are developmentally appropriate. The results of such research are of critical importance to physical activity programmes designed for authentic educational environments. The next challenge will be to determine whether physical activity interventions developed under laboratory conditions can be successfully adapted to school settings.

Educational applications

Given evidence suggesting that acute bouts of physical activity improve attention, information processing and decision making, it is easy to see its importance to academic performance. Neuroscience has much to offer schools and the sooner and more often its offerings are provided, the better it will be for children. The challenge, however, is how to apply research findings to school settings in meaningful ways. 'Translational research' is the term most often used to describe the application of laboratory research findings to natural environments. Several problems face translational researchers who are interested in using physical activity interventions to enhance children's academic performance and behaviour in school settings. These include: multiple constituencies; silos; finding a place; and redefining the gold standard.

Multiple constituencies

Schools are living, breathing organisms that have their own culture, politics and economics, and are governed by multiple layers of adults with different job responsibilities (McLaren, 2015). As with any large ecosystem, the chance for conflict between individuals is high. Getting scientists, funding agencies, school administrators, faculty and parents of school children to cooperate is a challenge.

Silos

The backgrounds and interests of basic and clinical researchers and those working in and for schools differ considerably. These differences often result in silos of expertise. Kretchmar (2008) has warned that some aspects of silos have merit and are essential, but those with walls that 'are lower and more permeable, whose spirit is more playful, and whose researchers and practitioners interact more democratically, with increasing levels of interdependence and humility and with a higher degree of mutual respect' (p. 3) are foundational to 'more collaboration, greater interdependency, and a deepened sense of mutual respect' (p. 11). This does not mean that it is the responsibility of researchers to reach out to those in schools or vice versa; it is simply a logistical condition that must be considered and addressed before any meaningful translational research can be done.

Finding a place

It is not enough for parties to leave their silos. Merely meeting and talking will not ensure that translational research can occur. Researchers with ideas are regularly met with realities in schools that seemingly prevent interventions from taking place. The focus of translational research is closely affiliated with 'play', and is often considered as ancillary to the purpose of schools. In such situations, acquiring support from school administrators can be difficult. Demands placed on school decision makers to improve children's academic performance have led to less scheduled time for children to be physically active during the school day.

Redefining the gold standard

The randomized controlled trial is viewed as the gold-standard method for determining the existence of a causal relation between an intervention and its outcomes. Few randomized controlled trials have been conducted in school settings, and those that have been conducted have typically had to alter school environments in ways that are not readily achievable in traditional school settings. What is needed for translational research in exercise science is a paradigm shift that allows for and accommodates reasonable methods for assessing the impact of an intervention on a wide number of outcome measures. The RE-AIM model introduced by Glasgow and his colleagues (Glasgow, Klesges, Dzewaltowski, Bull, & Eastbrooks, 2004) provides translational physical activity researchers with an alternative to the randomized controlled trial.

Despite these and other challenges that face successful implementation of translational research in authentic school settings, the message provided from neuroscience is clear. Physical activity alters brain health (Hillman, Erickson, & Kramer, 2008). Recently, Cairney and his colleagues (Cairney, Bedard, Dudley, & Kriellaars, 2016) evaluated the neuropsychological literature and proposed the need for a renewed interest in physical literacy that begins early in life and continues throughout the lifespan. National initiatives supported by educational agencies that emphasize physical literacy instruction may provide the traction needed to impact children's physical and mental development (Corbin, 2016).

References

Adolph, K. E. (2008). Learning to move. *Current Directions in Psychological Science, 17*(3), 213–218.

Amso, D., & Casey, B. J. (2006). Beyond what develops when. *Current Directions in Psychological Science, 15*(1), 24–29.

Atkinson, R., & Shiffrin, R. M. (1971). The control of short-term memory. *Scientific American, 225*, 82–90.

Audiffren, M. (2009). Acute exercise and psychological functions: A cognitive-energetic approach. In T. McMorris, P. D. Tomporowski, & M. Audiffren (Eds.), *Exercise and cognitive function* (pp. 3–39). Chichester, UK: John Wiley.

Baddeley, A. D. (2000). The episodic buffer: A new component of working memory? *Trends in Cognitive Sciences, 4*, 417–423.

Baddeley, A. D., & Hitch, G. J. (1974). Working memory. In G. Bower (Ed.), *The psychology of learning and motivation: Advances in research and theory* (Vol. 8, pp. 47–89). New York: Academic Press.

Battig, W. F. (1956). Transfer from verbal pretraining to motor performance as a function of task complexity. *Journal of Experimental Psychology, 51*(6), 371–378.

Baudry, S. (2016). Aging changes the contribution of spinal and corticospinal pathways to control balance. *Exercise and Sport Science Reviews, 44*(1), 104–109.

Belmont, J., & Butterfield, E. C. (1977). The instructional approach to developmental cognitive research. In R. Kail & J. W. Hagen (Eds.), *Perspectives on the development of memory and cognition* (pp. 437–481). Hillsdale, NJ: Erlbaum.

Best, J. R. (2010). Effects of physical activity on children's executive function: Contributions of experimental research on aerobic exercise. *Developmental Review, 30*(4), 331–351.

Best, J. R. (2013). Exergaming in youth. *Zeitschrift fur Psychologie, 221*(2), 72–78.

Bjorklund, D. F. (2005). *Children's thinking: Cognitive development and individual differences* (4th ed.). Pacific Grove, CA: Thomson-Wadsworth.

Black, J. E., Isaacs, K. R., Anderson, B. J., Alcantara, A. A., & Greenough, W. T. (1990). Learning causes synaptogenesis, whereas activity causes angiogenesis in cerebellar cortex of adult rats. *Proceedings of the National Academy of Science, 87*, 5568–5572.

Brocki, K. C., & Bohlin, G. (2004). Executive functions in children aged 6 to 13: A dimensional and developmental study. *Developmental Neuropsychology, 26*(2), 571–593.

Bunge, S. A., & Wright, S. B. (2007). Neurodevelopmental changes in working memory and cognitive control. *Current Opinion in Neurobiology, 17*, 243–250.

Cairney, J., Bedard, C., Dudley, D., & Kriellaars, D. (2016). Toward a physical literacy framework to guide the design, implementation and evaluation of early childhood movement-based interventions targeting cognitive development. *Annals of Sports Medicine and Research, 3*(4), 1073.

Campos, J. J., Anderson, D. I., Barbu-Roth, M.A., Hubbard, E. M., Hertenstein, M. J., & Witherington, D. (2000). Travel broadens the mind. *Infancy, 1*(2), 149–219.

Carlson, N. R. (2013). *Physiology of behavior* (11th ed.). Boston: Allyn and Bacon.

Casey, B. J., Amso, D., & Davidson, M. C. (2006). Learning about learning and development with modern imaging technology. In Y. Munakata & M. H. Johnson (Eds.), *Processes of change in brain and cognitive development: Attention and performance XXI* (Vol. 21, pp. 513–533). Oxford: Oxford University Press.

Casey, B. J., Galvan, A., & Hare, T. A. (2005). Changes in cerebral functional organization during cognitive development. *Current Opinion in Neurobiology, 15*(2), 239–244.

Casey, B. J., Giedd, J. N., & Thomas, K. M. (2000). Structural and functional brain development and its relation to cognitive development. *Biological Psychology, 54*, 241–257.

Chaddock, L., Erickson, K. I., Prakash, R. S., Kim, J. S., Voss, M. W., VanPatter, M., & Pontifex, M. B. (2010). A neuroimaging investigation of the association between aerobic fitness, hippocampal volume, and memory performance in preadolescent children. *Brain Research, 1358*, 172–183.

Chaddock, L., Hillman, C. H., Buck, S. M., & Cohen, N. J. (2011). Aerobic fitness and executive control of relational memory in preadolescent children. *Medicine and Science in Sports and Exercise, 43*(2), 344–349. doi: 10.1249/MSS.0b013e3181e9af48.

Chaddock-Heyman, L., Hillman, C. H., Cohen, N. J., & Kramer, A. F. (2014). III. The importance of physical activity and aerobic fitness for cognitive control and memory in children. *Monographs of the Society for Research in Child Development, 79*(4), 25–50.

Chang, Y-K., Labban, J. D., Gapin, J. I., & Etnier, J. L. (2012). The effects of acute exercise on cognitive performance: A meta-analysis. *Brain Research, 1453,* 87–101.

Chi, M. T. H. (1977). Age differences in memory span. *Journal of Experimental Child Psychology, 23,* 266–281.

Churchill, J. D., Galvez, R., Colcombe, S., Swain, R. A., Kramer, A. F., & Greenough, W. T. (2002). Exercise, experience and the aging brain. *Neurobiology of Aging, 23*(5), 941–955.

Corbin, C. B. (2016). Implications of physical literacy for research and practice: A commentary. *Research Quarterly for Exercise and Sport, 87*(1), 14–17.

Curlik, D. M., & Shors, T. J. (2012). Training your brain: Do mental and physical (MAP) training enhance cognition through the process of neurogenesis in the hippocampus? *Neuropharmacology, 64,* 506–514. doi: 10.1016/j.neuropharm.2012.07.027.

Dempster, F. N. (1981). Memory span: Sources of individual and developmental differences. *Psychological Bulletin, 89,* 63–100.

Diamond, A. (2000). Close interrelation of motor development and cognitive development and of the cerebellum and prefrontal cortex. *Child Development, 71*(1), 44–56.

Diamond, A. (2002). Normal development of prefrontal cortex from birth to young adulthood: Cognitive functions, anatomy, and biochemistry. In D. T. Stuss & R. T. Knight (Eds.), *Principles of frontal lobe function* (pp. 466–503). New York: Oxford University Press.

Diamond, A. (2012). Activities and programs that improve children's executive functions. *Current Directions in Psychological Sciences, 21*(5), 335–341.

Diamond, A. (2013). Executive functions. *Annual Review of Psychology, 64*(1), 135–168. doi: 10.1146/annurev-psych-113011-143750.

Diamond, A. (2015). Effects of physical exercise on executive functions: Going beyond simply moving to moving with thought. *Annals of Sports Medicine and Research, 2*(1), 1011.

Diamond, A., & Goldman-Rakic, P. S. (1989). Comparison of human infants and rhesus monkeys on Piaget's A-not-B task: Evidence for dependence on dorsolateral prefrontal cortex. *Experimental Brain Research, 74*(24–40).

Diamond, A., & Lee, K. (2011). Interventions shown to aid executive function development in children 4 to 12 years old. *Science, 959.* doi: 10.1126/science.1204529.

Diamond, A., & Ling, D. S. (2016). Conclusions about interventions, programs, and approaches for improving executive functions that appear justified and those that, despite hype, do not. *Developmental Cognitive Neuroscience, 18,* 34–38. doi: 10.1016/j.dcn.2015.11.005.

Dietrich, A., & Audiffren, M. (2011). The reticular-activating hypofrontality (RAH) model of acute exercise. *Neuroscience and Biobehavioral Reviews, 35,* 1305–1325.

Donnelly, J. E., Hillman, C. H., Castelli, D., Etnier, J. L., Lee, S., Tomporowski., P. D., . . . Szabo-Reed, N. (2016). Physical activity, cognitive function and academic achievement in children: American College of Sports Medicine position stand. *Medicine and Science in Sports and Exercise, 48*(6), 1197–1222. doi: DOI: 10.1249/MSS.0000000000000901.

Dornelles, A., de Lima, M. N. M., Grazziotin, M., Presti-Torres, J., Garcia, V. A., Scalco, F. S., . . . Schroder, N. (2007). Adrenergic enhancement of consolidation of object recognition memory. *Neurobiology of Learning and Memory, 88*(1), 137–142. doi: 10.1016/j.nlm.2007.01.005.

Ebbinghaus, H. (1885/1913). *On memory: An investigation to experimental psychology*. New York: Columbia University Press (original work published 1885).

Erickson, K. I., Voss, M. W., Prakash, R. S., Basak, C., Szabo, A., Chaddock, L., . . . Kramer, A. F. (2011). Exercise training increases size of hippocampus and improves memory. *Proceedings of the National Academy of Science, 108*(7), 3017–3022. doi: 10.1073/pnas.105950108/./DCSupplement.

Etnier, J. L., & Chang, Y-K. (2009). The effect of physical activity on executive function: A brief commentary on definitions, measurement issues, and the current state of the literature. *Journal of Sport and Exercise Psychology, 31*, 469–483.

Etnier, J. L., Labban, J. D., Piepmeier, A. T., Davis, M, E., & Henning, D. A. (2014). Effects of an acute bout of exercise on memory in 6th grade children. *Pediatric Exercise Science, 26*, 250–258.

Fabel, K., Wolf, S. A., Ehninger, D., Babu, H., Leal-Galicia, P., & Kempermann, G. (2009). Additive effects of physical exercise and environmental enrichment on adult hippocampal neurogenesis in mice. *Frontiers in Neuroscience, 3*, 50. doi: 10.3389/neuro.22.002.2009.

Fitts, P., & Posner, M. I. (1967). *Human performance*. Belmont, CA: Brooks/Cole.

Flavell, J. H. (1971). First discussant's comments: What is memory development the development of? *Human Development, 14*, 225–286.

Flavell, J. H. (2000). Development of children's knowledge about the mental world. *International Journal of Behavioral Development, 24*, 15–23.

Flavell, J. H., Beach, D. H., & Chinsky, J. M. (1966). Spontaneous verbal rehearsal in a memory task as a function of age. *Child Development, 37*, 283–299.

Gabbard, C. P. (2004). *Lifelong motor development* (4th ed.). New York: Pearson.

Gallese, V., & Metzinger, T. (2003). Motor ontology: The representational reality of goals, action and selves. *Philosophical Psychology, 16*(3), 365–388.

Gibson, E. J. (1969). *Principles of perceptual learning and development*. New York: Academic Press.

Glasgow, R. E., Klesges, L. M., Dzewaltowski, D. A., Bull, S. S., & Eastbrooks, P. (2004). The future of health behavior change research: What is needed to improve translation of research into health practice? *Annals of Behavioral Medicine, 27*(1), 3–12.

Gold, P. E. (2001). *Memory consolidation: Essays in honor of James L. McGaugh*. Washington, DC: American Psychological Association.

Gold, P. E., & van Buskirk, R. (1975). Facilitation of time-dependent memory processes with posttrial epinephrine injections. *Behavioral Biology, 13*, 145–153.

Gregory, R. L. (1970). *The intelligent eye*. London: Weidenfeld and Nicolson.

Guadagnoli, M. A., & Lee, T. D. (2004). Challenge point: A framework for conceptualizing the effects of various practice conditions in motor learning. *Journal of Motor Behavior, 36*(2), 212–224.

Hagen, J. W., & Stanovich, K. E. (1977). Memory: Strategies of acquisition. In R. Kail & J. W. Hagen (Eds.), *Perspectives on the development of memory and cognition* (pp. 89–111). Hillsdale, NJ: Erlbaum.

Hatfield, B. D., Haufler, A. J., Hung, T-M., & Spalding, T. W. (2004). Electroencephalographic studies of skilled psychomotor performance. *Journal of Clinical Neurophysiology, 21*, 144–156.

Hebb, D. O. (1949). *The organization of behavior*. New York: Wiley-Interscience.

Hergenhahn, B. R. (2001). *An introduction to the history of psychology* (4th ed.). Belmont, CA: Wadsworth.

Hillman, C. H., Erickson, K. I., & Kramer, A. F. (2008). Be smart, exercise your heart: Exercise effects on brain and cognition. *Nature Reviews Neuroscience, 9*(1), 58–65.

Hintzman, D. L. (1978). *The psychology of learning and memory*. New York: W. H. Freeman.

Howie, E. K., & Pate, R. R. (2012). Physical activity and academic achievement in children: A historical perspective. *Journal of Sport and Health Science, 1*, 160–169.

Huizinga, M. M., Dolan, C. V., & van der Molen, M. W. (2006). Age-related change in executive function: Developmental trends and a latent variable analysis. *Neuropsychologia, 44*, 2017–2036.

Hull, C. L. (1952). *A behavior system*. New York: Appleton-Century.

Jackson, P. L., & Decety, J. (2004). Motor cognition: A new paradigm to study self–other interactions. *Current Opinion in Neurobiology, 14*, 259–263.

James, W. (1981/1890). *The principles of psychology*. Cambridge, MA: Harvard University Press (originally published in 1890).

Kantak, S. S., & Winstein, C. J. (2011). Learning–performance distinction and memory processes for motor skills: A focused review and perspective. *Behavioural Brain Research, 228*, 219–231. doi: 10.1016/j.bbr.2011.11.028.

Kempermann, G. (2008). The neurogenic reserve hypothesis: What is adult hippocampal neurogenesis good for? *Trends in Neuroscience, 31*(4), 163–169.

Kempermann, G., Fabel, K., Ehninger, D., Babu, H., Leal-Galicia, P., Garthe, A., & Wolf, S. A. (2010). Why and how physical activity promotes experience-induced brain plasticity. *Frontiers in Neuroscience, 4*, 189. doi: 10.3389/fnins.2010.00189.

Kerick, S. E., Douglas, L. W., & Hatfield, B. D. (2004). Cerebral cortical adaptations assocoiated with visuomotor practice. *Medicine and Science in Sports and Exercise, 36*(1), 118–129.

Kontra, C., Goldin-Meadow, S., & Beilock, S. L. (2012). Embodied learning across the life span. *Topics in Cognitive Science, 4*, 731–739. doi: 10.1111/j.1756-8765.2012.01221.x.

Kontra, C., Lyons, D. J., Fischer, S. M., & Beilock, S. L. (2015). Physical experience enhances science learning. *Psychological Science, 26*(6), 737–749. doi: 10.1177/0956797615569355.

Koziol, L. F., Budding, D. E., & Chidekel, D. (2011). From movement to thought: Executive function, embodied cognition, and the cerebellum. *Cerebellum, 11*(2), 505–525.

Koziol, L. F., & Lutz, J. T. (2013). From movement to thought: The development of executive function. *Applied Neuropsychology: Child, 2*(2), 104–115.

Kramer, A. F., Hahn, S., McAuley, E., Cohen, N. J., Banich, M. T., Harrison, C. R., . . . Vakil, E. (2002). Exercise, aging, and cognition: Healthy body, healthy mind? In W. A. Rogers & A. D. Fisk (Eds.), *Human factors interventions for the health care of older adults* (pp. 91–120). Mahwah, NJ: Erlbaum.

Kretchmar, R. S. (2008). The utility of silos and bunkers in the evolution of kinesiology. *Quest, 60*(1), 3–12.

Labban, J. D., & Etnier, J. L. (2011). Effects of acute exercise on long-term memory. *Research Quarterly for Exercise and Sport, 82*(4), 712–721.

Lakes, K. D., Bryars, T., Sirisinahal, S., Salim, N., Arastoo, S., Emmerson, N., . . . Kang, C. J. (2013). The Healthy for Life Taekwondo pilot study: A preliminary evaluation of effects on executive function and BMI, feasibility, and acceptability. *Mental Health and Physical Activity, 6,* 181–188.

Lakes, K. D., & Hoyt, W. T. (2004). Promoting self-regulation through school-based martial arts training. *Applied Developmental Psychology, 25,* 283–302. doi: 10.1016/j.appdev.2004.04.002.

Lambourne, K., & Tomporowski, P. D. (2010). The effect of acute exercise on cognitive task performance: A meta-regression analysis. *Brain Research Reviews, 1341,* 12–24.

Luciana, M. (2003). The neural and functional development of human prefrontal cortex. In M. de Haan & M. H. Johnson (Eds.), *The cognitive neuroscience of development* (pp. 157–179). New York: Psychology Press.

Maguire, E. A., Gadian, D. G., Johnsrude, I. S., Good, C., Ashburner, J., Frackowiak, R. S. J., & Frith, C.D. (2000). Navigation-related structural change in the hippocampi of taxi drivers. *Proceedings of the National Academy of Science, 97*(8), 4398–4403.

Mang, C. S., Campbell, K. L., Ross, C. J. D., & Boyd, L. A. (2013). Promoting neuroplasticity for motor rehabilitation after stroke: Considering the effects of aerobic exercise and genetic variation on brain-derived neurotrophic factor. *Physical Therapy, 93,* 1707–1796.

McGaugh, J. L. (2004). The amygdala modulates the consolidation of memories of emotionally arousing experiences. *Annual Review of Neuroscience, 27,* 1–28.

McGaugh, J. L. (2015). Consolidating memories. *Annual Review of Psychology, 66,* 1–24. doi: 10.1146/annurev-psych-010814-014954.

McLaren, P. (2015). *Life in schools: An introduction to critical pedagogy in the foundations of education.* London: Routledge.

McMorris, T., Collard, K., Corbett, J., Dicks, M., & Swain, J. P. (2008). A test of the catecholamines hypothesis for acute exercise–cognition interaction. *Pharmacology, Biochemistry and Behavior, 89,* 106–115.

McMorris, T., & Graydon, J. (2000). The effect of incremental exercise on cognitive performance. *International Journal of Sport Psychology, 31,* 66–81.

McMorris, T., & Hale, B. J. (2015). Is there an acute exercise-induced physiological/ biochemical threshold which triggers increased speed of cognitive functioning? *Journal of Sport and Health Science, 4*(1), 4–13. doi: 10.1016/j.jshs.2014.08.003.

McMorris, T., Hale, B. J., Corbett, J., Robertson, K., & Hodgson, C. I. (2015). Does acute exercise affect the performance of whole-body, psychomotor skills in an inverted-U fashion? A meta-analytic investigation. *Physiology and Behavior, 141,* 180–189. doi: 10.1016/j.physbeh.2015.01.010.

Mirenowicz, J., & Schultz, W. (1994). Importance of unpredictability for reward responses in primate dopamine neurons. *Journal of Neurophysiology, 72,* 1024–1027.

Mithen, S. (1996). *The prehistory of the mind.* London: Thames and Hudson.

Miyake, A., Friedman, N. P., Emerson, M. J., Witzki, A. H., Howerter, A., & Wager, T. D. (2000). The unity and diversity of executive functions and their contributions to complex "frontal lobe" tasks: A latent variable analysis. *Cognitive Psychology, 41,* 49–100.

Miyashita, Y. (2004). Cognitive memory: Cellular and network machineries and their top-down control. *Science, 306,* 435–440.

Moreau, D., Morrison, A. B., & Conway, A. R. A. (2015). An ecological approach to cognitive enhancement: Complex motor training. *Acta Psychologica, 157,* 44–55.

Morris, R. (2013). Neurobiology of learning and memory. In D. W. Pfaff (Ed.), *Neuroscience in the 21st century* (pp. 2173–2211). New York: Springer.

Nelson, C. A. (2000). Neural plasticity and human development: The role of early experience in sculpting memory systems. *Developmental Science, 3,* 115–136.

Nelson, C. A., Monk, C. S., Lin, J., Carver, L. J., Thomas, K,. M., & Truwit, C. L. (2000). Functional neuroanatomy of spatial working memory in children. *Developmental Psychology, 36,* 109–116.

Newcombe, N. S., & Frick, A. (2010). Early education for spatial intelligence: Why, what, and how. *Mind, Brain and Education, 4*(3), 102–111.

Newell, A., & Rosenbloom, P. S. (1981). Mechanisms of skill acquisition and the law of practice. In J Anderson, R. (Ed.), *Cognitive skills and their acquisition* (pp. 1–55). Hillsdale, NJ: Erlbaum.

Olds, J., & Milner, P. (1954). Positive reinforcement produced by electrical stimulation of setal area and other regions of rat brain. *Journal of Comparative and Physiological Psychology, 47,* 419–427.

Pavlov, I. P. (1963). *Lectures on conditioned reflexes.* London: Lawrence and Wishart.

Pesce, C., Croce, R., Ben-Soussan, T. D., Vazou, S., McCullick, B., Tomporowski, P. D., & Horvat, M. (2016). Variability of practice as an interface between motor and cognitive development promotion. *International Journal of Sport and Exercise Psychology.* doi: 10.1080/1612197X.2016.1223421.

Pesce, C., Crova, C., Cereatti, L., Casella, R., & Bellucci, M. (2009). Physical activity and mental performance in preadolescents: Effects of acute exercise on free-recall memory. *Mental Health and Physical Activity, 2,* 16–22.

Pesce, C., Crova, C., Marchetti, M., Struzzolino, I., Masci, I., Vannozzi, G., & Forte, R. (2013). Searching for cognitively optimal challenge point in physical activity for children with typical and atypical motor development. *Mental Health and Physical Activity, 6,* 172–180.

Petzinger, G. M., Fisher, B. E., McEwen, S., Beeler, J. A., Walsh, J. P., & Jakowec, M. W. (2013). Exercise-enhanced neuroplasticity targeting motor and cognitive circuitry in Parkinson's disease. *Lancet Neurology, 12,* 716–726. doi: 10.1016/S14744422(13)70123-6.

Piaget, J. (1963). *The origins of intelligence in children* (M. Cook, trans.). New York: W. W. Norton.

Posner, M. I., & Rothbart, M. K. (2007). *Educating the human brain.* Washington, DC: American Psychological Association.

Prakash, R., Voss, M. W., Erickson, K. I., & Kramer, A. F. (2015). Physical activity and cognitive vitality. *Annual Review of Psychology, 66,* 769–797. doi: 10.1146/annurev-psych-010814-015249.

Proctor, R.W., Reeve, E. G., & Weeks, D. J. (1990). A triphasic approach to the acquisition of response-selection skill. In G. H. Bower (Ed.), *The psychology of learning: Advances in research and theory* (pp. 207–240). New York: Academic Press.

Puff, C. R. (Ed.). (1982). *Handbook of research methods in human memory and cognition*. New York: Academic Press.

Randall, L., & Tyldesley, K. (2016). Evaluating the impact of working memory training programmes on children: A systematic review. *Educational and Child Psychology, 33*(1), 34–50.

Roebers, C. M. (in press). Executive function and metacognition: Towards a unifying framework of cognitive self-regulation. *Developmental Review*.

Roig, M., Nordbrant, S., Geertsen, S. S., & Nielsen, J. B. (2013). The effects of cardiovascular exercise on human memory: A review with meta-analysis. *Neuroscience and Biobehavioral Reviews, 37*, 1645–1666. doi: 10.1016/j.neubiorev.2013.06.012.

Roig, M., Thomas, R., Mang, C. S., Snow, N. J., Ostadan, F., Boyd, L. A., & Lundbye-Jensen, J. (2016). Time-dependent effects of cardiovascular exercise on memory. *Exercise and Sport Science Reviews, 44*(2), 81–88. doi: 10.1249/JES.0000000000000078.

Roozendaal, B. (2000). Glucocorticoids and the regulation of memory consolidation. *Psychoneuroendocrinology, 25*, 213–238.

Roozendaal, B., Okuda, S., Van der Zee, E., & McGaugh, J. L. (2006). Glucocorticoid enhancement of memory requires arousal-induced noradrenergic activation in the basolateral amygdala. *Proceedings of the National Academy of Science, 103*(17), 6741–6746. doi: 01.1073/pnas.0601874103.

Scherf, K. S., Sweeney, J. A., & Liuna, B. (2006). Brain basis of developmental changes in visuo-spatial working memory. *Journal of Cognitive Neuroscience, 18*(7), 1045–1058.

Schmidt, R. A. (1975). A schema theory of discrete motor skill learning theory. *Psychological Review, 82*, 225–260.

Schmidt, R. A., & Wrisberg, C. A. (2008). *Motor learning and performance*. Champaign. IL: Human Kinetics.

Schneider, W. (2015). *Memory development from early childhood through emerging adulthood*. Cham, Switzerland: Springer International Publishers.

Schott, B. H., Sellner, D. B., Lauer, C-J., Habib, R., Frey, J. U., Guderian, S., . . . Duzel, E. (2004). Activation of midbrain structures by associative novelty and the formation of explicit memory in humans. *Learning and Memory, 11*, 383–387. doi: 10.1101/lm.75004.

Shors, T. J., Anderson, M. L., Curlik, D. M., & Nokia, M. S. (2012). Use it or lose it: How neurogenesis keeps the brain fit for learning. *Behavioural Brain Research, 227*, 450–458. doi: 10.1016/j.bbr.2011.04.023.

Sibley, B. A., & Etnier, J. L. (2003). The relationship between physical activity and cognition in children: A meta-analysis. *Pediatric Exercise Science, 15*, 243–256.

Skinner, B. F. (1938). *The behavior of organisms: An experimental analysis*. New York: Appleton-Century.

Skinner, B. F. (1990). Can psychology be a science of the mind? *American Psychologist, 45*, 1206–1210.

Sommerville, J. A., & Decety, J. (2006). Weaving the fabric of social interaction: Articulating developmental psychology and cognitive neuroscience in the domain of motor cognition. *Psychonomic Bulletin and Review, 13*(2), 179–200.

Song, S. (2009). Consciousness and the consolidation of motor learning. *Behavioural Brain Research, 196*, 180–186. doi: 10.1016/j.bbr.2008.09.034.

Squire, L. R. (2004). Memory systems of the brain: A brief history and current perspective. *Neurobiology of Learning and Memory, 82*, 171–177. doi: 10.1016/j.nlm.2004.06.005.

Stones, M. J., & Dawe, D. (1993). Acute exercise facilitates semantically cued memory in nursing home residents. *Journal of the American Geriatrics Society, 41*, 531–534.

Stoykov, M. E., & Madhavan, S. (2015). Motor priming in neurorehabiliation. *Journal of Neurologic Physical Therapy, 39*(1), 33–42. doi: 10.1097/NPT.0000000000000065.

Thelen, E. (1996). Motor development. *American Psychologist, 50*(2), 79–95.

Thomas, A. G., Dennis, A., Bandettini, P. A., & Johansen-Berg, H. (2012). The effects of aerobic activity on brain structure. *Frontiers in Psychology, 3*, 86. doi: 10.3389/fpsyg.2012.00086.

Thompson, R. A., & Nelson, C. A. (2001). Developmental science and the media. *American Psychologist, 56*(1), 6–15.

Thorndike, E. L. (1914). *Educational psychology: Briefer course.* New York: Columbia University Press.

Tomporowski, P. D. (2003a). Cognitive and behavioral responses to acute exercise in youth: A review. *Pediatric Exercise Science, 15*, 348–359.

Tomporowski, P. D. (2003b). Effects of acute bouts of exercise on cognition. *Acta Psychologica, 112*, 297–324.

Tomporowski, P. D., McCullick, B. A., & Horvat, M. (2010). *Role of contextual interference and mental engagement on learning.* New York: Nova Science.

Tomporowski, P. D., McCullick, B., Pendleton, D. M., & Pesce, C. (2015). Exercise and children's cognition: The role of task factors and a place for metacognition. *Journal of Sport and Health Science, 4*, 47–55. doi: 10.1016/j.jshs.2014.09.0.

van der Fels, I. M. J., te Wierike, S. C. M., Hartman, E., Elferink-Gemser, M. T., Smith, J., & Visscher, C. (2015). The relationship between motor skills and cognitive skills in 4–16 year old typically developing children: A systematic review. *Journal of Science and Medicine in Sport, 18*, 697–703.

van Pragg, H., Christie, B. R., Sejnowski, T. J., & Gage, F. H. (1999). Running enhances neurogenesis, learning, and long-term potentiation in mice. *Proceedings of the National Academy of Science, 96*(23), 13427–13431.

Voss, M. W., Vivar, C., Kramer, A. F., & Van Praag, H. (2013). Bridging animal and human models of exercise-induced brain plasticity. *Trends in Cognitive Sciences, 17*(10), 525–544. doi: 10.1016/j.tics.2013.08.001.

Willingham, D. B. (1999). The neural basis of motor-skill learning. *Current Directions in Psychological Sciences, 8*(6), 178–182.

Wilson, M. (2002). Six views of embodied cognition. *Psychonomic Bulletin and Review, 9*(4), 625–636.

Woodworth, R. S., & Schlosberg, H. (1954). *Experimental psychology.* New York: Holt.

Yerkes, R. M., & Dodson, J. D. (1908). The relation of strength of stimulus to rapidity of habit formation. *Journal of Comparative Neurology and Psychology, 18*, 459–482.

Chapter 3

Future directions

Rigorous research design and authentic application of neuroscience

Charles H. Hillman and Darla M. Castelli

Introduction

The number of research studies focused on the effects of physical activity participation on scholastic achievement and cognitive health has grown exponentially since the beginning of the 21st century (Castelli et al., 2014). As evident from previous chapters, there is a continued emphasis on standards-based achievement as a measure of school effectiveness, thus making the investigation of known facilitators of children's learning, a priority. Although the increased breadth of research related to this topic is valued, there is concern that the design of research studies remains largely cross-sectional, examining the relationship of physical activity within a small subject sample of a single demographic (Singh Uijtdewilligen, Twisk, van Mechelen, & Chinapaw, 2012). As such, while we have accumulated a wealth of descriptive evidence collectively, we have done little to advance the field in a novel and meaningful manner. Accordingly, the purpose of this chapter is to highlight some of the limitations of the existing research and to provide recommendations for future directions.

Background on the study of physical activity and cognitive performance

Intuitively, we have long believed that physical activity has both physical and cognitive health benefits that facilitate learning; however, the scientific evidence for such relationships has only recently emerged, first among non-human animals and older adults, and more recently in children. Such evidence and the interactions among the variables are complex and not easily interpreted; therefore, readers should critically scrutinize each study, despite the high volume of research resulting in null or positive findings.

Since the 1960s–1970s scholars (Gabbard & Barton, 1979; Ismail, 1967) have attempted to document the importance of physical activity during the school day by examining how participation in physical education (and other physical activity opportunities like recess) may have immediate benefits related to attention, memory and on-task behaviours. Several meta-analytic reviews have not only confirmed that there is a positive associa-tion between physical activity/physical fitness and scholastic achievement/cognitive performance/mental health (Biddle & Asare, 2011; Donnelly et al., 2016; Howie & Pate, 2012; Tomporowski, Davis, Miller, & Naglieri, 2008), but also dose–response effects between physical activity and scho-lastic achievement (Timmons, Naylor, Pfieffer, 2007; van Dusen, Kelder, Kohl, Ranjit, & Perry, 2011). Comprehensive reviews of literature can be found in the Institute of Medicine (2013) report, *Educating the Student Body: Taking Physical Activity and Physical Education to School* and the American College of Sports Medicine's position stand, "Physical activity, fitness, cognition function, and academic achievement in children: A sys-tematic review" (Donnelly et al., 2016). Such reviews have inherent value, as we want our children to minimize health risk and be successful learners, but often the studies included in the reviews are limited by the lack of matched control groups, consistent application of research methods (i.e. known con-founding variables are commonly not measured), as well as the small size and make-up of the sample.

A systematic review (Basch, 2010) of this line of inquiry has revealed the examination of the effects of physical activity and fitness on scholastic achieve-ment has been largely limited to Caucasian, middle-class to affluent commu-nities, where parents have high levels of education and an appreciation of the scientific inquiry. Few studies (Basch, 2011) have investigated the effects of physical activity among underprivileged children of colour in an urban setting. Further, across 50 years of study, the limitations of this field repeat-edly emerge: (1) lack of authentic application of neuroscience understanding; (2) few randomized controlled trials; and (3) no measurement of health risks.

Lab and classroom

One necessary future direction is the fusion of basic laboratory science with applied, real-world environments. To date, these areas have emerged as sep-arate research threads, with few examples to the contrary. On the one hand, laboratory studies, designed to establish relationships using internally valid methods, have determined that physical activity is related to select aspects of brain and cognition. However, while much has been learned regarding physical activity effects on brain and cognition, most findings derived from these studies are not directly applicable to the academic environment, rend-ing it difficult to determine how best to apply the findings (see Raine et al., 2013, for one exception).

On the other hand, school-based studies have demonstrated the effi-cacy of physical activity for scholastic performance and behaviours using externally valid approaches such as academic achievement outcomes and time-on-task behaviour. However, many of these findings have occurred with little understanding of neural networks, mechanisms or cognitive processes that underlie changes in scholastic performance, leading to a lack of understanding for how and why such a pattern of findings was observed, and at times, difficulty replicating the initial findings. Unfortunately, few efforts have ensued, which utilized a translational approach to research, taking basic laboratory findings and demonstrating their efficacy in a real-world environment. Further, few studies have measured the effects of the learning environment, including why teachers select specific instructional strategies; how opportunities for physical activity are structured; what incentivizes healthy student and teacher behaviours; what role other school personnel play in enhancing the learning environment; and how facilities/resources facilitate physical activity engagement.

Accordingly, future research should focus on outcomes that extend beyond the laboratory and plan experiments that focus on the promotion of cognitive health and learning in a manner in which children are likely to benefit from such findings. Similarly, school-based research should look to basic laboratory findings to guide not only matters surrounding physical activity administration (i.e. physical activity characteristics and environments that have demonstrated efficacy for a cognitive change) but also for expectations regarding the changes in cognition and learning that are reasonable to expect from intervention. Through this partnership, both long- and short-term goals could be established as a prioritization of research questions, guidelines for new researchers interested in undertaking a process of inquiry related to this topic and as a means of pooling existing data. Such a marriage of basic and applied research would likely benefit from the construction of transdisciplinary research teams that include kinesiologists, cognitive neuroscientists, developmental psychologists, physical educators and educators alike.

Lack of data

One challenge within the field thus far has been the rush to action in an attempt to implement change in children's physical activity in and out of school. That is, several examples of models, which in some cases appear commonsensical, have gained considerable appeal despite little empirical support. For example, Best (2010) has suggested that physical activity, which includes a cognitively engaging component, may have larger benefits to cognition and learning beyond those of more standard physical activity practices. Although there is considerable appeal to this hypothesis, little empirical evidence has been reported in the literature, and a considerably larger database exists that has used more traditional (i.e. so-called 'non-engaging') physical activity methods to demonstrate benefits to brain and cognition. As such, future research needs not only to determine whether there is evidence to support 'cognitively engaging physical activity' benefits to cognition (beyond that of typical or 'non-engaging' physical activity), but such determination needs to be made using the strongest study designs (i.e. randomized controlled trials). Given that randomized controlled trials have been used to establish an effect of 'non-engaging' physical activity on the brain, cognition and academic performance, a similar standard is required for future research on cognitively engaging physical activity to disentangle this relation fully from that of 'non-engaging' physical activity with brain and cognition. Such determination will be challenging, given that cognitively engaging physical activity includes similar physical characteristics to non-engaging physical activity. Thus, proper study design with the necessary control groups will be crucial toward determining the worth of this hypothesis. Such considerations, and programmes of research, are necessary prior to implementation in the classroom to ensure that physical activity is inserted into the school context in the best possible manner to achieve cognitive and learning outcomes.

To that end, similar future directions are needed for the rush to improve standard classroom practices using a wealth of different tools and techniques to improve physical activity and other health behaviours. Specifically, little empirical evidence exists at this time to support walking desks, active chairs and the myriad of classroom-based physical activity programmes (see Donnelly et al., 2009, for one exception). This is not to say that specific benefits for physical activity behaviour may be derived from these interventions, but a clear link to advantages in the domains of cognition and learning is not evident at this time. Accordingly, future research and public health recommendations must proceed cautiously, given the strong desire for the field to discover methods of physical activity to best improve children's lives.

Randomized controlled trials

Although several recent randomized controlled trials have investigated physical activity effects on brain and cognition (Davis et al., 2011; Hillman et al., 2014), additional research is needed to expand the knowledge base on the extent to which physical activity and other health behaviours may effect change. That is, to date, most randomized controlled trials have focused on executive control processes, which are mediated by a neural network involving the prefrontal cortex. However, the effect of physical activity across the breadth of executive control processes as well as other aspects of cognition remains unknown at this time.

While some studies have utilized epidemiologic designs as an attempt to capture dose–response effects (Timmons et al., 2007, children in preschool; van Dusen et al., 2011, school-aged children), what is unknown at this point is the optimal dose of physical activity in terms of intensity, duration and mode to optimize change, and whether the characteristics of the physical activity intervention must be modified as a function of age, sex and other relevant demographics (e.g. intelligence, socioeconomic status, pubertal timing). Further, knowledge is needed of whether various special populations (e.g. attention deficit-hyperactivity disorder, autism, metabolic syndrome) are similarly responsive to physical activity interventions, or whether modifications to the physical activity stimulus are required to promote benefits to brain and cognition better. Regardless, the ultimate goal is to inundate the field with findings in an attempt to bring about consensus of the effect of physical activity on brain and cognition, with the goal of understanding a dose–response relationship that brings about efficacious improvements in childhood cognition and learning.

The 'proper' control group

One difficulty thus far has been the determination of proper control groups or conditions for demonstrating the efficacy of the physical activity–cognition relationship. As such, several different comparisons have been employed in laboratory experiments, including wait-list control groups (Hillman et al., 2014) and non-activity attentional controls (i.e. board game and art projects; Krafft et al., 2014) in randomized controlled trials; quiet sitting and reading in acute exercise experiments (Hillman et al., 2009; Pontifex, Saliba, Raine, Picchietti, & Hillman, 2013); and typical physical education (Sallis et al., 1999) or non-activity breaks (Donnelly et al., 2009; Ma, Le Mare, & Gurb, 2014) within classroom environments in school-based research. Given that there is little continuity between studies it remains unclear which is the best means of comparison. Certain approaches such as wait-list controls or non-activity classroom breaks are appealing because they allow comparison with typical environments and behaviours. However, such an approach also raises concerns about a lack of control over factors unrelated to the physical activity intervention, such as social aspects of the intervention, or attention from experimenters and exercise leaders. Similarly, control groups that account for these factors, such as non-physically active environments (e.g. homework assistance) may alter children's typical behaviours, which may involve daily physical activity, and would thus call into question the directionality of group effects. As such, future research will need to account for not only the physical activity environments used to influence changes in cognition and learning but also the comparison groups or conditions to ensure the validity of the reported findings.

Which witch is which: creating a lexicon

Scholastic or academic achievement, executive function or control; these are just a few of the terms being inconsistently and sometimes inaccurately applied. Disciplinary jargon has existed for quite some time, but given the development of transdisciplinary and interdisciplinary research teams, it is now more important than ever to seek to understand one another's discipline. Neuroscience, psychology, kinesiology and education are blended in such study, but often only choose to publish research in their primary discipline. Greater dissemination of scientific evidence and theory needs to be decomposed and expressed in the terminology that educators use in their daily routines (Castelli, Centeio, & Nicksic, 2013) because relearning existing vocabulary is frustrating and time consuming for teachers. When we speak with a common language, the potential of transdisciplinary research is maximized.

Health risks and cognitive impairment

The cost to care for individuals with cardiovascular disease (CVD) has the potential to cripple the global economy, especially since both physical and cognitive function are affected, as dementia and other cognitive impairments are predicted to cost $600 billion (Kinsella & Wan, 2009). The magnitude of health care costs is concerning given the presence of known scientifically based prevention strategies (i.e. regular engagement in physical activity), as behavioural and environmental factors shape one's cognitive health (Ballesteros, Kraft, Santana, & Tziraki, 2015; Kramer, Bherer, Colcombe, Dong, & Greenough, 2004).

Adult CVD, a range of conditions related to the damage of vasculature, which inhibits blood circulation, often begins with physical inactivity and unhealthy eating during childhood and young adulthood. Prevalence of risk for CVD has increased globally, but most commonly in highly industrialized countries. Physical activity participation is one method for decreasing CVD risks, while also having the potential to improve cognitive performance, as health indicators have been directly and indirectly associated with scholastic achievement (Castelli et al., 2014; Janssen & LeBlanc, 2010). Dementia, memory loss due to ageing or a preliminary step in the progression of Alzheimer's disease is expected to impact over 100 million people by 2050 (Kinsella & Wan, 2009). Among the risk factors that have been associated with and indirectly related to cognitive performance are physical inactivity, poor physical fitness, obesity and high blood pressure.

Physical inactivity and low aerobic fitness

Aerobically fit children (Carlson et al., 2008; Castelli, Hillman, Buck, & Erwin, 2007; Chomitz et al., 2009; Etnier, Nowell, Landers, & Sibley, 2006; Wittberg, Northrup, & Cottrell, 2009, 2012) demonstrate enhanced scholastic performance over their inactive and unfit peers. Research findings exploring the relationship between physical activity and cognitive performance have been less robust, as previously stated, because different studies utilized differing volumes and types of physical activity. Physical activity intervention studies sometimes produce positive findings (Kamijo et al., 2011) and at other times, non-significant differences in cognitive performance when the groups were compared (Ahamed et al., 2007), despite using randomized controlled research designs. Despite the varying degree to which physical activity was directly or indirectly related to scholastic achievement, there is robust evidence that engagement in physical activity during childhood is necessary for health and normal development. Recently, comprehensive models have been created to align school personnel and the school-day schedule with opportunities for children to participate in physical activity (Castelli, Carson, & Kulinna, in press).

Childhood obesity

Today, youth are more sedentary and overweight than their parents were during childhood (Fontaine, Redden, Wang, Westfall, & Allison, 2013). When children enter school overweight or become overweight in their first few years of formalized schooling, they have lower scholastic performance than those who are of healthy body weight (Datar & Sturm, 2006; Datar, Sturm, & Magnabosco, 2004). Children who eat breakfast are more likely to have a healthy body weight and do well in school (Rampersaud, Pereira, Girard, Adams, & Metzl, 2005). As such, we should be examining big data that schools commonly collect (e.g. what type of food is consumed during school lunch, academic achievement, ethnicity, standardized testing, physical fitness, health screenings) to identify patterns of behaviour, productive environments and points in need of intervention.

High blood pressure

A longitudinal study conducted over 28–30 years revealed that high blood pressure was associated with increased risk for poor cognitive performance on visual memory tasks and even greater risk among hypertensive individuals (Elias et al., 1997). Specific to children, those with elevated blood pressure did not perform as well on memory tasks as those with healthy blood pressure (Lande, Kaczorowski, Auinger, Schwartz, & Weitzman, 2003). Linking annual wellness visits to the physician with school data has the greatest potential to help children maximize their potential for success. Until this collaboration occurs, individual education plans designed to customize the educational experience to the needs of the child will be something reserved for those individuals with a clinically diagnosed health or cognitive disorder.

Declarations

Since the authors or their colleagues have expressed many of the recommendations identified in this chapter previously, we are now entitling our assertions *declarations*, with the hope that our fellow scholars will act on the following before researching this topic. Given the paucity of studies in some research threads (e.g. neuroscience in authentic settings) and the overabundance in others (e.g. cross-sectional research on scholastic performance), we recommend the following ideas be considered before engaging in future research:

- apply rigorous experimental designs that include matched controls and understudied populations;
- measure and control for established confounding variables (i.e. physical fitness, IQ, school climate, socioeconomic status);
- replicate research findings in school settings, while accounting for the learning environment;
- promote physical activity, physical education and healthy eating within the school setting as strategies to prevent and decrease the prevalence of health risk factors related to CVD and cognitive impairment;
- disseminate findings and make recommendations within and beyond your discipline.

Implications

In sum, the advent of new technologies with enhanced sensitivity will continue to help us to understand how behavioural and environmental factors influence learning and cognitive health. New technology and high interest will advance the field, but a lack of rigorous research design, a lexicon of study and authentic ground truthing in the school settings (models that apply neuroscience in the schools that include an evaluation plan confirming the fidelity and effectiveness of such interventions) inhibit progress associated with such investments. Collaborative and collective efforts among scientists are necessary if comprehensive dose–response recommendations about physical activity are to become commonplace in schools.

References

Ahamed, Y., Macdonald, H., Reed, K., Naylor, P., Liu-Ambrose, T., & Mckay, H. (2007). Schoolbased physical activity does not compromise children's academic performance. *Medicine and Science in Sports and Exercise, 39*(2), 371–376. doi: 10.1249/01.mss.0000241654.45500.8e.

Ballesteros, S., Kraft, E., Santana, S., & Tziraki, C. (2015). Maintaining older brain functionality: A targeted review. *Neuroscience and Biobehavioral Reviews, 55*, 453–477.

Basch, C. E. (2010). *Healthier students are better learners: A missing link in efforts to close the achievement gap.* Equity Matters: Research Review No. 6. New York: The Campaign for Educational Equity.

Basch, C. E. (2011). Physical activity and the achievement gap among urban minority youth. *Journal of School Health, 81*(10), 626–634. doi: 10.1111/j.1746-1561.2011.00637.x.

Best, J. R. (2010). Effects of physical activity on children's executive function: Contributions of experimental research on aerobic exercise. *Developmental Review, 30,* 331–351.

Biddle, S. J. H., & Asare, M. (2011). Physical activity and mental health in children and adolescents: A review of reviews. *British Journal of Sports Medicine, 45*(11), 886–895. doi:10.1136/bjsports-2011-090185.

Carlson, S. A., Fulton, J. E., Lee, S. M., Maynard, L. M., Brown, D. R., Kohl, H. W., & Dietz, W. H. (2008). Physical education and academic achievement in elementary school: Data from the early childhood longitudinal study. *American Journal of Public Health, 98,* 721–727.

Castelli, D. M., Carson, R., & Kulinna, P.H. (in press). PETE programs creating teacher leaders to integrate Comprehensive School Physical Activity Programs. *Journal of Health, Physical Education, Recreation, and Dance.*

Castelli, D. M., Centeio, E. E., Hwang, J., Barcelona, J. M., Glowacki, E. M., Calvert, H. G., & Nicksic, H. (2014). The history of physical activity and academic performance research: Informing the future. *Society for Research in Child Development* – Monograph, 79(4), 119–148.

Castelli, D. M., Centeio, E. E., & Nicksic, H. M. (2013). Preparing educators to promote and provide physical activity in schools. *American Journal of Lifestyle Medicine, 7*(5), 324–332.

Castelli, D. M., Hillman, C. H., Buck, S. M., & Erwin, H. E. (2007). Physical fitness and academic achievement in third- and fifth-grade students. *Journal of Sport and Exercise Psychology, 29,* 239–352.

Chomitz, V. R., Slining, M. M., McGowan, R. J., Mitchell, S. E., Dawson, G. F., & Hacker, K. A. (2009). Is there a relationship between physical fitness and academic achievement? Positive results from public school children in the northeastern United States. *The Journal of School Health, 79,* 30–37.

Datar, A., & Sturm, R. (2006). Childhood overweight and elementary school outcomes. *International Journal of Obesity, 30,* 1449–1460.

Datar, A., Sturm, R., & Magnabosco, J. L. (2004). Childhood overweight and academic performance: national study of kindergartners and first-graders. *Obesity, 12,* 58–68.

Davis, C. L., Tomporowski, P. D., McDowell, J. E., Austin, B. P., Miller, P. H., Yanasak, N. E., Allison, J. D., & Naglieri, J. A. (2011). Exercise improves executive function and achievement and alters brain activation in overweight children: A randomized, controlled trial. *Health Psychology, 30,* 91–98.

Donnelly, J. E., Greene, J. L., Gibson, C. A., Smith, B. K., Washburn, R. A., Sullivan, D. K., . . . Williams, S. L. (2009). Physical Activity Across the Curriculum (PAAC): A randomized controlled trial to promote physical activity and diminish overweight and obesity in elementary school children. *Preventive Medicine, 49,* 336–341.

Donnelly, J. E., Hillman, C. H., Castelli, D., Etnier, J. L., Lee, S., Tomporowski, P., Lambourne, K., . . . Szabo-Reed, A. N. (2016). Physical activity, fitness, cognitive function, and academic achievement in children: A systematic review. *Medicine and Science in Sports and Exercise, 48*(6), 969–1225.

Elias, P. K., Elias, M. F., D'Agostino, R. B., Cupples, A., Wilson, P. W., Silbershatz, H., & Wolf, P. A. (1997). NIDDM and blood pressure as risk factors for poor cognitive performance: The Framingham Study. *Diabetes Care, 20*(9), 1388–1395.

Etnier, J. L., Nowell, P. M., Landers, D. M., & Sibley, B. A. (2006). A meta-regression to examine the relationship between aerobic fitness and cognitive performance. *Brain Research Reviews, 52*(1), 119–130.

Fontaine, K. R., Redden, D. T., Wang, C., Westfall, A. O., & Allison, D. B. (2003). Years of life lost due to obesity. *Journal of the American Medical Association, 289*, 187–193.

Gabbard, C., & Barton, J. (1979). Effects of physical activity on mathematical computation among young children. *Journal of Psychology, 103*, 287–288.

Hillman, C. H., Pontifex, M. B., Castelli, D. M., Khan, N. A., Raine, L. B., Scudder, M. R., . . . Kamijo, K. (2014). Effects of the FITKids randomized controlled trial on executive control and brain function in children. *Pediatrics, 134*, 1063–1071.

Hillman, C. H., Pontifex, M. B., Raine, L., Castelli, D. M., Hall, E. E., & Kramer, A. F. (2009). The effect of acute treadmill walking on cognitive control and academic achievement in preadolescent children. *Neuroscience, 159*, 1044–1054.

Howie, E. K., & Pate, R. R. (2012). Physical activity and academic achievement in children: A historical perspective. *Journal of Sport and Health Science, 1*(3), 160–169.

Institute of Medicine (IOM). (2013). *Educating the student body: Taking physical activity and physical education to school.* Washington, DC: Institute of Medicine.

Ismail, A. H. (1967). The effects of a well-organized physical education programme on intellectual performance. *Research in Physical Education, 1*, 31–38.

Janssen, I., & LeBlanc, A. G. (2010). Systematic review of the health benefits of physical activity and fitness in school-aged children and youth. *International Journal of Behavioral Nutrition and Physical Activity, 7*, 1–16.

Kamijo, K., Pontifex, M. B., O'Leary, K. C., Scudder, M. R., Chien-Ting, W., Castelli, D. M., & Hillman, C. H. (2011). The effects of an afterschool physical activity program on working memory in preadolescent children. *Developmental Science, 14*(5), 1046–1058.

Kinsella, K., & Wan, H. (2009). *Census Bureau, international population reports.* P95/09-1. An Aging World: 2008. Washington, DC: US Government Printing Office.

Krafft, C. E., Schwarz, N. F., Chi, L., Weinberger, A. L., Schaeffer, D. J., Pierce, J. E., . . . McDowell, J. E. (2014). An 8-month randomized controlled exercise trial alters brain activation during cognitive tasks in overweight children. *Obesity, 22*, 232–242.

Kramer, A. F., Bherer, L., Colcombe, S. J., Dong, W., & Greenough, W. T. (2004). Environmental influences on cognitive and brain plasticity during aging. *The Journal of Gerontology: Medical Sciences, 59*, 940–957.

Lande, M. B., Kaczorowski, J. M., Auinger, P., Schwartz, G. J., & Weitzman, M. (2003). Elevated blood pressure and decreased cognitive function among school-age children and adolescents in the United States. *The Journal of Pediatrics, 143*(6), 720–724.

Ma, J. K., Le Mare, L., & Gurb, B. J. (2014). Classroom-based high-intensity interval activity imrpoves off-task behaviour in primary school students. *Applied Physiology, Nutrition, and Metabolism, 39*, 1332–1337.

Pontifex, M. B., Saliba, B. J., Raine, L. B., Picchietti, D. L., & Hillman, C. H. (2013). Exercise improves behavioral, neurophysiologic, and scholastic performance in children with ADHD. *The Journal of Pediatrics, 162,* 543–551.

Raine, L. B., Lee, H. K., Saliba, B. J., Chaddock-Heyman, L., Hillman, C. H., & Kramer, A. F. (2013). The influence of childhood aerobic fitness on learning and memory. *PLOS One, 8,* 1–6.

Rampersaud, G. C., Pereira, M. A., Girard, B. L., Adams, J., & Metzl, J. D. (2005). Breakfast habits, nutritional status, body weight, and academic performance in children and adolescents. *Journal of the American Dietetic Association, 105*(5), 743–760.

Sallis, J. F., Mckenzie, T. L., Kolody, B., Lewis, M., Marshall, S., & Rosengard, P. (1999). Effects of health-related physical education on academic achievement: Project SPARK. *Research Quarterly for Exercise and Sports, 70,* 127–134.

Singh, A., Uijtdewilligen, L., Twisk, J. W. R., van Mechelen, W., & Chinapaw, M. J. M. (2012). Physical activity and performance in school: A systematic review of literature including a methodological quality assessment. *Archives of Pediatric and Adolescent Medicine, 166*(1), 49–55. doi: 10.1001/archpediatrics.2016.

Timmons, B. W., Naylor, P., & Pfeiffer, K. A. (2007). Physical activity for preschool children – how much and how? *Applied Physiology, Nutrition, and Metabolism, 32,* S122–S134. doi: 10.1139/H07-112.

Tomporowski, P. D., Davis, C. L., Miller, P. H., & Naglieri, J. A. (2008). Exercise and children's intelligence, cognition, and academic achievement. *Educational Psychology Review, 20,* 111–131. doi: 10.1007/s10648-007-9057-0.

van Dusen, D., Kelder, S. H., Kohl, H. W. III, Ranjit, N., & Perry, C. L. (2011). Associations of physical fitness and academic performance among school children. *Journal of School Health, 81*(12), 733–740.

Wittberg, R. A., Northrup, K. L., & Cottrel, L. A. (2009). Children's physical fitness and academic performance. *American Journal of Health Education, 40,* 30–36.

Wittberg, R. A., Northrup, K. L., & Cottrell, L. A. (2012). Children's aerobic fitness and academic achievement: A longitudinal examination of students during their fifth and seventh grade years. *American Journal of Public Health, 102,* 2303–2307.

Part II

Insights and innovations

Chapter 4

Exercise, neurotransmission and neurotrophic factors

Romain Meeusen, Cajsa Tonoli, Kristel Knaepen and Danusa Dias Soares

Introduction

Neurotransmitters govern the communication between neurons in different brain regions and neuronal pathways. Generally speaking, nerve cells in the brain are firing all the time, giving a massive 'background noise'. Probably none of the neurons in the brain are exposed only to excitation, and certainly no nerve cells are affected solely by inhibitory signals. Most brain functions such as learning, memory, cognition, control of movement and other mechanisms need the interaction of neurotransmitters and neuromodulators. In order to establish new memories and to encode, store and retrieve memories, cross-talk between several brain structures such as the hippocampus and interplay between several neurotransmitters and neuromodulators are important (Taylor et al., 2016). Understanding the function of various neurotransmitters and neuromodulators helps in understanding their role during whole-body exercise, fatigue, learning and memory.

In this chapter we will describe how different forms of exercise influence neurotransmission and how neurotrophic factors and especially brain-derived neurotrophic factor (BDNF) respond to an exercise stimulus, forming the basis for learning and memory.

Biosynthesis of monoamines

The biogenic amines include the catecholamines dopamine (DA), noradrenaline (norepinephrine: NA), adrenaline, and the indoleamine 5-hydroxytryptamine or serotonin (5-HT). Tyrosine is the common amino acid precursor of all catecholamines, while the precursor of 5-HT is the essential amino acid tryptophan. Monoaminergic neurons modulate a wide range of functions in the central nervous system. Noradrenergic neurons are involved in cardiovascular function, sleep and analgesic responses, while dopaminergic neurons are linked with motor function (Freed & Yamamoto, 1985) and serotonergic activity is associated with pain, fatigue, appetite and sleep (Dunn & Dishmann, 1991).

The dopaminergic system

Dopaminergic cell groups are found in the mesencephalon, the diencephalon and the telencephalon. The main ascending dopaminergic pathways include the nigrostriatal tractus, the ventral mesostriatal (or mesolimbic) pathway and the tuberoinfundibular system, which arises from cells located in the diencephalon (Meeusen & De Meirleir, 1995). The rate-limiting step in the biosynthesis of DA is the hydroxylation of tyrosine to dihydroxyphenylalanine (DOPA) by the enzyme tyrosine hydroxylase. The majority of tyrosine hydroxylase is located in catecholamine nerve terminals. DOPA is decarboxylated to DA by the enzyme DOPA decarboxylase (aromatic amino acid decarboxylase). The activity of this enzyme is not rate-limiting in the synthesis of the catecholamines, and is therefore no regulating factor in their formation. In normal physiological conditions DA is first metabolized to 3,4-dihydroxyphenylacetic acid (DOPAC) by monoamine oxidase (MAO) and aldehyde oxidase. DOPAC is then further metabolized into homovanillic acid by catechol-O-methyltransferase (COMT) (Meeusen & De Meirleir, 1995).

The noradrenergic system

The neurons that synthesize NA are restricted to the pontine and medullary tegmental region. The locus coeruleus is quantitatively the most important noradrenergic nucleus in the brain. Its efferent fibres constitute a major ascending pathway, the dorsal noradrenergic bundle. Along its course different branches emerge to innervate a large number of mesencephalic areas (dorsal raphe nucleus, thalamus, hypothalamus, hippocampus, septum, cortex). In the noradrenergic neurons DA is converted into NA through dopamine beta-hydroxylase. The enzymes responsible for the catabolism of noradrenaline are MAO and COMT (Meeusen & De Meirleir, 1995).

The serotonergic system

5-HT-containing neurons are present in the mesencephalon, pons and medulla oblongata. They are mainly located in the raphe nuclei. Efferent fibres innervate the substantia nigra, various thalamic centres, the nucleus caudatus, the putamen, the nucleus accumbens, the cortex and the hippocampus. Other serotoninergic cells innervate the ventral horn of the spinal cord and the medulla (Meeusen & De Meirleir, 1995). The synthesis of 5-HT requires two enzymatic steps. The dietary amino acid precursor tryptophan is first hydroxylated by a tryptophan hydroxylase to l-5-hydroxytryptophan and then decarboxylated to 5-HT. 5-HT itself is metabolized by two enzymes (aldehyde dehydrogenase and MAO) to 5-hydroxyindoleacetic acid (5-HIAA).

Exercise and neurotransmission

Acute and chronic exercise will influence neurotransmitter release, and therefore also several motor functions, movement initiation, and control of locomotion, as well as emotions and cognitive functions. The first studies examined the effects of exercise on brain homogenates post exercise. These studies showed that a single bout of exercise results in a depletion of brain NA, while chronic exercise or training, has been found to elevate brain NA levels (Meeusen & De Meirleir, 1995). The influence of acute or chronic exercise on brain DA concentrations is region-specific, with studies finding increases and decreases in DA concentrations following exercise (Meeusen & De Meirleir, 1995; Meeusen et al., 2001). Most of the studies agree that whole-brain 5-HT and 5-HIAA increase following an acute bout of exercise (Meeusen & De Meirleir, 1995). However, in trained rats it seems that brain 5-HT concentration is unaltered while the concentration of the metabolites increases, indicating a higher turnover. Although there are great discrepancies in experimental protocols, such as duration and intensity of exercise, the results indicate that there is evidence in favour of changes in synthesis and metabolism of monoamines during exercise (for review, see Meeusen & De Meirleir, 1995).

Because of shortcomings with postmortem methods, and in part because of the desire to be able to relate neurochemistry directly to behaviour, there has been considerable interest in the development of in vivo neurochemical methods. Since the chemical interplay between cells occurs in the extracellular fluid, there was a need to access this compartment in intact brain of living and freely moving animals (Meeusen et al., 2001). The microdialysis technique employs the dialysis (from Greek: to separate) principle in which a membrane, permeable to water and small solutes, separates two fluid compartments. The principle is based on the kinetic dialysis principle: the membrane is continuously flushed on one side with a solution that lacks the substances of interest, whereas the other side is in contact with the extracellular space. A concentration gradient is created causing diffusion of substances from the extracellular space into the dialysis probe; microdialysis makes it possible to sample continuously for hours or days in a single animal; in addition to other advantages, this decreases the number of animals needed in an experiment.

Most of the studies used treadmill-walking or running protocols to measure the exercise effects on extracellular neurotransmitter concentrations. It was shown that in most brain regions neurotransmitter levels increased, and that there seems to be a 'threshold speed' above which neurotransmitter release starts (Meeusen et al., 2001). It is clear that also the running duration will influence neuronal output; this was demonstrated by several authors (Meeusen et al., 1994, 1996, 1997, 2003; Pagliari & Peyrin, 1995a, b).

In order to clarify the influence of different exercise protocols on extracellular DA levels in rat striatum, Meeusen et al. (2003) found that extracellular DA levels are more likely to be linked to the exercise duration than to exercise speed, and that the perturbation of extracellular DA levels lasts longer when exercise duration is longer. Six weeks of exercise training on extracellular neurotransmitter levels showed that basal concentrations of DA, NA and glutamate were significantly lower for the trained compared to control animals Meeusen et al. (1997). Sixty minutes of exercise significantly increased extracellular DA, NA and glutamate levels in both control and trained animals, but there was no significant difference in the exercise-induced increase (expressed as percentage increase above baseline) between trained and control animals (Meeusen et al., 1997). The results indicate that exercise training appears to result in diminished basal activity of striatal neurotransmitters, while maintaining the necessary sensitivity for responses to acute exercise. These findings could be interesting for the therapeutic value of exercise, e.g. in patients with Parkinson's disease, showing that exercise training has a sparing effect on neurotransmitter release, therefore 'sparing' the little amount of DA that is left in cell bodies.

After these first studies, microdialysis became more routinely used, and several studies have tried to measure neurotransmitter release in specific brain areas in order to explain physiological adaptations that occur during exercise, such as thermoregulation. Hasegawa et al. (2011) investigated the relationship between thermoregulation and catecholamine release in the preoptic area and anterior hypothalamus during incremental treadmill running in the rat. They found that thermoregulatory responses are dependent on the intensity of the exercise and that these responses are associated with changes in NA and DA release, but not in 5-HT release in the preoptic area and anterior hypothalamus. Using the same method they also showed that the ergogenic effects of caffeine may be associated with the adenosine receptor blockade-induced increases in brain DA release (Zheng & Hasegawa, 2016).

The cross-talk between periphery and central neurotransmission was examined in different studies and set-ups. Gerin et al. (2008, 2011) implanted microdialysis probes in the spinal cord of rats in order to measure neurotransmitter release during exercise (60 minutes at 16 m/min), and found an increased release of 5-HT and a decrease in DA and NA. They further showed in spinal cord-lesioned animals that 5-HT release during neural regeneration might play an important role in neuronal network rearrangement, which later regulates variations of 5-HT release necessary to locomotion (Gerin et al., 2010).

Exercise and neurogenesis

The beneficial effect of exercise on cognitive function has been well documented. It is now clear from several studies and meta-analyses that exercise improves cognitive performance through the lifespan and especially decreases cognitive decline in older adults. A meta-analysis of Colcombe and Kramer (2003) clearly demonstrated the benefits of fitness training on several cognitive tasks in older adults. Furthermore, Erickson et al. (2011) performed a randomized controlled trial in two groups of older persons (65 years or older). One group performed 45 minutes of walking and jogging exercises three times per week, while the control group performed stretching exercises. The volume of the hippocampus increased during the year's intervention in the aerobic exercise group, while it decreased in the stretching control group, clearly demonstrating neurogenesis. Both aerobic exercise as well as resistance exercise (strength training) improve cognition in elderly people. Several randomized controlled trials that used strength training in older persons (65–75 years) used different longitudinal protocols (strength training for 24 weeks up to 52 weeks), one to three times per week (Cassilhas et al., 2007; Liu-Ambrose et al., 2010, 2012). All these studies clearly demonstrated improved cognitive performance in the older population after a strength-training programme. This is of interest because older persons are more likely to benefit from strength training as a preventive measure for muscle atrophy or sarcopenia.

Also in adults it is clear that exercise has a positive effect on brain health. In a recent controlled study we used cycling desks as a means of reducing sedentary time in the office (Torbeyns et al., 2016). We examined if people would be as efficient in performing their desk-based office work when combined with stationary cycling at 30% W_{max}. Typing performance, cognitive tests and accuracy on the Stroop test did not differ between conditions. Reaction times were shorter while cycling relative to sitting, while brain activity (measured by electroencephalogram) was similar. This study showed that typing performance and short-term memory do not deteriorate when people cycle at 30% W_{max}. Furthermore, cycling had a positive effect on response speed across tasks requiring variable amounts of attention and inhibition (Torbeyns et al., 2016).

Recent studies in school-aged children showed that regular physical activity and a better fitness level were associated with better memory and performance on cognitive tasks. A recent systematic review on physical fitness and academic performance in youth examined 35 cross-sectional studies and showed that there was strong evidence for a positive association between cardiovascular fitness and academic performance. The effect of strength training was uncertain, while there was no association with flexibility training. Also a cluster of physical fitness (several activities) showed a clear and positive association (Santana et al., 2016).

The neural mechanisms that underpin the effects of exercise on the brain are multiple. As for learning and memory it is clearly established that exercise will stimulate neurogenesis and cell proliferation (Van Praag et al., 1999). Numerous studies have shown that neurogenesis continuously occurs. The brain area in which this happens is the dentate gyrus of the hippocampus. Most of these newly generated cells differentiate into neurons and integrate into the existing brain circuitry, where they likely play a role in short-term memory and long-term associative memory (Lee et al., 2014).

Physical activity seems to be the key intervention to trigger the processes through which neurotrophins mediate neural plasticity. Of all neurotrophins, BDNF seems to be the most susceptible to regulation by exercise and physical activity (Knaepen et al., 2010). In search of mechanisms underlying plasticity and brain health, exercise is known to induce a cascade of molecular and cellular processes that support (brain) plasticity. BDNF could play a crucial role in these induced mechanisms. Therefore, from the early 1990s, studies started to investigate the effects of physical activity, acute exercise and/or training on levels of BDNF, first in animals, and later in humans.

The first human studies examined the effects of exercise on peripheral BDNF in subjects with a neurodegenerative disease (i.e. multiple sclerosis patients) in order to explore the restorative potential of exercise in this particular disease (e.g. Gold et al., 2003). Since then, many studies on the effects of acute exercise and/or training on BDNF in humans have been carried out, mostly on healthy subjects. Circulating BDNF originates from central and peripheral sources. Predominantly, the effect of acute exercise protocols on peripheral BDNF has been investigated in human subjects. There is a large variation in the protocols used to apply an acute exercise intervention. There is a tendency for acute high-intensity exercise protocols to have larger increases in BDNF concentrations than acute low-intensity exercise protocols. The increase in peripheral BDNF following an acute exercise protocol is transient. BDNF concentration returns to baseline levels within 10–60 minutes postexercise, showing a fast disappearance rate of BDNF after cessation of the exercise (Goekint et al., 2011). No effect of strength training on peripheral levels of BDNF can be found (Goekint et al., 2010).

The literature is consistent about the influence of chronic exercise (exercise training) on baseline BDNF levels. BDNF levels will be equal or slightly lower after an exercise training programme (Knaepen et al., 2010). A lower level of BDNF in trained subjects and athletes could indicate that BDNF clearance is more effective (i.e. has a higher disappearance rate), than in untrained subjects. It is also possible that lower levels of BDNF could represent the shift in blood volume instead of a true change in BDNF as plasma volume increases by 10–20% following regular physical training. No acute exercise or training protocol has a long-lasting influence on peripheral BDNF concentrations in healthy subjects or people with chronic diseases or disabilities.

As stated before, both aerobic (endurance) exercise and strength training will positively influence cognitive performance. However, strength training does not seem to influence BDNF, therefore there must be another mechanism involved. We evaluated the effects of resistance training on spatial memory and the signalling pathways of BDNF and insulin-like growth factor 1 (IGF-1), comparing these effects with those of aerobic exercise (Cassilhas et al., 2012). Adult male Wistar rats underwent 8 weeks of aerobic training on a treadmill (AERO group) or resistance training on a vertical ladder (RES group). After the training period, both AERO and RES groups showed improved learning and spatial memory in a similar manner. However, both groups presented distinct signalling pathways. Although the AERO group showed increased levels of IGF-1, BDNF, tyrosine receptor kinase B and calcium/calmodulin-dependent kinase II in the hippocampus, the RES group showed an induction of peripheral and hippocampal IGF-1 with concomitant activation of receptor for IGF-1 (IGF-1R) and AKT in the hippocampus. These distinct pathways culminated in an increase of synapsin 1 and synaptophysin expression in both groups. These findings demonstrated that both aerobic and resistance exercise can employ divergent molecular mechanisms but achieve similar results on learning and spatial memory (Cassilhas et al., 2012).

Exercise, pollution and the brain

So, exercise is good for the brain. It increases neurotransmission, stimulates neurogenesis and improves learning and memory. But are these positive effects also present when exercising in an polluted environment ?

Today, air pollution is a growing environmental problem worldwide and the high traffic density in urban environments and cities is a major cause of this problem. Recently, air pollution exposure has been linked to adverse effects on the brain such as cognitive decline, neuroinflammation and neuropathology (Bos et al., 2014). The link between urban air pollution and neuropathology emerged from studies that were carried out postmortem on animals and human postmortem studies that were exposed to the polluted urban environment of Mexico City (Calderon-Garciduenas et al., 2002, 2003, 2008). The brains showed ultrafine particle (UFP) deposition, oxidative stress, microglia activation, infiltration of inflammatory cells and an increase in inflammatory markers.

Long-term particle matter (PM) exposure has been linked to cognitive decline in children, adolescents and adults, and with mild cognitive impairment in the elderly (Bos et al., 2014). Ranft et al. (2009) found a significant reduction in cognitive function in elderly people who lived for more than 20 years within a distance of 50 metres from a busy road (traffic density more than 10,000 vehicles/day). Neuroinflammation seems to be the primary mechanism influencing brain. It is clear from animal studies that even after short periods (days to weeks) of PM exposure, functional impairments are found, such as disturbances in motor/exploratory behaviour and emotionality and impairments in spatial and non-spatial learning and memory (Win-Shwe et al., 2008). In addition to the early neuroinflammatory changes, microglia activation, a sign of neuroinflammation, is found in different brain regions, such as cerebral cortex and hippocampus in studies with PM exposure for 4 weeks and longer (Guerra et al., 2013).

Ventilation rate increases during exercise, and in polluted environments this will result in a substantial enhancement of air pollution inhalation (Int Panis et al., 2010). So the question can be raised of whether known benefits of regular physical activity on the brain also apply when physical activity is performed in polluted air.

We performed a series of studies to investigate the influence of PM on general and brain health. In a cross-over study in humans we investigated the acute effect of traffic-related air pollution exposure during exercise on serum BDNF levels. In this study, volunteers performed two identical cycling tests in terms of duration and intensity, but one in a clean room where particles were removed from the air and one along a busy road. We found increased BDNF levels in serum after a cycling test in the clean room. In contrast, the serum BDNF level was not elevated after cycling along the busy road with levels of PM10, PM2.5 and UFP that were moderate but substantially higher than in the clean room (Bos et al., 2011). The findings suggest that exposure to traffic-related air pollution during exercise inhibits the exercise-induced increase of BDNF levels in serum (Bos et al., 2011).

From this first study, it could be speculated that traffic-related air pollution exposure during exercise might inhibit the acute exercise-induced increase of central BDNF production/secretion. This hypothesis was explored in a controlled intervention study in rodents where the acute effect of UFP exposure during exercise on BDNF gene expression in the rat hippocampus was examined. The findings showed that the mRNA level of BDNF in the rat hippocampus was increased 24 hours after 90 minutes of treadmill running at a moderate speed in ambient air compared with the control group that rested in ambient air (Bos et al., 2012). In contrast, there was no increase of the BDNF mRNA level after the same running bout in air with high UFP levels, which suggests that there might be a negative effect of UFP exposure on the exercise-induced increase of BDNF gene expression. The absence of an exercise-induced increase in BDNF gene expression might be the result of a negative effect of UFP exposure on basal gene expression of BDNF. Since there was only a trend towards a decreased BDNF mRNA level in rats exposed to UFP during rest, here the increased ventilation rate could also play a role in the amount of particles inhaled.

Finally, we designed a study to investigate the effect of air pollution exposure during aerobic training on cognition. In this study, formerly untrained subjects participated in a 12-week aerobic training programme, one group in a rural environment and another in an urban environment. At the end of the training programme, performance in the Stroop Colour–Word test, a test to measure executive function, was improved in the group that had trained in the rural environment but not in the group that had trained in the urban environment, where UFP levels were significantly higher (Bos et al., 2013). The findings suggest that high exposure to traffic-related air pollution during exercise training inhibits the positive effects of exercise training on cognition. This indicates that air pollution exposure might have a negative effect on cognition, which is in accordance with previous studies that have shown an inverse link between air pollution exposure and cognition (Chen & Schwartz, 2009; Ranft et al., 2009). After 12 weeks, we did not observe a chronic effect of exercise or air pollution exposure on basal serum BDNF levels.

The evidence suggests that regular exercise in highly polluted air might not result in the same neurological benefits that are observed in non-polluted air.

Conclusions

Exercise influences neurotransmission, depending on the intensity and the duration of the exercise bout. Endurance exercise will increase the release of neurotransmitters in several brain nuclei. An endurance training programme has been shown to decrease the baseline output of neurotransmitters such as DA from the striatum. This decreased release could indicate that exercise induces an adaptation of the receptors. It is now well established that exercise is one of the most essential triggers to create neurogenesis. BDNF is one of the most important growth factors in the brain that help to establish neurogenesis. Both endurance and strength training will improve cognition, but through different pathways. Despite the positive effects of physical activity on brain health, evidence shows that when exercise is performed in a polluted environment, these positive effects are suppressed.

References

Bos, I., De Boever, P., Int Panis, L., et al. (2012). Negative effects of ultrafine particle exposure during forced exercise on the expression of brain-derived neurotrophic factor in the hippocampus of rats. *Neuroscience*, 223, 131–139.

Bos, I., De Boever, P., Int Panis, L., et al. (2014). Physical activity, air pollution and the brain. *Sports Medicine,* 44(11), 1505–1518.

Bos, I., De Boever, P., Vanparijs, J., et al. (2013). Subclinical effects of aerobic training in urban environment. *Medicine and Science in Sports and Exercise*, 45(3), 439–447.

Bos, I., Jacobs, L., Nawrot, T.S., et al. (2011). No exercise-induced increase in serum BDNF after cycling near a major traffic road. *Neuroscience Letter*, 500(2), 129–132.

Calderon-Garciduenas, L., Azzarelli, B., Acuna, H., et al. (2002). Air pollution and brain damage. *Toxicologic Pathology*, 30(3), 73–89.

Calderon-Garciduenas, L., Maronpot, R.R., Torres-Jardon, R., et al. (2003). DNA damage in nasal and brain tissues of canines exposed to air pollutants is associated with evidence of chronic brain inflammation and neurodegeneration. *Toxicologic Pathology*, 31(5), 941524–941538.

Calderon-Garciduenas, L., Solt, A.C., Henriquez-Roldan, C., et al. (2008). Long-term air pollution exposure is associated with neuroinflammation, an altered innate immune response, disruption of the blood–brain barrier, ultrafine particulate deposition, and accumulation of amyloid beta-42 and alpha-synuclein in children and young adults. *Toxicologic Pathology*, 36(2), 289–310.

Cassilhas, R., Fernandes, L., Oliveira, M., et al. (2012). Spatial memory is improved by aerobic and resistance exercise through divergent molecular mechanisms. *Neuroscience*, 309–317.

Cassilhas, R., Viana, V., Grassmann, V., et al. (2007). The impact of resistance exercise on the cognitive function of the elderly. *Medicine and Science in Sports and Exercise*, 39, 1401–1407.

Chen, J.C., Schwartz, J. (2009). Neurobehavioral effects of ambient air pollution on cognitive performance in US adults. *Neurotoxicology*, 30(2), 231–239.

Colcombe, S., Kramer, A.F. (2003). Fitness effects on the cognitive function of older adults: A meta-analytic study. *Psychological Science*, 14(2), 125–130.

Dunn, A., Dishmann, R. (1991). Exercise and the neurobiology of depression. *Exercise and Sport Sciences Reviews,* 19, 41–98.

Erickson, K.I., Voss, M.W., Prakash, R.S., et al. (2011). Exercise training increases size of hippocampus and improves memory. *Proceedings of the National Academy of Sciences of the United States of America*, 108(7), 3017–3022.

Freed, C., Yamamoto, B. (1985). Regional brain dopamine metabolism: A marker for the speed, direction and posture of moving animals. *Science*, 229, 62–65.

Gerin, C.G., Hill, A., Hill, S., et al. (2010). Serotonin release variations during recovery of motor function after a spinal cord injury in rats. *Synapse,* 64(11), 855–861.

Gerin, C.G., Smith, K., Hill, S., et al. (2011). Motor activity affects dopaminergic and noradrenergic systems of the dorsal horn of the rat lumbar spinal cord. *Synapse*, 65(12), 1282–1288.

Gerin, C.G., Teilhac, J.R., Smith, K., et al. (2008). Motor activity induces release of serotonin in the dorsal horn of the rat lumbar spinal cord. *Neuroscience Letter,* 436(2), 91–95.

Goekint, M., De Pauw, K., Roelands, B., et al. (2010). Strength training does not influence serum brain-derived neurotrophic factor. *European Journal of Applied Physiology*, 110(2), 285–293.

Goekint, M., Roelands, B., Heyman, E., et al. (2011). Influence of citalopram and environmental temperature on exercise-induced changes in BDNF. *Neuroscience Letter*, 494(2), 150–154.

Gold, S.M., Schulz, K., Hartmann, S., et al. (2003). Basal serum levels and reactivity of nerve growth factor and brain-derived neurotrophic factor to standardized acute exercise in multiple sclerosis and controls. *Journal of Neuroimmunology*, 183, 99–105.

Guerra, R., Vera-Aguilar, E., Uribe-Ramirez, M., et al. (2013). Exposure to inhaled particulate matter activates early markers of oxidative stress, inflammation and unfolded protein response in rat striatum. *Toxicology Letters,* 222(2), 146–154.

Hasegawa, H., Takatsu, S., Ishiwata, T., et al. (2011). Continuous monitoring of hypothalamic neurotransmitters and thermoregulatory responses in exercising rats. *Journal of Neuroscience Methods*, 202(2), 119–123.

Int Panis, L., de Geus, B., Vandenbulcke, G., et al. (2010). Exposure to particulate matter in traffic: A comparison of cyclists and car passengers. *Atmospheric Environment*, 44, 2263–2270.

Knaepen, K., Goekint, M., Heyman, E., et al. (2010). Neuroplasticity – Exercise-induced response of peripheral brain-derived neurotrophic factor: A systematic review of experimental studies in human subjects. *Sports Medicine*, 40(9), 765–801.

Lee, T., Wong, M., Lau, B., et al. (2014). Aerobic exercise interacts with neurotrophic factors to predict cognitive functioning in adolescents. *Psychoneuroendocrinology*, 39, 214–224.

Liu-Ambrose, T., Nagamatsu, L., Graf, P., et al. (2010). Resistance training and executive functions: A 12-month randomised controlled trial. *Archives of Internal Medicine*, 170(2), 170–178.

Liu-Ambrose, T., Nagamatsu, L., Voss, M., et al. (2012). Resistance training and functional plasticity of the aging brain: A 12-month randomized controlled trial. *Neurobiology of Aging*, 33, 1690–1698.

Meeusen, R., Chaouloff, F., Thorré, K., et al. (1996). Effects of tryptophan and/or acute running on extracellular 5-HT and 5-HIAA levels in the hippocampus of food-deprived rats. *Brain Research*, 740, 245–252.

Meeusen, R., De Meirleir, K. (1995). Exercise and brain neurotransmission. *Sports Medicine*, 20(3), 160–188.

Meeusen, R., Piacentini, M.F., De Meirleir, K. (2001). Brain microdialysis in exercise research. *Sports Medicine*, 31(14), 965–983.

Meeusen, R., Sarre, S., De Meirleir, K., et al. (2003). The effects of running speed and running duration on extracellular dopamine levels in rat striatum, measured with microdialysis. *Medicina Sportiva*, 7(1), 29–36.

Meeusen, R., Sarre, S., Michotte, Y., et al. (1994). The effects of exercise on neurotransmission in rat striatum, a microdialysis study. In: Louilot, A., Durkin, T., Spampinato, U., et al. (Eds.), *Monitoring molecules in neuroscience*. Bordeaux: Gradignan, pp. 181–182.

Meeusen, R., Smolders, I., Sarre, S., et al. (1997). Endurance training effects on striatal neurotransmitter release, an 'in vivo' microdialysis study. *Acta Physiologica Scandinavica*, 159, 335–341.

Pagliari, R., Peyrin, L. (1995a). Norepinephrine release in the rat frontal cortex under treadmill exercise: A study with microdialysis. *Journal of Applied Physiology*, 78(6), 2121–2130.

Pagliari, R., Peyrin, L. (1995b). Physical conditioning in rats influences the central and peripheral catecholamine responses to sustained exercise. *European Journal of Applied Physiology*, 71, 41–52.

Ranft, U., Schikowski, T., Sugiri, D., et al. (2009). Long-term exposure to traffic-related particulate matter impairs cognitive function in the elderly. *Environmental Research*, 109(8), 1004–1011.

Santana, C.C., Azevedo, L.B., Cattuzzo, M.T., et al. (2016). Physical fitness and academic performance in youth: A systematic review. *Scandinavian Journal of Medicine and Science in Sports*, 27(6), 579–603. doi: 10.1111/sms.12773.

Taylor, J., Amann, M., Duchateau, J., et al. (2016). Neural contributions to muscle fatigue: From the brain to the muscle and back again. *Medicine and Science in Sports and Exercise*, 48(11), 2294–2306.

Torbeyns, T., de Geus, B., Bailey, S., et al. (2016). Cycling on a bike desk positively influences cognitive performance. *PLoS One,* 11(11), e0165510.

Van Praag, H., Kempermann, G., Gage, F. (1999). Running increases cell proliferation and neurogenesis in the adult mouse dentate gyrus. *Nature Neuroscience,* 2(3), 266–270.

Win-Shwe, T.T., Yamamoto, S., Fujitani, Y., et al. (2008). Spatial learning and memory function-related gene expression in the hippocampus of mouse exposed to nanoparticle-rich diesel exhaust. *Neurotoxicology,* 29(6), 940–947.

Zheng, X., Hasegawa, H. (2016). Administration of caffeine inhibited adenosine receptor agonist-induced decreases in motor performance, thermoregulation, and brain neurotransmitter release in exercising rats. *Pharmacology Biochemistry and Behavior,* 140, 82–89.

Chapter 5

The development of the acute exercise–catecholamines–cognition interaction theory

Implications for learning and memory

Terry McMorris

Introduction

The catecholamines hypothesis, as an explanation of the underlying processes that affect cognition, was first posited by Cooper (1973) and later added to by Chmura, Nazar, and Kaciuba-Uścilko (1994). While being able to account for some of the empirical research results, it was inadequate with respect to others. In recent articles, my colleagues and I (McMorris, 2016a, b; McMorris et al., 2016) have drawn on animal studies to develop the hypothesis further and provide some explanation of the probable mechanisms underlying most of the changes found in the acute exercise–cognition empirical literature. It is not the purpose of this chapter to replicate those studies but to provide an outline of how the hypothesis has been developed since Cooper and, more importantly, to show how these developments have implications for learning and memory, and how they can guide our practical utilization of physical activity to aid academic achievement.

The original catecholamines hypothesis

Cooper's (1973) hypothesis followed an empirical study (Davey, 1973), which showed that acute exercise affected cognition in an inverted-U manner, similar to that shown by Yerkes and Dodson (1908) for arousal–performance interaction. Although several studies examining acute exercise–cognition interaction had been undertaken at this time, no one had attempted to provide any theoretical input. Cooper pointed to two basic but very important factors. Firstly, he highlighted that there was evidence to show that exercise induces increases in peripheral concentrations of the neurohormone noradrenaline, also known as norepinephrine (Vendsalu, 1960), which, along with adrenaline, also known as epinephrine, and dopamine makes up a class of aromatic amines called catecholamines. Secondly, Cooper pointed to evidence from animal studies which showed that increases in arousal level were dependent on activation of the brain reticular formation by noradrenaline (Kasamatsu, 1970; Podvoll & Goodman, 1967; Reis & Fuxe, 1968, 1969). Thus, Cooper believed that the exercise-induced increases in peripheral noradrenaline concentrations somehow affected brain concentrations, which in turn resulted in increased arousal levels and hence improved cognitive performance. However, he had to explain how this could occur.

Although peripheral noradrenaline is circulating in plasma, it is prevented from crossing into the brain by the blood–brain barrier. Brain endolethial cells differ from other endolethial cells in that they have tight junctions, which prevent transcapillary movement of molecules. Nor do they contain transendolethial pathways, hence they form a barrier (Butt, Jones, & Abbott, 1990). Although the blood–brain barrier is selective, e.g. substances with high lipid solubility can cross by simple diffusion (Lund-Andersen, 1979), and diffusion of neutral L-amino acids, such as tyrosine, which is the precursor of catecholamines, is mediated by facilitative transporters (Hawkins, O'Kane, Simpson, & Viña 2006), catecholamines do not readily cross (Cornford, Braun, Oldendorf, & Hill, 1982; Oldendorf, 1977). However, Cooper (1973) pointed to evidence from research with mice that showed that high concentrations of catecholamines in the periphery were able to cross the blood–brain barrier (Samorajaski & Marks, 1962), probably in the median eminence at the base of the hypothalamus and in the anterior pituitary gland. Thus, if exercise were intense enough, peripheral noradrenaline would cross into the brain. Moreover, based on the work of Rushmer, Smith, and Lasher (1960), Cooper was aware that higher centres of the brain were able to feed forward to the hypothalamus, due to anticipation of undertaking exercise, and this resulted in the synthesis and release of dopamine and noradrenaline in the brain by the sympathoadrenal system. This, alone, would result in increased activation of the reticular formation and hence higher levels of arousal.

The final stage of Cooper's (1973) hypothesis was to explain the inverted-U effect that Davey (1973) had found, and how this related to noradrenaline and dopamine. He stated that at low concentrations of central catecholamines (low levels of exercise and arousal), brain activity is limited because the appropriate sequence of neuronal activation cannot be obtained as a result of neurons being at such a low level of excitation that they cannot be stimulated to an adequate level of summation. Hence cognitive performance is poor. Moderate-intensity exercise and the resultant increase in central catecholamines (moderate levels of exercise and arousal) mean that excitation levels are such that summation is facilitated and the appropriate sequence occurs. However, as catecholamine concentrations rise even higher (high levels of exercise and arousal), neurons which are not required are also activated, producing neural 'noise' and hence poor cognitive performance.

Developments in the catecholamines hypothesis

The interaction between acute exercise, catecholamines and cognition begins with the role of the catecholamines in the periphery during exercise.

During low-intensity exercise, noradrenaline and adrenaline aid lipolysis by activating receptors in adipose tissue, resulting in the mobilization of free fatty acids as fuel, stimulating receptors in muscle, activating receptors in the pancreas to suppress insulin release and stimulating secretion of the hormones glucagon, growth hormone and cortisol (Arakawa et al., 1995). As exercise intensity increases hypoglycaemia occurs, which results in large increases in plasma noradrenaline concentrations. Adrenaline concentrations rapidly increase when there is a decline in hepatic glucose concentrations. At this stage, adrenaline stimulates glycogenolysis and hepatic glucose release in the liver, and glycogenolysis in muscle. Adrenaline and, to a lesser extent, noradrenaline also act on the cardiovascular system by activating receptors responsible for increasing heart rate and contractile force, while stimulating arteriolar constriction in renal, splanchnic and cutaneous vascular beds (Arakawa et al., 1995).

The points at which the sudden rises in noradrenaline and adrenaline plasma concentrations are demonstrated are known as the noradrenaline and adrenaline thresholds. They generally show moderate to high correlations (Podolin, Munger, & Mazzeo, 1991), therefore they are often referred to as the catecholamines thresholds (CT). It is generally thought that intensity needs to be ~75% of maximum volume of oxygen uptake ($\dot{V}o_{2max}$) (Podolin et al., 1991), which, according to Arts and Kuipers (1994) equates to ~65% maximum power output ($\dot{W}_{max}$), but there are large interindividual variations (Urhausen, Weiler, Coen, & Kindermann, 1994). Moreover, blood lactate concentrations follow a similar exponential profile and the lactate threshold (LT) also shows moderate to high correlations with CT (Podolin et al., 1991). If exercise intensity increases beyond the threshold, plasma catecholamine concentrations continue to rise and soon reach very high levels. However, I would argue that it is unlikely that, with humans in normoxia, concentrations of peripheral catecholamines induced by even very heavy exercise would result in the blood–brain barrier being compromised. However, comparatively recent research (Miyashita & Williams, 2006) provides the answer to the issue of how these peripherally circulating neurohormones affect brain concentrations.

Miyashita and Williams (2006), in a well-controlled experiment with rodents, found that circulating adrenaline and, to a lesser extent, noradrenaline activate β-adrenoceptors on the afferent vagus nerve, which runs from the abdomen through the chest, neck and head, and terminates in the nucleus tractus solitarii (NTS) within the blood–brain barrier. The excitatory neurotransmitter glutamate mediates synaptic communication between the vagal afferents and the NTS. Noradrenergic cells in the NTS project into the locus coeruleus, which is the main source of noradrenaline synthesis and release to other parts of the brain (McGaugh, Cahill, & Roozendaal, 1996). Moreover, Grenhoff, and Svensson (1993) have shown that stimulation of α_1-adrenoceptors potentiates the firing of dopamine neurons in the ventral tegmental area of the brain, probably due to α_1-adrenoceptor activation inducing enhanced glutamate release, which affects the excitability of dopamine neurons (Velásquez-Martinez, Vázquez-Torres, & Jiménez-Riveira, 2012). Thus, acute exercise-induced increases in peripheral adrenaline and noradrenaline concentrations can directly affect brain synthesis and release of the catecholamine brain neurotransmitters, dopamine and noradrenaline.

Significance of noradrenergic and dopaminergic pathways for cognition

The stimulation of the locus coeruleus, via the NTS, and the subsequent activation of the dorsal bundle of the noradrenergic pathway is key to acute exercise–cognition interaction, as is the resulting activation of the mesocorticolimbic dopaminergic pathway (Figure 5.1). Noradrenaline and dopamine act as neurotransmitters in the brain (see Chapter 4). Once synthesized they are held in vesicles and, when released, innervate the noradrenergic and dopaminergic pathways. The dorsal bundle of the noradrenergic pathway is served by the locus coeruleus and has axons ending in the spinal cord, cerebellum, entire cerebral cortex and hippocampus. Thus it is very important with regard to cognition, including learning and memory. Dopaminergic neurons in the ventral tegmental area form the mesolimbic and mesocortical pathways. The former serves the ventral striatum, which is part of the basal ganglia (Carr & Sesack, 2000; Sogabe, Yagasaki, Onozawa, & Kawakami, 2013), while the latter transmits to the frontal cortex (Tritsch & Sabatini, 2012); both areas are important for cognition, especially the frontal cortex.

Exercise intensity and activation of the nucleus tractus solitarii

Cooper (1973) realized that the key issue, with regard to how acute exercise results in improved cognition, was the induced increase in brain concentrations of dopamine and noradrenaline. As we have seen, he placed his faith in exercise compromising the blood–brain barrier, but this idea was superseded by Miyashita and Williams' (2006) finding that peripherally circulating adrenaline and noradrenaline activate the locus coeruleus via β-adrenoceptors on the vagus nerve, which in turn stimulates NTS activity. At first sight, this appears to solve the problem with Cooper's original hypothesis concerning the interaction between peripheral catecholamines and central catecholamines. However, a question raised in a seminal paper (Tomporowski & Ellis, 1986) still needed to be answered. These authors wanted to know the exercise intensity required to induce increased arousal, which means increased brain concentrations of dopamine and noradrenaline. They were particularly concerned with the fact

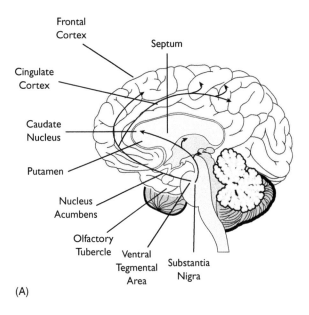

(A)

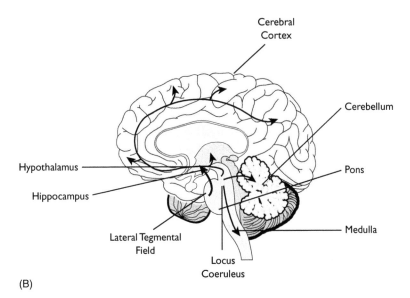

(B)

Figure 5.1 Schematic representation of (A) the dopaminergic and (B) noradrenergic pathways. (Reproduced with permission from McMorris, T., Turner, A., Hale, B. J., & Sproule, J. (2016). Beyond the catecholamines hypothesis for an acute exercise–cognition interaction: A neurochemical perspective. In T. McMorris (Ed.), *Exercise–cognition interaction: Neuroendocrine perspectives* (pp. 65–104). New York: Elsevier Academic Press.)

that the term 'moderate' was freely used, but with different definitions. More importantly, this 'moderate'-intensity exercise was not producing unequivocal results in empirical studies.

The first to attempt to solve this problem scientifically, and indeed the first to develop Cooper's (1973) hypothesis, were Chmura et al. (1994), who hypothesized that the point at which CT was achieved was the key factor. Moreover, they provided evidence of support for their hypothesis. My colleagues and I (McMorris et al., 1999) supported Chmura et al.'s claims and, following Miyashita and Williams' (2006) findings, we were convinced that CT was the key factor. It made sense that a significant increase in peripherally circulating catecholamines would activate the β-adrenoceptors on the vagus nerve and thus initiate increased synthesis and release of noradrenaline from the locus coeruleus (McMorris & Hale, 2012; McMorris, Sproule, Turner, & Hale, 2011).

However, our confidence proved to be a little misplaced. In a meta-analysis, we (McMorris & Hale, 2015) calculated the mean effect size for speed of response in cognitive tests undertaken at, or immediately following, CT or one of the two other similar threshold measures, LT and ventilatory threshold (VT), the point at which ventilatory carbon dioxide shows a greater increase than ventilatory oxygen (Beaver, Wasserman, & Whipp, 1986); LT and VT are highly correlated with CT (Podolin et al., 1991; Yamamoto et al., 1991). We compared this effect size to the mean effect size for studies where the exercise intensity was $\geq 40\%$ $\dot{V}o_{2max}$ but $< 80\%$ $\dot{V}o_{2max}$, which was below the thresholds or where the thresholds had not been measured. We found no significant difference ($g = 0.58$, SE $= 0.20$ vs. $g = 0.54$, SE $= 0.11$).

We attempted to explain these data by pointing to Mason's (1975a, b) claims concerning the nature of stress. Mason argued that, if the individual perceives the situation as being unpredictable and/or one in which he/she is not in control, higher centres of the brain, e.g. the prefrontal cortex and limbic system, may initiate activation of the sympathoadrenal system, which will induce increased synthesis and release of noradrenaline and dopamine in the brain. Indeed, Cooper (1973) made similar claims based on the work of Rushmer et al. (1960). He argued that feedforward, due to anticipation of undertaking exercise, led to the initiation of the sympathoadrenal system by the hypothalamus, which would induce increased activation of the reticular formation and hence higher levels of arousal. The prefrontal cortex and limbic system (Barbas, Saha, Rempel-Clower, & Ghashghaei, 2003; Myers, Dolgas, Kasckow, Cullinan, & Herman, 2014) project to the hypothalamus, which projects to the locus coeruleus (Aston-Jones, Ennis, Pieribone, Nickell, & Shipley, 1986; Cedarbaum & Aghajanian, 1978). These projections would result in the release of noradrenaline to the prefrontal cortex and hippocampus by the locus coeruleus, thus affecting cognition, including learning and long-term memory. However, one must question the extent to which undertaking moderate-intensity exercise would be perceived as stressful by participants, therefore questions arise as to whether these processes would be initiated. As a result, observation of the rodent literature on acute exercise-induced neural plasticity led me to propose a more likely explanation (McMorris, 2016a, b).

Rodent studies have shown that acute exercise below as well as above LT, and hence CT, induces c-Fos expression, which is indicative of neuronal activity, in noradrenergic neurons in the NTS (Ohiwa et al., 2006). Dahlströem and Fuxe (1964) termed these A1 and A2 eurons. Although the effect on noradrenergic neurons in the locus coeruleus (Dahlström and Fuxe's A6 neurons) was not measured, it would not be unreasonable to expect similar activation of these neurons, especially as A2 neurons project to the locus coeruleus and are thought to modulate A6 activity (Ferrucci, Giorgi, Bartalucci, Busceti, & Fornai, 2013; Rinaman, 2011). A1, A2, A5 and locus coeruleus neurons also project to the ventral tegmental area (Mejías-Aponte, Drouin, & Aston-Jones, 2009), where they activate α_1-adrenoceptors, which induce enhanced glutamate release by an interaction with extracellular calcium influx, thus potentiating the firing of dopaminergic neurons (Velásquez-Martinez et al., 2012). Also, these noradrenergic neurons, along with the adrenergic C1 neurons, project to the retrorubral field in the reticular formation and stimulate dopamine activation there (Rinaman, 2011). The ventral tegmental area and retrorubral field are brain regions involved in cognitive functioning, with projections to the frontal cortex and cingulate cortex. Activation of the NTS at sub-LT/CT intensities is extremely unlikely to have been the result of an increase in circulating plasma catecholamine concentrations activating β-adrenoceptors on the vagus nerve. However, the vagus nerve also contains mechanoreceptors, baroreceptors and nociceptors. Information from mechanoreceptors, or more accurately, stretch receptors, in the heart and lungs, is fed back to the NTS via the vagus nerve (Berthoud & Neuhuber, 2000; Moor et al., 2005). Similarly, arterial baroreceptors provide feedback concerning blood pressure to the NTS via the glossopharyngeal and vagus nerves (Kougias, Weakley, Yao, Lin, & Chen, 2010). Heart rate, tidal volume and blood pressure begin to increase immediately exercise begins (Watson, 1974), and the feedback allows the hypothalamus to initiate activation of the sympathoadrenal system, culminating in the synthesis and release of catecholamines, in anticipation of increased exercise intensity. Thus, it is not surprising to see c-Fos expression in A1 and A2 neurons in the NTS prior to CT. We should note that, although sub-LT exercise induced increased c-Fos expression in A1 and A2 neurons, supra-LT exercise demonstrated significantly greater expression (Ohiwa et al., 2006). Nevertheless, the resultant increase in brain concentrations in noradrenaline and dopamine concentrations is probably enough to induce improved cognitive function (see Robbins & Roberts, 2007, for a review of the effects of catecholamines on cognitive performance).

Short- to moderate-duration, moderate-intensity exercise effects on cognition

Before outlining the effects of acute moderate-intensity exercise on cognition, I will present a working definition of moderate-intensity exercise. Above and in previous studies, my colleagues and I (McMorris, 2016b; McMorris & Hale, 2012; McMorris et al., 2011) have defined moderate-intensity exercise as being $\geq 40\%$ $\dot{V}_{O_{2max}}$ but $< 80\%$ $\dot{V}_{O_{2max}}$. This is based on the work of Borer (2003), an exercise endocrinologist. It is open to criticism, as is any definition that generalizes, but it provides a science-based working definition at the very least. It should also be noted that the duration of such exercise influences its effect on cognition (see McMorris 2016a, b; McMorris et al., 2016). In this subsection, we will deal with short- to moderate-duration exercise which, based on the work of Hodgetts, Coppack, Frayn, and Hockaday (1991), we have interpreted as being 10–20 minutes, possibly as long as 30 minutes, depending on individuals' fitness levels (McMorris, 2016b).

In general, short- to moderate-duration, acute moderate-intensity exercise has a beneficial effect on speed of performance of cognitive tasks (see McMorris & Hale, 2012, for a meta-analysis), with the possible exception of learning/long-term memory tasks (see McMorris et al., 2016, for a review of the empirical data). It is thought that this is due to increased noradrenaline release from the locus coeruleus stimulating the reticular formation, which increases arousal. This was the major part of Cooper's (1973) original hypothesis for acute moderate-intensity exercise-induced facilitation of cognitive performance. Effects on accuracy of performance are less clear but this is probably due to the fact that most of the tasks used in such studies were designed to measure task efficiency by speed rather than accuracy (see McMorris & Hale, 2012; McMorris et al., 2016). There may be some benefits for learning and memory during the acquisition and retrieval phases due to increased arousal aiding attention (Gagnon & Wagner, 2016). Although most types of task appear to benefit from exercise of this duration and intensity, central executive tasks (see below for a description), which are dependent on a large input from the prefrontal cortex, benefit the most (McMorris & Hale, 2012). Studies with rodents and non-human primates have shown that stress (of all kinds, including exercise) induces moderate increases in brain concentrations of noradrenaline and dopamine, which benefit prefrontal cortex activity (Arnsten, 2009, 2011). Noradrenaline activates firing of the high-affinity α_{2A}-noradrenergic receptors (Roth, Tam, Ida, Yang, & Deutch, 1988), which increases the strength of neural signalling in the preferred direction, i.e. to the desired stimulus (Deutch & Roth, 1990; Wang et al., 2007). Similarly, the high-affinity dopaminergic D_1-receptors are activated by dopamine, which dampens the 'noise' by inhibiting firing to non-preferred stimuli (Finlay, Zigmond, & Abercrombie, 1995). So dopamine and noradrenaline, working together, improve the signal-to-noise ratio. This is particularly positive for central executive tasks as they require a great deal of prefrontal cortex activation (Barbas, 2000; Leh, Petrides, & Strafella, 2010), but most other tasks also involve some prefrontal cortex activation (see below).

Long-duration, moderate-intensity and heavy exercise effects on cognition

As we saw earlier, CT marks the exercise intensity at which there is a significant increase in plasma catecholamine concentrations. From this point onwards, there is an exponential rise in plasma concentrations and Cooper (1973) argued that high brain concentrations of noradrenaline would result in increased neural 'noise', hence poor cognitive performance. The situation is exacerbated by the fact that at $\sim$80% $\dot{V}o_{2max}$, there are also increases in plasma cortisol concentrations. More importantly for the acute exercise–cognition interaction effect, rodent studies have shown evidence of increases in corticotrophin-releasing factor (CRF) messenger ribonucleic acid (mRNA) expression, in the paraventricular nucleus of the hypothalamus, immediately following acute exercise (Jiang et al., 2004; Kawashima et al., 2004; Yanagita, Amemiya, Suzuki, & Kita, 2007). CRF interacts with noradrenaline neurons in the locus coeruleus to increase noradrenaline release. Furthermore, when exercise is of moderate intensity but for a long duration ($\gtrsim$45 minutes), plasma cortisol concentrations are also increased (Bridge, Weller, Rayson, & Jones, 2003; Shojaei, Farajov, & Jafari, 2011) but more importantly, exercise of this duration and intensity induces increased release of 5-hydroxytryptamine (5-HT), also known as serotonin, from the raphe nuclei (Chen et al., 2008; Chennaoui et al., 2001). Activation of the 5-HT_{1A} and 5-HT_{2A} serotonergic receptors in the locus coeruleus facilitates noradrenaline release, while activation of these receptors in the medial prefrontal cortex stimulates release of dopamine from the ventral tegmental area (Díaz-Mataix et al., 2005). Thus, in both long-duration, moderate-intensity and heavy exercise, there is excess noradrenaline and dopamine in the brain. Cooper (1973) saw this as being detrimental to cognition but more recent research, with humans, non-human primates and rodents, shows that all is dependent on the nature of the tasks to be undertaken.

Central executive tasks

Central executive tasks are part of what Baddeley (1986) termed working memory. He described the process as the interactive functioning of three separate but interdependent parts, the central executive mechanism, and two short-term memory subsystems, the phonological loop, encoding of acoustic and verbal information, and the visuospatial sketch pad, processing of visual and visuospatial information. The role of the central executive is to oversee and control the whole process. It ensures that there is integration of perceptual input and comparison of the present situation (held in short-term memory) with recalled information from long-term memory. Miyake, Friedman, Emerson, Witzki, and Howerter (2000) described central executive processes as ones involving several functions, which include shifting between tasks or mental sets; updating and monitoring working-memory representations, which involves the removal of redundant information and replacing it with new, relevant information; inhibition of prepotent responses; planning; and the coordination of multiple tasks. Leh et al. (2010) provided other examples, e.g. abstract thinking, cognitive flexibility and selecting relevant sensory information. Central executive tasks primarily activate the prefrontal cortex but also draw on information recalled from other parts of the brain (see Barbas, 2000; Leh et al., 2010, for reviews).

As we saw earlier, these tasks are facilitated by increased α_{2A}-adrenoreceptor and D_1-receptor activation during moderate levels of stress (Arnsten, 2009, 2011). However, when stress levels are high, noradrenaline and dopamine concentrations become excessive and noradrenaline activates the lower-affinity α_1- and β-adrenoceptors (Roth et al., 1988). Activation of α_1-adrenoceptors results in reduced neuronal firing in the prefrontal cortex, while excessive stimulation of D_1-receptors and β-adrenoceptors induces excess activity of the second messenger cyclic adenosine monophosphate (cAMP), which dampens all neuronal activity, thus weakening the signal-to-noise ratio (Arnsten, 2011). Hence, during heavy and long-duration, moderate-intensity exercise, performance of central executive tasks is inhibited, although the stop signal task and the attentional set-shifting tasks can be facilitated by high concentrations of noradrenaline (Eagle et al., 2010; Lapiz & Morilak, 2006).

Perceptual ability and short-term memory tasks

As we saw above, short-term memory is part of working memory and plays an important role in central executive task performance. In this context, these tasks activate the prefrontal cortex and the dorsal frontoparietal attention network (Braunlich, Gomez-Lavin, & Seger, 2015; Gordon, Stollstorff, & Vaidya, 2012); however, when tasks require simply acquiring the information and immediately recalling it, they are processed similarly to perceptual ability tasks or, rather, 'bottom-up' or externally driven perceptual ability tasks. Perception and attention are issues in all types of task, including central executive tasks, which are top-down tasks. As with the short-term memory tasks, top-down perceptual ability tasks are controlled by the dorsal frontoparietal attention network (Corbetta & Shulman, 2002). An example of such tasks would be tasks where there is competition for attention (Goltz et al., 2015). In the 'bottom-up' tasks, which have been commonly used in acute exercise–cognition research, such as simple and choice reaction time, the dorsal frontoparietal attention network does not appear to affect behaviour (Molenberghs, Mesulam, Peeters, & Vandenberghe, 2007). In these cases, the task activates the relevant sensory cortex, which passes information to the sensory association cortices and prefrontal cortex where it is integrated and interpreted. The level of integration and interpretation varies between tasks but is less demanding than the processes involved in central executive tasks.

Stress research with animals has shown that, in contrast to the prefrontal cortex, high concentrations of noradrenaline, which activate α_1- and β-adrenoceptors, have a positive effect on signal detection (Waterhouse, Moises, & Woodward, 1980, 1981). Moreover, research has also shown that the effect can be stimulated by CRF acting on the locus coeruleus–noradrenergic system. CRF causes tonic firing of locus coeruleus noradrenergic neurons, which results in suppression of somatosensory signal transmission within the somatosensory thalamus and cortex (Devilbiss, Waterhouse, Berridge, & Valentino, 2012). This appears to reduce detectability of low-intensity stimuli without affecting high-intensity stimuli (Devilbiss & Waterhouse, 2002; Moore, 2004). At this moment in time, empirical research support for this, when exercise is the stressor, is somewhat equivocal (McMorris & Hale, 2012; McMorris et al., 2016). However, a limited number of studies have examined the effect of long-duration, moderate-intensity and heavy exercise on cognition in such tasks.

Learning/long-term memory tasks

Learning is generally divided into three stages: encoding, storage and retrieval. Encoding consists of two substages, acquisition and consolidation. Acquisition is really part of short-term memory and refers to the registering and sensory analysis of information. Consolidation is the creation of a stronger representation and takes place over a period of time. The second stage is storage, which is the creation and maintenance of a permanent record in long-term memory. The final stage, retrieval, refers to using the stored information to recall facts. Memory can be declarative, also known as explicit memory, which is consciously encoded and recalled; or non-declarative, also known as implicit memory, which refers to subconsciously or implicitly learned information. Consolidation of declarative information appears to be primarily undertaken by the hippocampus and requires the process of long-term potentiation (LTP), the strengthening of synaptic connections between neurons (Bliss & Lømo, 1973). Processes of consolidation in implicit memory are less well understood. The basal ganglia are thought to be important in implicit learning (Poldrack et al., 2001; Reber & Squire, 1994). Although there are some common brain activations during explicit and implicit learning, distinct neural mechanisms serve explicit versus implicit learning/memory (Yang & Li, 2012).

Consolidation is generally divided into two phases, early and late. Early-LTP (E-LTP) lasts for about 4–6 hours, while late-LTP (L-LTP) has a duration of more than 4–6 hours (Straube, Korz, Balschun, & Frey, 2003). The E-LTP process is dependent on the fact that during long-duration, moderate-intensity exercise and heavy exercise (and indeed other forms of exercise, which increase force, such as resistance training), nitric oxide is released from the endothelium (Tanaka et al., 2015), where it is produced from the amino acid L-arginine, with cyclic guanosine monophosphate (cGMP) as the second messenger. Nitric oxide signalling is mostly mediated by soluble guanylyl cyclase (Arnold, Mittal, Katsuki, & Murad, 1977) and this leads to the activation of cGMP-dependent protein kinase. Protein kinase, in turn, enhances neurotransmitter release (Hawkins, Kandel, & Siegelbaum, 1993; Hawkins, Son, & Arancio, 1998) and this forms the basis of E-LTP.

As we can see from the above, catecholamines play little part in E-LTP and the process is independent of protein synthesis (Bailey, Kandell, & Harris, 2015; Kennedy, 2016). However, both catecholamines and the synthesis of the protein brain-derived neurotrophic factor (BDNF) are vital for L-LTP. When the exercise intensity and/or duration induce high concentrations of noradrenaline in the hippocampus, it activates β-adrenoceptors, which are guanosine triphosphate (GTP)-binding proteins and stimulate cAMP activation. Acute exercise also results in increases in serum or plasma BDNF concentrations in humans (Ferris, Williams, & Shen, 2007; Rasmussen et al., 2009), while animal studies have demonstrated strong evidence for acute exercise inducing increased BDNF and/or BDNF mRNA expression in the brain, in particular in the hippocampus (Berchtold, Castello, & Cotman, 2010; Gomez-Pinilla, Vaynman, & Ying, 2008). It is the interaction between BDNF and noradrenaline via cAMP activity that is vital for L-LTP.

The synaptic actions of BDNF are regulated by cAMP, as it modulates the signaling and trafficking of the BDNF receptor tropomyosin-related kinase B (Trk B) (Ji, Pang, Feng, & Lu, 2005; Yamada & Nabeshima, 2003). The binding of BDNF to Trk B initiates a number of intracellular signalling cascades, including calcium/calmodulin kinase II and mitogen-activated protein kinase, resulting in the phosphorylation of cAMP-response element-binding protein (CREB) (Binder & Scharfman, 2004; Waterhouse & Xu, 2009). The whole process modulates synaptic transmission in a lasting manner by modifying synaptic protein composition via local protein synthesis (Waterhouse & Xu, 2009), thus facilitating synaptic transmission.

So far we have been discussing research undertaken on explicit or declarative long-term memory tasks. However, LTP occurs also during implicit learning (Bailey et al., 2015; Horvitz, 2009), but there are some differences. The hippocampus is thought to play a part in the implicit learning of some, but not all, tasks (Albouy et al., 2008), but the basal ganglia, in particular the striatum, are heavily involved in many implicit learning tasks (Poldrack et al., 2001; Reber & Squire, 1994). While β-adrenoceptors are present in the basal ganglia (Reznikoff, Manaker, Rhodes, Winokur, & Rainbow, 1986) and may regulate BDNF/Trk B activity, the dopaminergic system is dominant and high concentrations of dopamine have been shown to aid learning in this region (Wickens, Horvitz, Costa, & Killcross, 2007). Like β-adrenoceptors, dopaminergic D_1-receptors are GTP-binding proteins, with cAMP as the second messenger. cAMP activates protein kinase A, which, in turn, activates CREB and thus LTP occurs (Tritsch & Sabatini, 2012).

Conclusion

Evidence from rodent and non-human primates shows that, during moderate-intensity exercise, feedback, both pre- and post-CT, from the cardiorespiratory system activates stretch receptors, baroreceptors and chemoreceptors

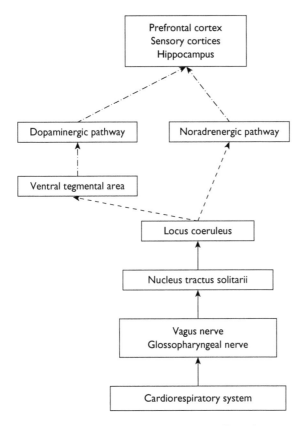

Figure 5.2 Schematic diagram outlining the effect of acute exercise on the synthesis and release of catecholamines. Unbroken arrows represent chemical and electrophysiological feedback. Dashes represent movement of noradrenaline and dashes with dots represent dopamine movement.

on the vagus and glossopharyngeal nerves. In turn, these stimulate the synthesis and release of noradrenaline from the locus coeruleus, which, via the dorsal noradrenergic pathway, activates the prefrontal cortex, limbic system and sensory cortices. It also triggers the synthesis and release of dopamine from neurons in the ventral tegmental area and this activates the mesocorticolimbic dopaminergic pathway. In the prefrontal cortex, this results in an optimal signal-to-noise ratio and hence optimal performance of central executive tasks.

In general, activation of the reticular formation and increased catecholamines release in the sensory cortices and their association areas result in improved performance of perceptual ability tasks and possibly short-term memory. However, heavy exercise induces excessive catecholamine concentrations in the prefrontal cortex, which results in an increase in noise at the expense of the signal (Figure 5.2). Many perceptual ability tasks are, however, facilitated as the signal for the salient stimulus becomes sharper due to repression of noise. Declarative, learning/long-term memory tasks are also facilitated due to β-adrenoceptor-initiated cAMP modulation of signalling and trafficking of Trk B activity. Implicit learning is aided by D_1 dopaminergic receptor-initiated cAMP modulation of signalling and trafficking of Trk B activity. These effects are enhanced by 5-HT and CRF acting on noradrenergic neurons, especially in the locus coeruleus, to stimulate further release of noradrenaline.

Practical implications for learning and memory

In this text there are many examples of how chronic exercise aids cognition and academic performance. In this short subsection, I will focus on how we can utilize acute exercise to augment the beneficial effects of chronic exercise. The fact that chronic and acute exercise aid cognition leads to the obvious conclusion that daily physical activity should be undertaken in schools. There is empirical support for this (Reed, Maslow, Long, & Hughey, 2013). An issue with this is simply the timetabling of the physical activity. From what we have covered with regard to central executive tasks, which include problem solving, planning and creativity, they would probably benefit from short- to moderate-duration, moderate-intensity exercise early in the school day, the positive effects of which have been shown in some research (Chen, Yan, Yin, Pan, & Chang, 2014; Janssen et al., 2014; Soga, Shishido, & Nagatomi, 2015). Parents could help by having children walk to school, at least part of the way. In many boarding schools, the day begins with a run but this is not possible in most schools. It should be noted that the positive effects of such exercise can last for a long time. Cooper, Bandelow, Nute, Morris, and Nevill (2015) found positive effects of acute exercise on cognition as long as 1 hour following cessation of the activity. Although the half-life of catecholamines in the periphery is only ~3 minutes (Genuth, 2004), Eisenhofer, Kopin, and Goldstein (2004) reported the half-life of brain catecholamines as being in the range of 8–12 hours, while Kadzierski, Aguila-Mansilla, Kozlowski, and Porter (1994) stated that the half-life of tyrosine hydroxylase mRNA was 14 ± 1 hour.

With regard to rote learning or the learning of facts, a different approach may be more beneficial. Short-duration, moderate-intensity exercise would aid attention during the acquisition phase, which would be beneficial, but the timing of exercise to aid consolidation is more problematic. Roig, Nordbrandt, Geertsen, and Nielsen (2013) claimed that heavy exercise closely following the acquisition phase is more beneficial for consolidation than when there has been a substantial gap between acquisition and exercise. There is a need for far more such research, but the key issue appears, to me, to be the exercise intensity. As we saw in the last section, heavy and long-duration, moderate-intensity exercise is best for aiding L-LTP formation. It makes some sense to think that the exercise could take place at the end of the day. Indeed, the child's participation in a physical activity outside of school could facilitate this. Given that sleep is also essential for neurogenesis and L-LTP (Alkadhi, Zagaar, Alhaider, Salim, & Aleisa, 2013), exercise before bed could be beneficial. However, I am not aware of any research which has looked at undertaking heavy exercise early in the school day and how that affects learning and other forms of cognition later in the day. When I was a physical education teacher in schools, many colleagues complained that the children were too tired to concentrate when they came back from some physical education lessons. Whether that affected learning, however, is another issue.

References

Albouy, G., Sterpenich, V., Balteau, E., Vandewalle, G., Desseilles, M., Thanh, D-V., . . . Maquet, P. (2008). Both the hippocampus and striatum are involved in consolidation of motor sequence memory. *Neuron, 58,* 261–272.

Alkadhi, K., Zagaar, M., Alhaider, I., Salim, S., & Aleisa, A. (2013). Neurobiological consequences of sleep deprivation. *Current Neuropharmacology, 11,* 231–249.

Arakawa, K., Miura, S., Koga, M., Kinoshita, A., Urata, H., & Kiyonaga, A. (1995). Activation of renal dopamine system by physical exercise. *Hypertension Research, 18,* S73–S77.

Arnold, W. P., Mittal, C. K., Katsuki, S., & Murad F. (1977). Nitric oxide activates guanylate cyclase and increases guanosine 3':5'-cyclic monophosphate levels in various tissue preparations. *Proceedings of the National Academy of Sciences U. S. A., 74,* 3203–3207.

Arnsten, A. F. T. (2009). Stress signalling pathways that impair prefrontal cortex structure and function. *Nature Reviews Neuroscience, 10,* 410–422.

Arnsten, A. F. T. (2011). Catecholamine influences on dorsolateral prefrontal cortical networks. *Biological Psychiatry, 69,* e89–e99. doi: 101016/jbiopsych201101027.

Arts, F. J. P., & Kuipers, H. (1994). The relation between power output, oxygen uptake and heart rate in male athletes. *International Journal of Sports Medicine, 15,* 228–231.

Aston-Jones, G., Ennis, M., Pieribone, V. A., Nickell, W. T., & Shipley, M. T. (1986). The brain nucleus locus coeruleus: Restricted afferent control of a broad efferent network. *Science, 234,* 734–737.

Baddeley, A. D. (1986). *Working memory.* New York: Oxford University Press.

Bailey, C. H., Kandell, E. R., & Harris, K. M. (2015). Structural components of synaptic plasticity and memory consolidation. *Cold Spring Harbor Perspectives in Biology, 7,* a021758. doi: 10.1101/cshperspect.a021758.

Barbas, H. (2000). Connections underlying the synthesis of cognition, memory, and emotion in primate prefrontal cortices. *Brain Research Bulletin, 52,* 319–330.

Barbas, H., Saha, S., Rempel-Clower, N., & Ghashghaei, T. (2003). Serial pathways from primate prefrontal cortex to autonomic areas may influence emotional expression. *BMC Neuroscience, 4,* 25. doi: 101186/1471-2202-4-25.

Beaver, W. L., Wasserman, K., & Whipp, B. J. (1986). A new method for detecting anaerobic threshold by gas exchange. *Journal of Applied Physiology, 60,* 2020–2027.

Berchtold, N. C., Castello, N., & Cotman, C. W. (2010). Exercise and time-dependent benefits to learning and memory. *Neuroscience, 167,* 588–597.

Berthoud, H. R., & Neuhuber, W. L. (2000). Functional and chemical anatomy of the afferent vagal system. *Autonomic Neuroscience: Basic and Clinical, 85,* 1–17.

Binder, D. K., & Scharfman, H. E. (2004). Brain-derived neurotrophic factor. *Growth Factors, 22,* 123–131.

Bliss, T., & Lømo, T. (1973). Long-lasting potentiation of synaptic transmission in the dentate area of the anaesthetized rabbit following stimulation of the perforant path. *Journal of Physiology (Lond.), 232,* 331–356.

Borer, K. T. (2003). *Exercise endocrinology.* Champaign, IL: Human Kinetics.

Braunlich, K., Gomez-Lavin, J., & Seger, C. A. (2015). Frontoparietal networks involved in categorization and item working memory. *NeuroImage, 107,* 146–162.

Bridge, M. W., Weller, A. S., Rayson, M., & Jones, D. A. (2003). Ambient temperature and the pituitary hormone responses to exercise in humans. *Experimental Physiology, 88,* 627–635.

Butt, A. M., Jones, H. C., & Abbott, N. J. (1990). Electrical resistance across the blood–brain barrier in anaesthetized rats: A developmental study. *Journal of Physiology, 429,* 47–62.

Carr, D. B., & Sesack, S. R. (2000). GABA-containing neurons in the rat ventral tegmental area project to the prefrontal cortex. *Synapse, 38,* 114–123.

Cedarbaum, J. M., & Aghajanian, G. K. (1978). Afferent projections to the rat locus coeruleus as determined by a retrograde tracing technique. *Journal of Comparative Neurology, 178,* 1–16.

Chen, A-G., Yan, J., Yin, H-C., Pan, C-Y., & Chang, Y-K. (2014). Effects of acute aerobic exercise on multiple aspects of executive function in preadolescent children. *Psychology of Sport and Exercise, 15,* 627–636.

Chen, H. I., Lin, L. C., Yu, L., Liu, Y. F., Kuo, Y. M., Huang, A. M., . . . Jen, C. J. (2008). Treadmill exercise enhances avoidance learning in rats: The role of down-regulated serotonin system in the limbic system. *Neurobiology of Learning and Memory, 89,* 489–496.

Chennaoui, M., Drogou, C., Gomez-Merino, D., Grimaldi, B., Fillion, G., & Guezennec, C. Y. (2001). Endurance training effects on 5-HT(1B) receptors mRNA expression in cerebellum, striatum, frontal cortex and hippocampus of rats. *Neuroscience Letters, 307,* 33–36.

Chmura, J., Nazar, H., & Kaciuba-Uścilko, H. (1994). Choice reaction time during graded exercise in relation to blood lactate and plasma catecholamine thresholds. *International Journal of Sports Medicine, 15,* 172–176.

Cooper, C. J. (1973). Anatomical and physiological mechanisms of arousal with specific reference to the effects of exercise. *Ergonomics, 16,* 601–609.

Cooper, S. B., Bandelow, S., Nute, M. L., Morris, J. G., & Nevill, M. E. (2015). Breakfast glycaemic index and exercise: Combined effects on adolescents' cognition. *Physiology and Behavior, 139,* 104–111.

Corbetta, M., & Shulman, G. L. (2002). Control of goal-directed and stimulus-driven attention in the brain. *Nature Reviews Neuroscience, 3,* 201–215.

Cornford, E. M., Braun, L. D., Oldendorf, W. H., & Hill, M. A. (1982). Comparison of lipid-related blood–brain barrier penetrability in neonates and adults. *American Journal of Physiology, 243,* C161–C168.

Dahlström, A., & Fuxe, K. (1964). Evidence for the existence of monoamine-containing neurons in the central nervous system. I. Demonstration of monoamines in the cell bodies of brain stem neurons. *Acta Physiologica Scandinavica, 62* (Suppl 232), 3–55.

Davey, C. P. (1973). Physical exertion and mental performance. *Ergonomics, 16,* 595–599.

Deutch, A. Y., & Roth, R. H. (1990). The determinants of stress-induced activation of the prefrontal cortical dopamine system. *Progress in Brain Research, 85,* 367–403.

Devilbiss, D. M., & Waterhouse, B. D. (2002). Determination and quantification of pharmacological, physiological, or behavioral manipulations on ensembles of simultaneously recorded neurons in functionally related neural circuits. *Journal of Neuroscience Methods, 121,* 181–198.

Devilbiss, D. M., Waterhouse, B. D., Berridge, C. W., & Valentino, R. (2012). Corticotropin-releasing factor acting at the locus coeruleus disrupts thalamic and cortical sensory-evoked responses. *Neuropsychopharmacology, 37,* 2020–2030.

Díaz-Mataix, L., Scorza, M. C., Bortolozzi, A., Toth, M., & Celada, P., & Artigas, F. (2005). Involvement of 5-HT$_{1A}$ receptors in prefrontal cortex in the modulation of dopaminergic activity: Role in atypical antipsychotic action. *Journal of Neuroscience, 25,* 10831–10843.

Eagle, D. M., Davies, K. R., Towse, B. W., Keeler, J. F., Theobald, D. E., & Robbins, T. W. (2010). Beta-adrenoceptor-mediated action of atomoxetine during behavioral inhibition on the stop-signal task in rats. *Society of Neuroscience Abstracts, 508,* 510. Cited by Arnsten, A. F. T. (2011). Catecholamine influences on dorsolateral prefrontal cortical networks. *Biological Psychiatry, 69,* e89–e99. doi: 101016/jbiopsych201101027.

Eisenhofer, G., Kopin, I. J., & Goldstein, D. S. (2004). Catecholamine metabolism: A contemporary view with implications for physiology and medicine. *Pharmacological Reviews, 56,* 331–348.

Ferris, L. T., Williams, J. S., & Shen, C. (2007). The effect of acute exercise on serum brain-derived neurotrophic factor levels and cognitive function. *Medicine and Science in Sports and Exercise, 39,* 728–734.

Ferrucci, M., Giorgi, F. S., Bartalucci, A., Busceti, C. L., & Fornai, F. (2013). The effects of locus coeruleus and norepinephrine in methamphetamine toxicity. *Current Neuropharmacology, 11*, 80–94.

Finlay, J. M., Zigmond, M. J., & Abercrombie, E. D. (1995). Increased dopamine and norepinephrine release in medial prefrontal cortex induced by acute and chronic stress: Effects of diazepam. *Neuroscience, 64*, 619–628.

Gagnon, S. A., & Wagner, A. D. (2016). Acute stress and episodic memory retrieval: Neurobiological mechanisms and behavioral consequences. *Annals of the New York Academy of Science, 1369*(1), 55–75. doi: 10.1111/nyas.12996.

Genuth, S. M. (2004). The endocrine system. In R. M. Berne, M. Levy, N. B. Koepen, & B. A. Stanton (Eds.), *Physiology* (5th ed., pp. 719–978). St. Louis, MO: Mosby.

Goltz, D., Gundlach, C., Nierhaus, T., Villringer, A., Müller, M., & Pleger, B. (2015). Connections between intraparietal sulcus and a sensorimotor network underpin sustained tactile attention. *Journal of Neuroscience, 35*, 7938–7949.

Gomez-Pinilla, F., Vaynman, S., & Ying, Z. (2008). Brain-derived neurotrophic factor functions as a metabotrophin to mediate the effects of exercise on cognition. *European Journal of Neuroscience, 28*, 2278–2287.

Gordon, E. M., Stollstorff, M., & Vaidya, C. J. (2012). Using spatial multiple regression to identify intrinsic connectivity networks involved in working memory performance. *Human Brain Mapping, 33*, 1536–1552.

Grenhoff, J., & Svensson, T. H. (1993). Prazosin modulates the firing pattern of dopamine neurons in rat ventral tegmental area. *European Journal of Pharmacology, 233*, 79–84.

Hawkins, R. A., O'Kane, R. L., Simpson, I. A., & Viña, J. R. (2006). Structure of the blood–brain barrier and its role in the transport of amino acids. *Journal of Nutrition, 136*, 218S–226S.

Hawkins, R. D., Kandel, E. R., & Siegelbaum, S. A. (1993). Learning to modulate transmitter release: Themes and variations in synaptic plasticity. *Annual Review of Neuroscience, 16*, 625–665.

Hawkins, R. D., Son, H., & Arancio, O. (1998). Nitric oxide as a retrograde messenger during long-term potentiation in hippocampus. *Progress in Brain Research, 118*, 155–172.

Hodgetts, V., Coppack, S. W., Frayn, K. N., & Hockaday, T. D. R. (1991). Factors controlling fat mobilization from human subcutaneous adipose-tissue during exercise. *Journal of Applied Physiology, 71*, 445–451.

Horvitz, J. C. (2009). Stimulus–response and response–outcome learning mechanisms in the striatum. *Behavioural Brain Research, 199*, 129–140.

Janssen, M., Chinapaw, M. J. M., Rauh, S. P., Toussaint, H. M., van Mechelen, W., & Verhagen, E. A. L. M. (2014). A short physical activity break from cognitive tasks increases selective attention in primary school children aged 10–11. *Mental Health and Physical Activity, 7*, 129–134.

Ji, Y. Y., Pang, P. T., Feng, L. Y., & Lu, B. (2005). Cyclic AMP controls BDNF-induced TrkB phosphorylation and dendritic spine formation in mature hippocampal neurons. *Nature Neuroscience, 8*, 164–172.

Jiang, Q. Y., Kawashima, H., Iwasaki, Y., Uchida, K., Sugimoto, K., & Itoi, K. (2004). Differential effects of forced swim-stress on the corticotropin-releasing hormone and vasopressin gene transcription in the paravocellular division of the paraventricular nucleus of rat hypothalamus. *Neuroscience Letters, 358*, 201–204.

Kadzierski, W., Aguila-Mansilla, N., Kozlowski, G. P., & Porter, J. C. (1994). Expression of tyrosine hydroxylase gene in cultured hypothalamic cells: roles of protein kinase A and C. *Journal of Neurochemistry, 62,* 431–437.

Kasamatsu, T. (1970). Maintained and evoked unit activity in the mesencephalic reticular formation of the freely behaving cat. *Experimental Neurology, 28,* 450–470.

Kawashima, H., Saito, T., Yoshizato, H., Fujikawa, T., Sato, Y., McEwen, B. S., & Soya, H. (2004). Endurance treadmill training in rats alters CRH activity in the hypothalamic paraventricular nucleus at rest and during acute running according to its period. *Life Sciences, 76,* 763–774.

Kennedy, M. B. (2016). Synaptic signaling in learning and memory. *Cold Spring Harbor Perspective in Biology, 8,* a016824.

Kougias, P., Weakley, S. M., Yao, Q., Lin, P. H., & Chen, C. Y. (2010). Arterial baroreceptors in the management of systemic hypertension. *Medical Science Monitor, 16,* RA1–RA8.

Lapiz, M. D., & Morilak, D. A. (2006). Noradrenergic modulation of cognitive function in rat medial prefrontal cortex as measured by attentional set shifting capability. *Neuroscience, 137,* 1039–1049.

Leh, S. E., Petrides, M., & Strafella, A. P. (2010). The neural circuitry of executive functions in healthy subjects and Parkinson's disease. *Neuropsychopharmacology, 35,* 70–85.

Lund-Andersen, H. (1979). Transport of glucose from blood to brain. *Physiological Reviews, 59,* 305–352.

Mason, J. W. (1975a). A historical view of the stress field: Part I. *Journal of Human Stress, 1,* 6–12.

Mason, J. W. (1975b). A historical view of the stress field: Part II. *Journal of Human Stress, 1,* 22–36.

McGaugh, J. L., Cahill, L., & Roozendaal, B. (1996). Involvement of the amygdala in memory storage: Interaction with other brain systems. *Proceedings of the National Academy of Sciences of the United States of America, 93,* 13508–13514.

McMorris, T. (2016a). Re-appraisal of the acute, moderate intensity exercise–catecholamines interaction effect on speed of cognition: Role of the vagal/NTS afferent pathway. *Journal of Applied Physiology, 120,* 657–658.

McMorris, T. (2016b). Developing the catecholamines hypothesis for the acute exercise–cognition interaction in humans: Lessons from animal studies. *Physiology and Behavior, 165,* 291–299.

McMorris, T., & Hale, B. J. (2012). Differential effects of differing intensities of acute exercise on speed and accuracy of cognition: A meta-analytical investigation. *Brain and Cognition, 80,* 338–351.

McMorris, T., & Hale, B. J. (2015). Is there an acute exercise-induced physiological/biochemical threshold which triggers increased speed of cognitive functioning? A meta-analytic investigation. *Journal of Sport and Health Science, 4,* 4–13.

McMorris, T., Myers, S., MacGillivary, W. W., Sexsmith, J. R., Fallowfield, J., Graydon, J., & Forster, D. (1999). Exercise, plasma catecholamine concentration and decision-making performance of soccer players on a soccer-specific test. *Journal of Sport Science, 17,* 667–676.

McMorris, T., Sproule, J., Turner, A., & Hale, B. J. (2011). Acute, intermediate intensity exercise, and speed and accuracy in working memory tasks: A meta-analytical comparison of effects. *Physiology and Behavior, 102,* 421–428.

McMorris, T., Turner, A., Hale, B. J., & Sproule, J. (2016). Beyond the catecholamines hypothesis for an acute exercise–cognition interaction: A neurochemical perspective. In T. McMorris (Ed.), *Exercise–cognition interaction: Neuroscience perspectives* (pp. 65–104). New York: Elsevier Academic Press.

Mejías-Aponte, C. A., Drouin, C., & Aston-Jones, G. (2009). Adrenergic and noradrenergic innervation of the midbrain ventral tegmental area and retrorubral field: Prominent inputs from medullary homeostatic centers. *Journal of Neuroscience, 29,* 3613–3626.

Miyake, A., Friedman, N. P., Emerson, M. J., Witzki, A. H., & Howerter, A. (2000). The unity and diversity of executive functions and their contributions to complex "frontal lobe" tasks: A latent variable analysis. *Cognitive Psychology, 41,* 49–100.

Miyashita, T., & Williams, C. L. (2006). Epinephrine administration increases neural impulses propagated along the vagus nerve: Role of peripheral beta-adrenergic receptors. *Neurobiology of Learning and Memory, 85,* 116–124.

Molenberghs, P., Mesulam, M. M., Peeters, R., & Vandenberghe, R. R. C. (2007). Remapping attentional priorities: Differential contribution of superior parietal lobule and intraparietal sulcus. *Cerebral Cortex, 17,* 2703–2712.

Moor, T., Mundorff, L., Bohringer, A., Philippsen, C., Langewitz, W., Reino, S. T., & Schachinger, H. (2005). Evidence that baroreflex feedback influences long-term incidental visual memory in men. *Neurobiology of Learning and Memory, 84,* 168–174.

Moore, C. I. (2004). Frequency-dependent processing in the vibrissa sensory system. *Journal of Neurophysiology, 91,* 2390–2399.

Myers, B., Dolgas, C. M., Kasckow, J., Cullinan, W. E., & Herman, J. P. (2014). Central stress-integrative circuits: Forebrain glutamatergic and GABAergic projections to the dorsomedial hypothalamus, medial preoptic area, and bed nucleus of the stria terminalis. *Brain Structure and Function, 219,* 1287–1303.

Ohiwa, N., Saito, T., Chang, H., Omoria, T., Fujikawa, T., Asada, T., & Soya, H. (2006). Activation of A1 and A2 noradrenergic neurons in response to running in the rat. *Neuroscience Letters, 395,* 46–50.

Oldendorf, W. H. (1977). The blood–brain barrier. *Experimental Eye Research, 25,* 177–190.

Podolin, D. A., Munger, P. A., & Mazzeo, R. S. (1991). Plasma-catecholamine and lactate response during graded-exercise with varied glycogen conditions. *Journal of Applied Physiology, 71,* 1427–1433.

Podvoll, E. M., & Goodman, S. J. (1967). Averaged neural electrical activity and arousal. *Science, 155,* 223–225.

Poldrack, R. A., Clark, J., Paré-Blagoev, E. J., Shohamy, D., Creso Moyano, J., Myers, C., & Gluck, M. A. (2001). Interactive memory systems in the human brain. *Nature, 414,* 546–550.

Rasmussen, P., Brassard, P., Adser H., Pedersen, M. V., Leick, L., Hart, E., . . . Pilegaard, H. (2009). Evidence for release of brain-derived neurotrophic factor from the brain during exercise. *Experimental Physiology, 94,* 1062–1069.

Reber, P. J., & Squire, L. R. (1994). Parallel brain systems for learning with and without awareness. *Learning and Memory, 1,* 217–229.

Reed, J. A., Maslow, A. L., Long, S., & Hughey, M. (2013). Examining the impact of 45 minutes of daily physical education on cognitive ability, fitness performance, and body composition of African American youth. *Journal of Physical Activity and Health, 10,* 185–197.

Reis, D. J., & Fuxe, K. (1968). Depletion of noradrenaline in the brainstem neurons during sham rage behaviour produced by acute brainstem transmission in cat. *Brain Research, 7,* 448–451.

Reis, D. J., & Fuxe, K. (1969). Brain norepinephrine: Evidence that neuronal release is essential for sham rage behavior following brainstem transection in the cat. *Proceedings of the National Academy of Science, 84,* 108–112.

Reznikoff, G. A., Manaker, S., Rhodes, C. H., Winokur, A., & Rainbow, T. C. (1986). Localization and quantification of beta-adrenergic receptors in human brain. *Neurology, 36,* 1067–1073.

Rinaman, L. (2011). Hindbrain noradrenergic A2 neurons: Diverse roles in autonomic, endocrine, cognitive, and behavioral functions. *American Journal of Physiology-Regulatory, Integrative and Comparative Physiology, 300,* R222–R235.

Robbins, T. W., & Roberts, A. C. (2007). Differential regulation of fronto-executive function by the monoamines and acetylcholine. *Cerebral Cortex, 17,* i151–i160.

Roig, M., Nordbrandt, S., Geertsen, S. S., & Nielsen, J. B. (2013). The effects of cardiovascular exercise on human memory: A review with meta-analysis. *Neuroscience and Biobehavioral Review, 37,* 1645–1666.

Roth, R. H., Tam, S-Y., Ida, Y., Yang, J-X., & Deutch, A. Y. (1988). Stress and the mesocorticolimbic dopamine systems. *Annals of the New York Academy of Science, 537,* 138–147.

Rushmer, R. F., Smith, O. A., Jr, & Lasher, E. P. (1960). Neural mechanisms of cardiac control during exertion. *Physiological Review, 40*(Suppl 4), 27–34.

Samorajaski, T., & Marks, B. H. (1962). Localization of tritiated norepinephrine in mouse brain. *Journal of Histochemistry and Cytochemistry, 10,* 393–399.

Shojaei, E. A., Farajov, A., & Jafari, A. (2011). Effect of moderate aerobic cycling on some systemic inflammatory markers in healthy active collegiate men. *International Journal of General Medicine, 4,* 79–84.

Soga, K., Shishido, T., & Nagatomi, R. (2015). Executive function during and after acute moderate aerobic exercise in adolescents. *Psychology of Sport and Exercise, 16,* 7–17.

Sogabe, S., Yagasaki, Y., Onozawa, K., & Kawakami, Y. (2013). Mesocortical dopamine system modulates mechanical nociceptive responses recorded in the rat prefrontal cortex. *BMC Neuroscience, 14,* 65. doi: 10.1186/1471-2202-14-65.

Straube, T., Korz, V., Balschun, D., & Frey, J. U. (2003). Requirement of β-adrenergic receptor activation and protein synthesis for LTP-reinforcement by novelty in rat dentate gyrus. *Journal of Physiology (Lond), 552,* 953–960.

Tanaka, L. Y., Bechara, L. R. G., dos Santos, A. M., Jordao, C. P., de Sousa, L. G. O., Bartholomeu, T., . . . Ramires, P. R. (2015). Exercise improves endothelial function: A local analysis of production of nitric oxide and reactive oxygen species. *Nitric Oxide, 45,* 7–14.

Tomporowski, P. D., & Ellis, N. R. (1986). Effects of exercise on cognitive processes: A review. *Psychological Bulletin, 99,* 338–346.

Tritsch, N. X., & Sabatini, B. L. (2012). Dopaminergic modulation of synaptic transmission in cortex and striatum. *Neuron, 76,* 33–50.

Urhausen, A., Weiler, B., Coen, B., & Kindermann, W. (1994). Plasma catecholamines during endurance exercise of different intensities as related to the individual anaerobic threshold. *European Journal of Applied Physiology, 69,* 16–20.

Velásquez-Martinez, M. C., Vázquez-Torres, R., & Jiménez-Riveira, C. A. (2012). Activation of alpha1-adrenoreceptors enhances glutamate release onto ventral tegmental area dopamine cells. *Neuroscience, 216,* 18–30.

Vendsalu, A. (1960). Studies on adrenaline and noradrenaline in human plasma. *Acta Physiologia Scandinavica, 49,* 1–123.

Wang, M., Ramos, B., Paspalas, C., Shu, Y., Simen, A., Duque, A., . . . Arnsten, A. F. (2007). Alpha2A-adrenoceptors strengthen working memory networks by inhibiting cAMP-HCN channel signaling in prefrontal cortex. *Cell, 129,* 397–410.

Waterhouse, B. D., Moises, H. C., & Woodward, D. J. (1980). Noradrenergic modulation of somatosensory cortical neuronal responses to iontophoretically applied putative transmitters. *Experimental Neurology, 69,* 30–49.

Waterhouse, B. D., Moises, H. C., & Woodward, D. J. (1981). Alpha-receptor-mediated facilitation of somatosensory cortical neuronal responses to excitatory synaptic inputs and iontophoretically applied acetylcholine. *Neuropharmacology, 20,* 907–920.

Waterhouse, E. G., & Xu, B. (2009). New insights into the role of brain-derived neurotrophic factor in synaptic plasticity. *Molecular Cell Neuroscience, 42,* 81–89.

Watson, A. W. S. (1974). The relationship between tidal volume and respiratory frequency during muscular exercise. *British Journal of Sports Medicine, 8,* 87–90.

Wickens, J. R., Horvitz, J. C., Costa, R. M., & Killcross, S. (2007). Dopaminergic mechanisms in actions and habits. *Journal of Neuroscience, 27,* 8181–8183.

Yamada, K., & Nabeshima, T. (2003). Brain-derived neurotrophic factor/TrkB signaling in memory processes. *Journal of Pharmacological Sciences, 91,* 267–270.

Yamamoto, Y., Miyashita, M., Hughson, R. L., Tmura, S., Shiohara, M., & Mutoh, Y. (1991). The ventilatory threshold gives maximal lactate steady state. *European Journal of Applied Physiology, 63,* 55–59.

Yanagita, S., Amemiya, S., Suzuki, S., & Kita, I. (2007). Effects of spontaneous and forced running on activation of hypothalamic corticotropin-releasing hormone neurons in rats. *Life Sciences, 80,* 356–363.

Yang, J., & Li, P. (2012). Brain networks of explicit and implicit learning. *PLoS One, 7,* e42993. doi: 101371/journalpone0042993.

Yerkes, R. M., & Dodson, J. D. (1908). The relation of strength of stimulus to the rapidity of habit formation. *Journal of Comparative Neurology and Psychology, 18,* 459–482.

Chapter 6

The motor–cognitive connection

Indicator of future developmental success in children and adolescents?

Nadja Schott and Thomas Klotzbier

Introduction

Recent studies suggest that motor and cognitive development are more closely related than previously assumed, depending on movement experiences, skills, age and gender. In particular, gross motor performance such as functional goal-oriented locomotion is not a merely automatic process, but requires higher-level cognitive input, highlighting the relationship between cognitive function and fundamental motor skills across the lifespan. Motor and cognitive development might even share similar trajectories and characteristics across the lifespan (Figure 6.1).

Similarly, Roebers et al. (2014) reported that fine motor skills, non-verbal intelligence and executive functioning are significantly interrelated. Additional findings show a strong relationship between age-related changes in motor and cognitive performance and motor skill acquisition (Favazza & Siperstein, 2016). Motor and cognitive functions appear to be even more strongly correlated in children with motor and/or cognitive impairment (e.g. developmental coordination disorder (DCD), Down's syndrome, autism) compared to typically developing children (Schott & Holfelder, 2015; Schott, El-Rajab, & Klotzbier, 2016).

To investigate the nature of motor and cognitive development, researchers have studied components mostly independently. While on a behavioural level, an elegant approach to assess the interdependence of motor and cognitive function comes from *cognitive–motor interference* (CMI) research using *dual-task* (DT) conditions (Schott et al., 2016), recent developments in neuroimaging methods support the notion that the brain is embodied, meaning that bodily experience underlies thinking, feeling and action (Wilson, 2002). To support the multifaceted aspects of motor and cognitive changes across the lifespan several frameworks were proposed to investigate interactions between the structure and function of the brain, cognition, motor learning, physical activity and lifestyle factors (Prado & Dewey, 2014; Ren, Wu, Chan, & Yan, 2013; Reuter-Lorenz & Park, 2014). However, they focus on cognitive ageing or on the effect of cognitive ageing on skill acquisition, or more generally on the impact of nutrition on brain development in early life.

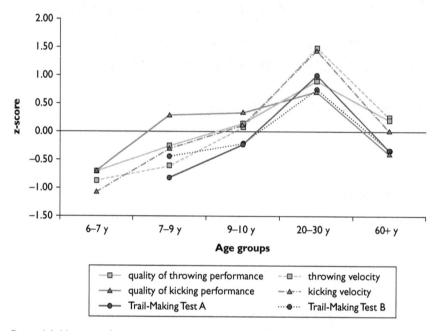

Figure 6.1 Motor performance (kicking, throwing) increases from childhood
(6–10 years) to young adulthood (20–30 years) and decreases from
young adulthood (20–30 years) to old age (60–85 years), mirroring the results
from cognitive performance of the Trail-Making Test (version A examines
attention, visual scanning, motor speed and coordination, while version B
examines in addition mental flexibility and working memory)
(n = 120; unpublished data).

In this chapter we first review cross-sectional studies using the DT
approach in children and adolescents, particularly in the areas of gait and
postural stability. Second, we will present an integrative framework for the
interaction of cognition, motor performance and life-course factors.

Current state of the art on the cognitive–motor interference during walking tasks in children and adolescents

Typically, practice of a new motor skill results in progressive improvement
of performance following a power–function curve. During the first learning phase, performance increases rapidly and attentional demands are high.
In an advanced (automatization) phase, which reflects procedural memory
consolidation processes, a performance plateau is reached, allowing the
motor task to be performed in a range of contexts with limited demands

on attentional resources (Magill & Anderson, 2014). The paradigm used to study the procedural learning and automatization of skills involves testing subjects under both single-task and DT conditions (Doyon et al., 2009). CMI refers to the phenomenon in which carrying out simultaneously a motor and a cognitive task interferes with the performance of one or both tasks. Where the motor task is adequately learned, few attentional resources are needed to perform the task, thereby leaving sufficient resources for the performance of concurrent attention-demanding tasks. However, an overload of attentional resources during DT may disrupt both cognitive and motor performance in children and adolescents with or without motor and/or cognitive impairments.

Methodological considerations

Due to the enormous number of studies published in late adulthood it can be seen that previous research efforts are characterized by the absence of a standardized DT paradigm, which significantly complicates the interpretation of results. Balance and locomotion tasks are often used as the primary motor task. Mostly the aim is to predict future falls and to show the association with cognitive functions (Muir, Gopaul, & Montero Odasso, 2012). Due to the enormous methodological heterogeneity, the secondary cognitive tasks in those studies are difficult to compare in qualitative and quantitative terms (Table 6.1). Al-Yahya et al. (2011) highlighted the immense problem of methodological variability in the DT literature, and classified the secondary cognitive tasks into five categories, namely, mental tracking, verbal fluency, working memory, reaction time and discrimination and decision making.

However, most previous studies in children have employed only one executive function. The use of general, non-specific tasks and the broad variability in the choice of secondary tasks have contributed to ongoing ambiguity regarding the relative contribution of specific higher-level processes to postural control and locomotion (Walshe, Patterson, Commins, & Roche, 2015). In a study from our own lab we investigated the relative effects of higher-level executive function tasks (n-back, serial subtraction, clock task, Stroop task, Trail-Walking Test, numbers and letters) in comparison to non-executive distracter tasks (simple reaction time task) while walking on a straight pathway or a zig-zag course (Trail-Walking Test; Schott et al., 2016). During normal straight walking we identified only significant differences between the non-executive distracter tasks and the higher-level executive function tasks; however, we failed to identify any significant differences in gait velocity between the higher-level executive function tasks (Figure 6.2). On the other hand, accuracy rates differed between tasks. While participants produced high accuracy rates on the serial subtraction and the Stroop task with no differences between the single-task or DT conditions, children – especially girls – improved their performance on the clock and the Stroop task when walking.

Table 6.1 Overview of the heterogeneity of study protocols and methodological variations of dual-task paradigms used in typically developing children and adolescents

Author (year)	Sample	Motor task	Cognitive task	Performance under dual-task condition	Calculation of DTEs
Whitall (1991)	$n = 32$, 2–10 years $n = 8$, 18–34 years (only girls)	Running and galloping	Recitation of a nursery rhyme and memorization of alphabetical letters	↓ Gait speed	No
Huang et al. (2003)	$n = 27$, 5–7 years	Free walking at preferred pace	Visual identification task, auditory identification task and memorization task	↓ Gait speed, cadence, step length, ↘↗ Cognitive performance	No
Cherng et al. (2007)	$n = 48$, 4–6 years	Free walking at preferred pace	Repeating a series of numbers forwards (easy) or backwards (difficult)	↓ Gait speed, cadence, stride length, ↑ DTC for more complex tasks	Yes
Schaefer al. (2010)	$n = 32$, age ∅ 9.0 ± 0.2 $n = 32$, age ∅ 25.3 ± 2.9	Treadmill walking at preferred speed or 2.5 km/h	n-back (1–4, auditory)	Children: ↑ walking variability with high cognitive load, ↑ cognitive performance	No
Krampe et al. (2011)	$n = 30$, 9 years $n = 30$, 11 years $n = 30$, age ∅ 24.3 ± 2.2 $n = 30$, age ∅ 64.3 ± 2.4	Walk a narrow track	Word Fluency Task	↓ Walking distance, children: ↓ cognitive performance, ↑ DTC	Yes
Boonyong et al. (2012)	$n = 20$, 5–6 years $n = 20$, 7–16 years	Level walking and obstacle crossing	Auditory Stroop task	yTD ↓ gait speed; oTD ↘ gait speed; ↓ cognitive performance DTC yTD > oTD	Yes

Study	Sample	Walking task	Cognitive task	DTE effects	oTD/yTD diff.
Beurskens et al. (2015)	n = 20, 7–9 years	Free walking at preferred pace	Serial subtraction (3s)	↓ Gait speed; ↑ walking variability	No
Schaefer et al. (2015)	n = 18, 7 years n = 18, 9 years n = 18, 20–30 years	Treadmill walking at different speeds	2-back, 3-back (auditory)	Easy cognitive task: ↑ gait regularity, hard cognitive task: ↓ gait regularity → cognitive performance	No
Hagmann-von Arx et al. (2016)	n = 138, 6.7–13.2 years	Free walking at preferred pace	Digits task	↓ Gait speed; ↑ walking variability, → cognitive performance	No
Howell et al. (2016)	n = 24, age ∅ 15.5 ± 1.1 n = 21, age ∅ 21.2 ± 4.5	Free walking at self-selected speed	Auditory Stroop task, spelling a five-letter word backwards, subtracting continually from a given numeral by 6s or 7s, reciting the months in reverse order, starting with a random month	↑ DTC for more complex tasks	Yes

∅, mean; DTE = dual-task effects: negative values for DTE indicate that performance deteriorated under dual-task conditions (i.e. dual-task cost, DTC), and positive values represent an improvement in the dual-task condition relative to single-task performance (i.e. dual-task benefit); yTD: young typically developing; oTD: older typically developing.

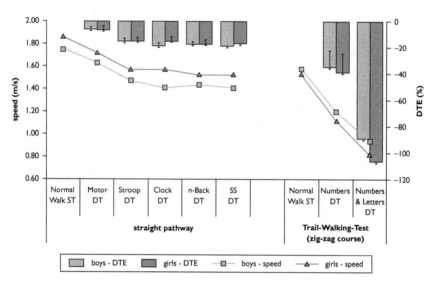

Figure 6.2 Speed (m/s; lines) and dual-task effects (DTE, % + se; bars) for seven
concurrent tasks (information-processing speed (motor task; Trail-
Walking Test numbers), executive working memory (serial subtraction,
SS; auditory 2-back task), visuospatial working memory (clock task; Trail-
Walking Test numbers and letters), inhibition (Stroop) by walking path
(straight vs. zig-zag) (*n* = 72; age range: 10–14 years; unpublished data).
ST, single task; DT, dual task.

Normal walking trials are relatively simple to perform, particularly in
the controlled environment of a laboratory. Recently, we have introduced
a complex walking task (higher demands for visual scanning) in combination with an increasing complexity of the cognitive task. Participants are
instructed to: (1) follow a line of connecting circles (single task); (2) step
on numbered targets in a sequential order (i.e. 1-2-3; DT); and (3) step
on targets with increasing sequential numbers and letters (i.e. 1-A-2-B-3-C;
DT) (Trail-Walking Test; Schott, 2015; Schott et al., 2016). On this more
challenging pathway, we were able to detect significant differences between
cognitive task difficulties (Figure 6.2).

Usually, participants have to complete two different tasks simultaneously for processing. The aim is to explore DT interferences, as evidence
of the capacity limitation of the human information-processing system
(Koch, 2008). In a DT, there is an interfering interaction in the processing
of the single tasks. This can be seen mostly in a decline in processing speed
or in an increase of errors in the respective tasks. Lindenberger, Marsiske,
and Baltes (2000) emphasize that an investigation of the resource conflict
(motor–cognitive interference) requires that pre-existing differences in the

performance of each task are taken into account. One possibility is to calculate relative costs (*DT effects,* DTE). This means, when calculating DTE, performance in each task under DT condition is related to the performance under single-task conditions (Doumas, Smolders, & Krampe, 2008). To obtain more detailed patterns of motor–cognitive interferences, and to calculate DTEs it is therefore important to assess the performance of both, the primary and the secondary task. Unfortunately, CMI is often measured inadequately or simply not calculated (Table 6.1). The DT results from the above-mentioned experiment (Figure 6.2) show that specific executive function tasks have a greater effect on gait regardless of motor difficulty. However, again, the Stroop, clock, n-back and serial subtraction task did not differ from each other as did the DTEs for the Trail-Walking Test numbers and Trail-Walking Test numbers and letters. It is important to note that all DTs effected a change in gait performance relative to single-task walking.

Overall, studies suggest that visually demanding secondary tasks are particularly sensitive for the production of DTEs (Lindenberger et al., 2000). It also can be concluded that walking performance is most affected by internal disturbances, as they occur in simultaneously performed mental tracking tasks (Al-Yahya et al., 2011). For external disturbing factors (e.g. reaction time tasks), this relationship could not be confirmed.

Studies with children with motor and/or cognitive impairments suggest that these children have even more difficulties in handling multiple tasks. For instance, children with cerebral palsy as well as children with attention deficit-hyperactivity disorder or DCD walk slower compared to typically developing children and exhibited higher DT costs (Katz-Leurer, Rotem, & Meyer, 2013; Leitner et al., 2007; Schott et al., 2016). Supported by the fact that the cerebellum is centrally involved in the ability to automate motor skills, Visser (2007) and Tsai, Pan, Cherng, and Wu (2009) have proposed that the *automatization deficit hypothesis* (Fawcett & Nicolson, 1992) is one possible explanation for the deficits related to motor functions, executive functions, visuospatial regulation and visuoperceptual functions in these children. *Automaticity* in the context of fine and gross motor control refers to the ability of the nervous system to control successfully, for example, typical steady-state walking effortlessly even when attention is directed elsewhere (e.g. DT), and without paying attention to the movements being produced (Clark, 2015). Therefore, the calculation of DTEs can then be used as an index of automaticity.

Age and gender effects on gait in single- and dual-task conditions

Regarding age-related differences in DT gait, the effects of concurrent tasks on walking are stronger for younger compared to older typically developing children or adolescents. For example, Boonyong, Siu, van Donkelaar, Chou, and Woollacott (2012) examined the effect of an auditory concurrent task[1] on spatiotemporal gait parameters in young (5–6 years) and older children (7–16 years) and compared both age groups with younger adults from a previous study with the same paradigm (Siu, Chou, Mayr, van Donkelaar, & Woollacott, 2008). Their results suggest a developmental trend in attentional resources used to control gait in typical children. However, young adults still outperform adolescents; this is probably caused by the problem that the parallel processing networks are not as efficient in children as in adults and thus parallel processing is less evident within their brain systems (Boonyong et al., 2012). Hagmann-von Arx et al. (2016) investigated the effect of a memory task on gait parameters in children and adolescents aged 6.7–13.2 years. The authors also found that DT gait decrements decreased with increasing age under the cognitive DT condition. However, the majority of studies on CMI while walking included rather small age ranges; to our knowledge there is no longitudinal study examining the development of CMI.

Although DT paradigms have been used to study gender differences in various human functions such as navigation strategies (Saucier, Bowman, & Elias, 2003) and object location memory (Postma, Izendoorn, & De Haan, 1998), gender differences in children and adolescents in gait under DT walking paradigms have gained minimal attention in past research. That said, neither the studies from Schaefer, Lövdén, Wieckhorst, and Lindenberger (2010), and Boonyong et al. (2012) nor our own studies (Figure 6.2) were able to identify gender-related differences regardless of the motor or cognitive difficulties of the tasks.

Correlates of cognitive–motor interference

While a great deal of research regarding CMI in typically developing children and adolescents has focused on the observation of the phenomenon itself under various testing conditions, to date there is only one study investigating the possible factors related to DT changes. Hagmann-von Arx, Manicolo, Lemola, and Grob (2016) examined the relationship between DT performance and cognitive performance, motor behaviour (i.e. higher sports participation), injury risk and injuries, as well as psychosocial functioning (i.e. physical and psychological well-being, mood and emotions, self-perception and autonomy, parent relation, financial resources, social support, school environment, as well as social acceptance) in children and adolescents (age range: 6.7–13.2 years). The authors found no significant associations between mean change values in gait parameters and other aspects of children's development, indicating that subtle DT effects on gait do not go along with other aspects of development in typically developing children during middle childhood. However, in this study the measures for motor and cognitive performance were short (~10 seconds) and fairly simple (10-metre walking with and without listening to and recalling digits). Other complex measures addressing cognitive processes such as cognitive flexibility while following a zig-zag course might result in larger DTEs, and therefore in stronger relationships to possible explanatory factors for DT decrements.

In search of a more general explanation for the development of the motor–cognitive connection we will introduce an *integrative conceptual framework* for the interaction of cognition, motor performance and life-course factors.

Integrative conceptual framework for the interaction of cognition, motor performance and life-course factors

The integrated conceptual framework of the scaffolding theory of maturation/ biological ageing, cognition, motor performance and motor skill acquisition (SMART COMPASS) can be used to evaluate and predict human performance in children and adolescents (Figure 6.3). The components and features of the proposed model come from three different streams of research. It combines the scaffolding theory of ageing (Reuter-Lorenz & Park, 2014), which examines how different brain variables are related to cognitive function with particular regard to lifestyle factors with the framework for the development of cognition, motor learning and skills from early to late adulthood (Ren et al., 2013). They postulate that significant changes in motor performance and learning can be accounted for by cognitive functions. Furthermore, our proposed framework is influenced by a recent research programme, embodied cognition, which assumes that the body functions as a constituent of the mind rather than a passive perceiver and actor serving the mind (Dijkstra & Post, 2015).

Maturation (as well as biological ageing), neural resource enrichment, as well as neural resource depletion, lead to structural and functional changes in the brain. Unique changes in brain structure and function, such as an increased participation of the dorsal anterior cingulate cortex with age during inhibitory control tasks, the role of the dorsal anterior cingulate cortex as a hub for the interconnectivity of networks (ability to monitor tasks) and a greater strength of short-range connections and weaker long-range connections in children compared to adults, suggest that, with development, there is a shift in predominance of local to distributed circuit engagement. Furthermore, the concurrent development of dopaminergic and γ-aminobutyric acid (GABA)ergic neurotransmission during adolescence may underlie the refinement of network architecture supporting the connectivity of components of control (for an excellent overview, see Luna, Marek, Larsen, Tervo-Clemmens, & Chahal, 2015).

Reuter-Lorenz and Park (2014) address the question how *life-course influences* (physical and social environment) can contribute to neural health or

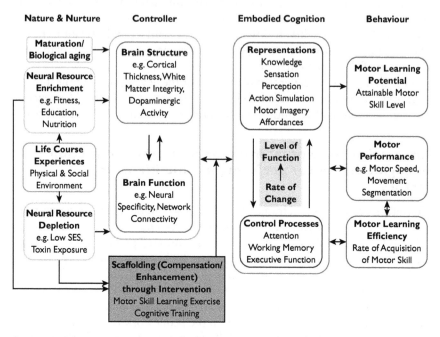

Figure 6.3 An integrated conceptual framework of the scaffolding theory of maturation/ biological ageing, cognition, motor performance and motor skill acquisition (SMART COMPASS). SES, socioeconomic status.

dysfunction. Life-course refers to the age-related sequence of roles, opportunities and constraints an individual experience across the lifespan, e.g. researchers examine how young people select personal experiences, interpersonal relationships and social settings in ways that reflect their past and contribute to their future (Johnson, Crosnoe, & Elder, 2011). The authors categorize these experiences further into neural resource enrichment and neural resource depletion factors. A considerable number of studies not only support the notion that children and adolescents who exhibit a higher fitness level, a healthy body mass index, and participate in intellectual activities perform better on cognitive tasks (Bustamante, Williams, & Davis, 2016; Tandon et al., 2016; Wass, 2015), but for example also show larger volumes of the dorsal striatum, greater activation in the prefrontal and parietal cortex, as well as a greater ability to upregulate neural processes involved in executive control to meet task demands and maintain performance (Hillman & Schott, 2013; Khan & Hillman, 2014).

Likewise, neural resource depletion represents negative influences on brain structure, neural function and cognition. Cognitive and educational performance vary with socioeconomic status, prenatal factors such as maternal smoking and drinking, perinatal factors such as birth weight or neonatal complications and postnatal factors such as exposure to environmental toxins and maternal stress (Christensen, Schieve, Devine, & Drews-Botsch, 2014). Reuter-Lorenz and Park (2014) also propose indirect effects in that life-course factors could increase or decrease the capacity for scaffolding enhancement (or compensation in individuals with diseases or older adults). Scaffolding is a process that characterizes neural dynamics such as when the brain is confronted with novel, unanticipated or increased levels of task demand of a motor skill. Petersen, Van Mier, Fiez, and Raichle (1998) demonstrate that when participants first encounter a novel task, a set of brain regions categorized as scaffolding regions (mainly prefrontal cortex, anterior cingulate cortex and posterior parietal cortex) are used to perform the task. As learning proceeds, performance becomes less effortful and, with enough practice, becomes automatic. Processes or associations are more efficiently stored and accessed and the scaffolding network falls away, displayed by decreased activation in the 'scaffolding' attentional and control areas, and an increase in task-specific areas such as representational cortex — primary and secondary sensory or motor cortex, or in areas related to the storage of those representations, such as parietal or temporal cortex (Kelly & Garavan, 2005).

Motor performance and learning (relatively permanent behavioural changes associated with practice or experience) depend on the level of cognitive function (individual's overall cognitive status) and the rate of possible change (metric of steepness of cognitive improvement in childhood and adolescents) in different cognitive domains (Jongbloed-Pereboom, Janssen, Steenbergen, & Nijhuis-van der Sanden, 2012). Longitudinal studies suggest that the rate of change is driven by both age and performance changes over time. For example, Koolschijn, Schel, De Rooij, Rombouts, and Crone (2011) demonstrated that performance in a task similar to the Wisconsin Card Sorting Task increased rapidly in childhood and early adolescence (8–14 years), after which it stabilized.

In another recent study Boelema et al. (2014) revealed developmental trajectories for the maturation of different executive function tasks during adolescence. While inhibition reached mature levels first, information-processing speed, working memory and shift attention exhibited largest change rates and therefore most maturation between the transitions from childhood to adulthood. However, evidence for the maturational timeline of executive function during childhood and adolescence is inconsistent, with findings of the rate of improvement varying considerably between individuals (Shanmugan & Satterthwaite, 2016).

Furthermore, important for *motor action planning* and *control* is the functional association between action representations, sensation, perception, feed-forward or feedback control strategies, internal models and the ability to represent actions mentally (Wolpert, Ghahramani, & Jordan, 1995). The integration of information about position and velocity of a limb in space based on sensory feedback as well as past experiences will allow individuals to control their movement more accurately and successfully complete the movement to achieve a desired outcome. If a child cannot plan or execute a motor movement effectively, this will decrease the efficiency with which this individual can build links between motor movements and other information such as emotions or cognitive tasks (e.g. maths, reading, problem solving). Specifically, this individual will experience a different way of how the body affects cognition, or that the body plays a meaningful role in it (whether that be through changes in perception and attention, differences in behaviour or the activation of neural motor systems) or, in other words, a difference influence of *embodiment* (Eigsti, 2013). It is well known that children display less coordinated movements than young adults, and children with motor and/or cognitive impairments (e.g. DCD, autism, Down's syndrome) exhibit, for example, more temporal and spatial variability, fewer anticipatory adjustments and differences in the ability to generate and detect information about affordances and invariant structures (Adams, Lust, Wilson, & Steenbergen, 2014; Elliott et al., 2010; Hellendoorn, Wijnroks, & Leseman, 2015). Because the body and brain are subject to physical, physiological and cognitive changes across childhood and adolescence it can be expected that the representation of the own body and therefore action representations and its affordances also change with age.

Motor imagery (MI) is a widely used experimental paradigm for the study of cognitive aspects of action planning and control and embodied cognition (Gabbard, 2012). It is described as an active cognitive process during which the representation of a specific action is internally reproduced in working memory without any overt motor output from a first-person perspective (Decety & Grèzes, 1999). Several studies suggest that MI processes are likely present in early childhood, evidenced by the speed–accuracy trade-off in imagined movements (e.g. hand laterality judgement paradigm) of young children aged approximately 7 years, although this relationship is more evident in older children (Funk, Brugger, & Wilkening, 2005). Imagined movement durations become closer to actual execution durations as a child ages (Caeyenberghs, Wilson, van Roon, Swinnen, & Smits-Engelsman, 2009; Smits-Engelsman & Wilson, 2013) and MI accuracy is gradually refined during development, with 11-year-olds significantly more accurate than 7- and 8-year-olds (Toussaint, Tahej, Thibaut, Possamai, & Badets, 2013), suggesting that there is ongoing refinement of action simulation processes in childhood.

While many have studied the effect of aerobic exercise on cognitive function, less is known about the causal relationships between motor and cognitive control processes and motor learning (Magallón, Narbona, & Crespo-Eguílaz, 2016), and how children and adolescents develop the ability to acquire an automatized motor skill with little or no interference by a demanding secondary task. The capability to achieve certain levels of performance with extended practice (motor learning potential) seems not to change much across the lifespan (Ren et al., 2013). However, most developmental studies of skill learning have not identified associations between working-memory performance assessed with digit-span tasks and measures of learning (Lejeune, Catale, Schmitz, Quertemont, & Meulemans, 2013; Savion-Lemieux et al., 2009); however, Julius and Adi-Japha (2015) demonstrated that kindergarteners' changes in performance were associated with a graphomotor task of sequential short-term memory.

Another recent study demonstrated that preadolescent children automatize the execution of longer movement sequences to a lesser extent than young adults, but exhibit similar performance gains with practice (Ruitenberg, Abrahamse, & Verwey, 2013). The authors explain their results with the dominance of a so-called cognitive processor in the execution of movement sequences; adults learn to use motor chunks which are dominated by an autonomous motor processor, while children still rely on the cognitive processor. Studies also show that children and adolescents with dysfunctions in the basal ganglia and cerebellum – as key players in motor adaptation and sequence learning – as is in DCD or autism, display learning difficulties for complex motor tasks, difficulties employing additional cognitive functions, such as explicit learning processes, and identifying related cues in the environment (Bo, Lee, Colbert, & Shen, 2016; Cantin, Ryan, & Polatajko, 2014).

The embodiment research is not only concerned with the involvement of sensorimotor processes in learning how to walk or avoid obstacles, eye–hand–object coordination, but how visuomotor processes are related to higher-level cognition such as word learning, how gestures and body movements influence thought and mathematics (see also Chandler & Tricot, 2015). Embodied theories suggest that cognitive representations of symbols such as numbers and letters are based on sensorimotor codes within a generalized system that was originally developed to control an organism's motor behaviour and perceive the world around it (Barsalou, 1999; Paas & Sweller, 2012). The idea that the mind and body are two interrelated entities has prompted research to determine how bodily movements can be incorporated in education to improve the effectiveness of learning environments (Moreau, 2015). For instance, Ruiter, Loyens, and Paas (2015) examined the effects of task-related body movements by employing a combination of big, medium and small steps on 118 first-graders' (around 6 years of age) learning of two-digit numbers (e.g. the number 36 was construed by saying out loud 10, 20, 30, 35, 36, while making three big steps, one medium and one small step on a ruler across the floor). Results revealed that using body movements can be highly beneficial for basic mathematical achievement compared to simply studying instruction.

Conclusion

As can be seen from this review of the state of the art in this paper, as well as the discussion of the open questions, the development of the motor–cognitive association in children and adolescents is a maturing field where we introduced a framework to explain underlying mechanisms, yet there remain many opportunities for further research and applications in specific interventions. The validation of this framework is necessary, but it offers insights into the association between maturation, life-course factors, brain development, cognition and motor performance. To date most studies have been based on cross-sectional comparisons of individuals at different ages as well as on some, but not all, components. However, relatively little work has addressed the motor–cognitive association and its influencing factors within individuals longitudinally. Some applications, such as in the educational field, have been discussed, but few have been explored in depth.

Can we answer the question of whether the motor–cognitive connection can be used as an indicator of future developmental success in children and adolescents? Not yet. Movement performance and motor learning can have wide-reaching benefits in cognitive development and learning. However, the associations between motor and cognitive performance are complex, the mechanisms are still unclear and vary between approaches, so bridging this gap in knowledge is a central challenge for future research.

Note

1 Auditory Stroop task: subjects are required to judge the pitch of the words 'high' and 'low' as quickly and accurately as possible by saying 'high' or 'low' while ignoring the actual word presented.

References

Adams, I., Lust, J., Wilson, P., & Steenbergen, B. (2014). Compromised motor control in children with DCD: A deficit in the internal model? A systematic review. *Neuroscience and Biobehavioral Reviews, 47,* 225–244.

Al-Yahya, E., Dawes, H., Smith, L., Dennis, A., Howells, K., & Cockburn, J. (2011). Cognitive motor interference while walking: A systematic review and meta-analysis. *Neuroscience and Biobehavioral Reviews, 35*(3), 715–728.

Barsalou, L. W. (1999). Perceptual symbol systems. *The Behavioral and Brain Sciences, 22*(4), 577–609.

Beurskens, R., Muehlbauer, T., & Granacher, U. (2015). Association of dual-task walking performance and leg muscle quality in healthy children. *BMC Pediatrics, 15*(2). doi: 10.1186/s12887-015-0317-8.

Bo, J., Lee, C. M., Colbert, A., & Shen, B. (2016). Do children with autism spectrum disorders have motor learning difficulties? *Research in Autism Spectrum Disorders, 23,* 50–62.

Boelema S. R., Harakeh Z., Ormel J., Hartman C. A., Vollebergh W. A. M., & van Zandvoort, M. J. E. (2014). Executive functioning shows differential maturation from early to late adolescence: Longitudinal findings from a TRAILS study. *Neuropsychology, 28*, 177–187.

Boonyong, S., Siu, K.-C., van Donkelaar, P., Chou, L.-S., & Woollacott, M. H. (2012). Development of postural control during gait in typically developing children: The effects of dual-task conditions. *Gait and Posture, 35*(3), 428–434.

Bustamente, E. E., Williams, C. F., & Davis, C. L. (2016). Physical activity interventions for neurocognitive and academic performance in overweight and obese youth: A systematic review. *Pediatric Clinics of North America, 63*(3), 459–480.

Caeyenberghs, K., Wilson, P. H., van Roon, D., Swinnen, S. P., & Smits-Engelsman, B. C. M. (2009). Increasing convergence between imagined and executed movement across development: Evidence for the emergence of movement representations. *Developmental Sciences, 12*(3), 474–483.

Cantin, N., Ryan, J., & Polatajko, H. J. (2014). Impact of task difficulty and motor ability on visual-motor task performance of children with and without developmental coordination disorder. *Human Movement Science, 34*, 217–232.

Chandler, P., & Tricot, A. (Eds.) (2015). Mind your body: The essential role of body movements in children's learning (special edition). *Educational Psychology Review, 27*(3), 365–558.

Cherng, R.-J., Liang, L.-Y., Hwang, S., & Chen, J.-Y. (2007). The effect of a concurrent task on the walking performance of preschool children. *Gait and Posture, 26*(2), 231–237.

Christensen, D. L., Schieve, L. A., Devine, O., & Drews-Botsch, C. (2014). Socioeconomic status, child enrichment factors, and cognitive performance among preschool-age children: Results from the Follow-Up of Growth and Development Experiences study. *Research in Developmental Disabilities, 35*, 1789–1801.

Clark, D. J. (2015). Automaticity of walking: Functional significance, mechanisms, measurement and rehabilitation strategies. *Frontiers in Human Neuroscience, 9*, 246. doi: 10.3389/fnhum.2015.00246.

Decety, J., & Grèzes, J. (1999). Neural mechanisms subserving the perception of human actions. *Trends Cognitive Sciences, 3*(5), 172–178.

Dijkstra, K., & Post, L. (2015). Mechanisms of embodiment. *Frontiers in Psychology, 6*, 1525. doi: http://doi.org/10.3389/fpsyg.2015.01525.

Doumas, M., Smolders, C., & Krampe, R. T. (2008). Task prioritization in aging: Effects of sensory information on concurrent posture and memory performance. *Experimental Brain Research, 187*(2), 275–281.

Doyon, J., Bellec, P., Amsel, R., Penhune, V., Monchi, O., Carrier, J., . . . Benali, H. (2009). Contributions of the basal ganglia and functionally related brain structures to motor learning. *Behavioral Brain Research, 199*, 61–75.

Eigsti, I. M. (2013). A review of embodiment in autism spectrum disorders. *Frontiers in Psychology, 4*, 224. doi: 10.3389/fpsyg.2013.00224.

Elliott, D., Hansen, S., Grierson, L. E., Lyons, J., Bennett, S. J., & Hayes, S. J. (2010). Goal-directed aiming: Two components but multiple processes. *Psychological Bulletin, 136*, 1023–1044.

Favazza, P. C., & Siperstein, G. N. (2016). Motor skill acquisition for young children with disabilities. In B. Reichow, B. A. Boyd, E. E. Barton, & S. L. Odom

(Eds.), *Handbook of early childhood special education* (pp. 225–245). Basel, Switzerland: Springer.

Fawcett, A. J., & Nicolson, R. I. (1992). Automatisation deficits in balance for dyslexic children. *Perceptual and Motor Skills, 75*(2), 507–529.

Funk, M., Brugger, P., & Wilkening, F. (2005). Motor processes in children's imagery: The case of mental rotation of hands. *Developmental Sciences, 8*(5), 402–408.

Gabbard, C. (2012). The role of mental simulation in embodied cognition. *Early Child Development and Care, 183*(5), 643–650.

Hagmann-von Arx, P., Manicolo, O., Lemola, S., & Grob, A. (2016). Walking in school-aged children in a dual-task paradigm is related to age but not to cognition, motor behavior, injuries, or psychosocial functioning. *Frontiers in Psychology, 7,* 352. doi: http://doi.org/10.3389/fpsyg.2016.00352.

Hellendoorn, A., Wijnroks, L., & Leseman, P. P. M. (2015). Unraveling the nature of autism: Finding order amid change. *Frontiers in Psychology, 6,* 359. doi: 10.3389/Fpsyg.2015.00359.

Hillman, C. H., & Schott, N. (2013). Der Zusammenhang von Fitness, kognitiver Leistungsfähigkeit und Gehirnzustand im Schulkindalter: Konsequenzen für die schulische Leistungsfähigkeit. *Zeitschrift für Sportpsychologie, 20*(1), 33–41.

Howell, D. R., Osternig, L. R., & Chou, L.-S. (2016). Consistency and cost of dual-task gait balance measure in healthy adolescents and young adults. *Gait and Posture, 49,* 176–180.

Huang, H.-J., Mercer, V. S., & Thorpe, D. E. (2003). Effects of different concurrent cognitive tasks on temporal-distance gait variables in children. *Pediatric Physical Therapy, 15*(2), 105–113.

Johnson, M. K., Crosnoe, R., & Elder, G. H. (2011). Insights on adolescence from a life course perspective. *Journal of Research on Adolescence: The Official Journal of the Society for Research on Adolescence, 21*(1), 273–280.

Jongbloed-Pereboom, M., Janssen, A. J., Steenbergen, B., & Nijhuis-van der Sanden, M. W. (2012). Motor learning and working memory in children born preterm: A systematic review. *Neuroscience and Biobehavioral Reviews, 36,* 1314–1330.

Julius M. S., & Adi-Japha E. (2015). Learning of a simple grapho-motor task by young children and adults: Similar acquisition but age-dependent retention. *Frontiers in Psychology, 6,* 225. doi: 10.3389/fpsyg.2015.00225.

Katz-Leurer, M., Rotem, H., & Meyer S. (2013). Effect of concurrent cognitive tasks on temporo-spatial parameters of gait among children with cerebral palsy and typically developed controls. *Developmental Neurorehabilitation, 17*(6), 363–367.

Kelly, A. M. C., & Garavan, H. (2005). Human functional neuroimaging of brain changes associated with practice. *Cerebral Cortex, 15,* 1089–1102.

Khan, N. A., & Hillman, C. H. (2014). The relation of childhood physical activity and aerobic fitness to brain function and cognition: A review. *Pediatric Exercise Science, 26,* 138–146.

Koch, I. (2008). Mechanismen der Interferenz in Doppelaufgaben. *Psychologische Rundschau, 59*(1), 24–32.

Koolschijn, P. C., Schel, M. A., De Rooij, M., Rombouts, S. A. R. B., & Crone, E. A. (2011). A 3-year longitudinal fMRI study on performance-monitoring and test-retest reliability from childhood to early adulthood. *Journal of Neuroscience, 31,* 4204–4212.

Krempe, R. T., Schaefer, S., Lindenberger, U., & Baltes, P. B. (2011). Lifespan changes in multi-tasking: Concurrent walking and memory search in children, young, and older adults. *Gait and Posture, 33*(3), 401–405.

Leitner, Y., Barak, R., Giladi, N., Peretz, C., Eshel, R., Gruendlinger, L., & Hausdorff, J. M. (2007). Gait in attention deficit hyperactivity disorder. *Journal of Neurology, 254,* 1330–1338.

Lejeune, C., Catale, C., Schmitz, X., Quertemont, E., & Meulemans, T. (2013). Age-related differences in perceptuomotor procedural learning in children. *Journal of Experimental Child Psychology, 116,* 157–168.

Lindenberger, U., Marsiske, M., & Baltes, P. B. (2000). Memorizing while walking: Increase in dual-task costs from young adulthood to old age. *Psychology and Aging, 15*(3), 417.

Luna, B., Marek, S., Larsen, B., Tervo-Clemmens, B., & Chahal, R. (2015). An integrative model of the maturation of cognitive control. *Annual Review of Neuroscience, 38,* 151–170.

Magallón, S., Narbona, J., & Crespo-Eguílaz, N. (2016). Acquisition of motor and cognitive skills through repetition in typically developing children. *PLoS One, 11*(7), e0158684. doi: http://doi.org/10.1371/journal.pone.0158684.

Magill, R. A., & Anderson, D. (2014). *Motor learning and control* (10th ed.). New York: McGraw-Hill.

Moreau, D. (2015). Brains and brawn: Complex motor activities to maximize cognitive enhancement. *Educational Psychology Review, 27*(3), 475–482.

Muir, S. W., Gopaul, K., & Montero Odasso, M. M. (2012). The role of cognitive impairment in fall risk among older adults: A systematic review and meta-analysis. *Age and Ageing, 41*(3), 299–308.

Paas, F., & Sweller, J. (2012). An evolutionary upgrade of cognitive load theory: Using the human motor system and collaboration to support the learning of complex cognitive tasks. *Educational Psychology Review, 24*(1), 27–45.

Petersen, S. E., Van Mier, H., Fiez, J. A., & Raichle, M. E. (1998). The effects of practice on the functional anatomy of task performance. *Proceedings of the National Academy of Sciences, 95,* 853–860.

Postma, A., Izendoorn, R., & De Haan, E. H. (1998). Sex differences in object location memory. *Brain and Cognition, 36,* 334–345.

Prado, E. L., & Dewey, K. G. (2014). Nutrition and brain development in early life. *Nutrition Reviews, 72*(4), 267–284.

Ren, J., Wu, Y. D., Chan, J. S. Y., & Yan, J. H. (2013). Cognitive aging affects motor performance and learning. *Geriatrics and Gerontolology International, 13,* 19–27.

Reuter-Lorenz, P. A., & Park, D. C. (2014). How does it STAC up? Revisiting the Scaffolding Theory of Aging and Cognition. *Neuropsychology Review, 24*(3), 355–370.

Roebers, C. M., Roethlisberger, M., Neuenschwander, R., Cimeli, P., Michel, E., & Jaeger, K. (2014). The relationship between cognitive and motor performance and their relevance for children's transition to school: A latent variable approach. *Human Movement Science, 33,* 284–287.

Ruitenberg, M. F. L., Abrahamse, E. L., & Verwey, W. B. (2013) Sequential motor skill in preadolescent children: The development of automaticity. *Journal of Experimental Child Psychology, 115*(4), 607–623.

Ruiter, M., Loyens, S., & Paas, F. (2015). Watch your step children! Learning two-digit numbers through mirror-based observation of self-initiated body movements. *Educational Psychology Review, 27*(3), 457–474.

Saucier, D., Bowman, M., & Elias, L. (2003). Sex differences in the effect of articulatory or spatial dual-task interference during navigation. *Brain and Cognition, 53*, 346–350.

Savion-Lemieux, T., Bailey, J. A., & Penhune, V. (2009). Developmental contributions to motor sequence learning. *Experimental Brain Research, 195*, 293–306.

Schaefer, S., Jagenow, D., Verrel, J., & Lindenberger, U. (2015). The influence of cognitive load and walking speed on gait regularity in children and young adults. *Gait and Posture, 41*, 258–262.

Schaefer, S., Lövdén, M., Wieckhorst, B., & Lindenberger U. (2010). Cognitive performance is improved while walking: Differences in cognitive–sensorimotor couplings between children and young adults. *European Journal of Developmental Psychology, 7*, 371–389.

Schott, N. (2015). Trail Walking Test zur Erfassung der motorisch-kognitiven Interferenz bei älteren Erwachsenen: Entwicklung und Überprüfung der psychometrischen Eigenschaften des Verfahrens [Trail walking test for assessment of motor cognitive interference in older adults: Development and evaluation of the psychometric properties of the procedure]. *Zeitschrift fuer Gerontologie und Geriatrie, 48*(8), 722–733.

Schott, N., El-Rajab, I., & Klotzbier, T. (2016). Cognitive-motor interference during fine and gross motor tasks in children with developmental coordination disorder (DCD). *Research in Developmental Disabilities, 57*, 136–148.

Schott, N., & Holfelder, B. (2015). Relationship between motor skill competency and executive function in children with Down's syndrome. *Journal of Intellectual Disability Research, 9*(59), 860–872.

Shanmugan, S., & Satterthwaite, T. D. (2016). Neural markers of the development of executive function: Relevance for education. *Current Opinion in Behavioral Sciences, 10*, 7–13.

Siu, K.-C., Chou, L.-S., Mayr, U., van Donkelaar, P., & Woollacott, M. H. (2008). Does inability to allocate attention contribute to balance constraints during gait in older adults? *The Journals of Gerontology Series A: Biological Sciences and Medical Sciences, 63*(12), 1364–1369.

Tandon, P. S., Tovar, A., Jayasuriya, A. T., Welker, E., Schober, D. J., Copeland, K., . . . Ward, D. S. (2016). The relationship between physical activity and diet and young children's cognitive development: A systematic review. *Preventive Medicine Reports, 3*, 379–390.

Toussaint, L., Tahej, P.-K., Thibaut, J.-P., Possamai, C.-A., & Badets, A. (2013). On the link between action planning and motor imagery: A developmental study. *Experimental Brain Research, 231*(3), 331–339.

Tsai, C. L., Pan, C. Y., Cherng, R. J., & Wu, S. K. (2009). Dual-task study of cognitive and postural interference: A preliminary investigation of the automatization deficit hypothesis of developmental co-ordination disorder. *Child: Care, Health and Development, 35*, 551–560.

Visser, J. (2007). Subtypes and co-morbidities. In R. H. Geuze (Ed.), *Developmental coordination disorder: A review of current approaches* (pp. 83–110). Marseille, France: Solal.

Walshe, E. A., Patterson, M. R., Commins, S., & Roche, R. (2015). Dual-task and electrophysiological markers of executive cognitive processing in older adult gait and fall-risk. *Frontiers in Human Neuroscience, 9*, 200. doi: 10.3389/fnhum.2015.00200.

Wass, S. V. (2015). Applying cognitive training to target executive functions during early development. *Child Neuropsychology, 21*(2), 150–166.

Whitall, J. (1991). The developmental effect of concurrent cognitive and locomotor skills: Time-sharing from a dynamical perspective. *Journal of Experimental and Child Psychology, 51*(2), 245–266.

Wilson, M. (2002). Six views of embodied cognition. *Psychonomic Bulletin and Review, 9.4*, 625–636.

Wolpert, D. M., Ghahramani, Z., & Jordan, M. I. (1995). An internal model for sensorimotor integration. *Science (New York, N.Y.), 269*(5232), 1880–1882.

Chapter 7

Psychological responses to stress and exercise on students' lives

Eduardo Matta Mello Portugal

Introduction

Students have several challenges during their academic life. Academic demands, self-expectations and external factors such as family pressure are kinds of stress. The stress generates physiological adaptations and affective changes that can compromise the student's mental health. For example, there is evidence linking the relationship between academic performance and symptoms of depression and anxiety. In this context, exercise seems to be a great strategy to improve mental health and academic performance. Improvements in resilience, coping strategies, mood and affective response are positive responses to stress that are generated by molecular and structural neuronal changes. The aim of this chapter is to discuss the effects generated by academic stress on psychological variables such as affective response, mood, resilience, motivation and how exercise can contribute to a better academic life by a positive modulation of these variables. The role of exercise on the student's life is very important for people who work in education.

Stress at school age

Schools are an optimal place for children and adolescents to improve their knowledge. However, many negative aspects can occur at school age (Figure 7.1). Following the Johns Hopkins Bloomberg School of Public Health guide to healthy adolescent development, adolescents have different stressors (causes of stress) such as pressure for career decisions, for clothes and style choices, and for experimenting with drugs, alcohol and sex, dating and friendship relationships (McNeely & Blanchard, 2010). In addition, they can have problems with their body image, physical and cognitive changes of puberty, conflicts with parents, violence and others things related to social life (McNeely & Blanchard, 2010). Although sports in school can be an optimal tool for improving several health aspects, academic achievement and social life, amongst others that will be discussed

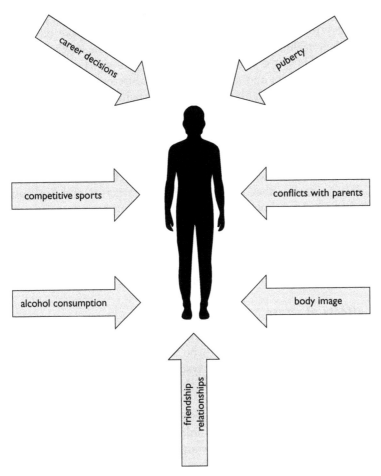

Figure 7.1 Stressors in children and adolescents. Children and adolescents suffer from the effects of many different stressors.

in this chapter, there is a small scientific background in youth sport guidelines, rules and regulations (Merkel, 2013). Some competitive teams can stimulate intense psychological pressure to achieve positive results and then very stressful training has to be done, aiming for optimal performance during competition. These and other factors can explain the increased rate of sports injuries (Adirim & Cheng, 2003).

It is clear that children and adolescents can suffer from high loads of psychological or physiological (i.e. competitive sports) stress. To detect an injury generated by inappropriate stressful exercises and sports set-up can be easy (Zoref-Shani, Kessler-Icekson, Wasserman, & Sperling, 1984).

Nevertheless, according to the American Psychological Association, the effects of high amounts of psychological stress on children and adolescents are not easy to detect, because the young people can have difficulties discussing their feelings and emotional state (American Psychological Association, 2009). Thus, it is important to look out for signs of the effects of stress. Although children and adolescents have different ways of manifesting the effects of stress, both may show different behaviour in their social life and physical effects such as stomach aches and headaches (American Psychological Association, 2009).

Psychologists can have an important role in stress management in children and adolescents who suffer from severe stress effects. Professionals with a sports and exercise science background can work in stress management, prescribing exercises that will improve body structure and function (i.e. physiological and psychological). Before discussing how exercise can improve students' life by alleviating stress, the biological mechanism caused by stress will be discussed.

Physiological and psychological stress effects

Biological effects of stress

Following Everly and Lating (2013), there are two kinds of stress. The first is biogenic stress that does not need to be interpreted by high cognitive processes to induce autonomic nervous system (ANS) and hypothalamic–pituitary–adrenal (HPA) axis activation (Vander, Sherman, & Luciano, 2001). For example, young athletes can suffer with this kind of stress, because they need to train hard in the hope of an optimal performance. In the meantime, however, several physiological adjustments have to be done. Consequently, muscles, leukocytes and other cells release molecules that reach the brain and so active a stress response (Maier, Watkins, & Fleshner, 1994). Decreased mood and affective response can be an acute manifestation of stress on brain. The second kind of stress is caused by psychosocial stressors that have to be processed by brain areas such as prefrontal cortex, amygdala and hippocampus that send inputs to activate the ANS and HPA axis.

Independently of the kind of stressors, whether biogenic (puberty, injuries and physiological effects of competitive sports) or psychosocial (pressure for career decisions, challenges in social life) (Everly & Lating, 2013), the organism will generate similar mechanisms to adapt to the stress. The study on the HPA axis helps to understand the stress effects on the organism (Figure 7.2). The hypothalamus is located above the thalamus and both structures are part of the diencephalon. Several functions are attributed to the different cell groups and pathways that are inside the hypothalamus, such as mood, appetite, thirst, temperature, sleep and sex (Vander et al., 2001). These responses

Stress mechanisms

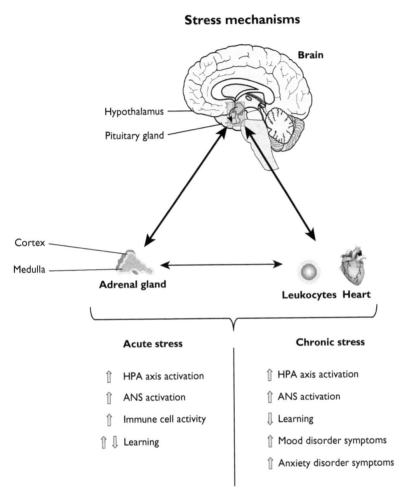

Figure 7.2 Biological mechanism of stress. HPA, hypothalamic–pituitary–adrenal; ANS, autonomic nervous system.

occur because the hypothalamus works as a master command centre, getting neural, endocrine and immune input and controlling different body systems (Vander et al., 2001).

The small pituitary gland is situated above the hypothalamus and releases hormones to activate or inhibit the release of other hormones. The paraventricular nucleus in hypothalamus parvocellular neurons releases corticotrophin-releasing hormone that stimulates the release of adrenocorticotrophic hormone (ACTH) by the pituitary gland (Goncharova, 2013). This hormone is released into the blood and reaches the adrenal glands, adrenal medulla and adrenal cortex, situated near the kidney (Goncharova, 2013). The adrenal medulla produces adrenaline (epinephrine) and noradrenaline (norepinephrine) which play a pivotal role in preparing the body for a stress situation. These hormones signal increased metabolism (i.e. glycogenolysis and beta oxidation), cardiovascular activity, increasing heart rate and blood pressure and immune cell activity. On the other hand, the adrenal cortex releases glucocorticoid, mainly cortisol in humans, that has anabolic functions (i.e. gluconeogenesis) (Khani & Tayek, 2001), and mostly catabolic functions (i.e. beta oxidation) (Brillon, Zheng, Campbell, & Matthews, 1995). Furthermore, cortisol seems to inhibit proinflammatory immune cell activation and HPA axis activation.

Although the HPA axis is an essential circuit for keeping the body in a homeostatic state, persistent activation of this axis generates negative effects. Chronic stress can modulate HPA activity at rest and during stress and compromise coping mechanisms (Faravelli, Lo Sauro, Lelli, et al., 2012). For example, at rest and during stress a high concentration of cortisol can occur in individuals who suffer from chronic stress. A possible reason for this response is that some brain areas, such as the hippocampus and prefrontal cortex, may have decreased glucocorticoid receptor expression, so cortisol increases as a compensatory mechanism (Herman et al., 2016). In addition, Herman et al. (2016), revising several consequences of chronic stress, showed that the adrenal gland could grow up and become more responsive to ACTH.

Stress effects on learning

Studying memory, learning and stress response relationships, Vogel and Schwabe (2016) considered that biological response during stress can operate in two different pathways. The first is the fast release of adrenaline and noradrenaline activation that can positively affect memory and learning by activating cells from the hippocampus, amygdala and prefrontal cortex (Vogel & Schwabe, 2016). This response can be a positive stimulus for memory only when it occurs close to presentation of a new information. When a stress occurs long before new information, learning may be compromised. This may be related to the cortisol response, since cortisol levels can be even higher during testing. Chronic stress causes a learning impairment (Schwabe, Dalm, Schachinger, & Oitzl, 2008).

Diseases related to stress

Repetitive exposure to a stressor will stimulate the above-mentioned stress mechanisms. Unfortunately, eventually the organism may not support the stress load and becomes sick. Although parents have a great responsibility to mediate stress in the child and adolescent (Grant et al., 2006), the challenge of the school environment may contribute to add stress. Mood and anxiety disorders are not diseases exclusive to older people; children and adolescents can also suffer from these diseases. The prevalence of depression in these populations varies from 0.9% to 3.4% depending on the study design and population analysed (Merikangas, Nakamura, & Kessler, 2009). In adulthood, some anxiety disorders are associated to early stressful events that increase the risk for other psychopathologies, including mood disorders (Faravelli, Lo Sauro, Godini, et al., 2012). The prevalence of anxiety disorders varies between 2.2% and 9.9% approximately in children and adolescents: the most prevalent forms are generalized anxiety disorder and social anxiety disorder (Merikangas et al., 2009).

The interactions between stressors and genetic predisposition are key components for risk of mood disorders (Grant et al., 2006). Some hypotheses have been created in an attempt to explain the pathophysiology of depression. One of these is the monoaminergic theory that consists of an imbalance in monoaminergic transmission (i.e. serotonin, adrenaline, noradrenaline and serotonin neurotransmitters). Another theory posits hyperactivity of the HPA axis that generates an extensive release of cortisol that works to change behaviour (Nestler et al., 2002). In this context, the most common drug therapies act by increasing levels of monoamines at the synaptic cleft (the space between neurons). The pathophysiology of anxiety disorders may be similar to mood disorders in some respects. Older individuals with generalized anxiety disorder can exhibit activitation of the HPA axis and, consequently, greater cortisol concentration than healthy individuals (Lenze et al., 2011). Furthermore, it seems that early stress can cause deleterious effects on the HPA axis and this has a role in the pathophysiology of anxiety disorder (Faravelli, Lo Sauro, Godini, et al., 2012).

Stress stimulates bidirectional communication between the ANS and HPA axis with the immune system and other cells both acutely and chronically. This activation can generate positive or negative effects on learning and on disease symptoms.

Exercise as a strategy for stress management

Exercise-induced stress: is it positive or negative?

As mentioned above, chronic stress can generate negative effects on the body. Some of these negative effects are related to hyperactivation of the HPA axis. Most evidence on exercise-induced HPA activity is based on experimental trials in animals, mainly rodents. The HPA axis of both rodents and humans works very similarly, so it is reasonable to infer that in this context animal evidence can help us to understand humans.

Exercise can change HPA function in different ways, for example, by reducing ACTH during the morning, increasing corticosterone levels during dark phase, and other responses (Droste et al., 2003). HPA axis response can also be changed when trained animals are faced with different kinds of stress (Droste et al., 2003). In summary, it is difficult to understand the complex adjustment of the HPA by chronic effects of exercise. In this context, it is very interesting to note that exercise activates the HPA axis in a similar way to other stressors. However, some stressors (i.e. social stress) have a negative impact on our body, while exercise can have a positive impact. The differentiation between these positive and negative effects is not clear. Stranahan, Lee, and Mattson (2008) discussed that exercise generates positive effects because it is predictable, controllable and a rewarding stimulus. The reward system is composed of many brain areas (for review, see Arias-Carrion et al., 2014) that when stimulated work to reinforce stimuli for a repetitive behaviour. Thus, exercise-activated reward system can be the key to stress management, because exercise will be tolerated and will generate positive effects in the organism.

Some evidence shows that repeated exercise possibly does not activate a reward response. First of all, the low rates of exercise adherence and the negative affective response caused by high-intensity exercises show that exercise can be a potent negative stressor (Ekkekakis, Hall, & Petruzzello, 2008; Portugal, Lattari, Santos, & Deslandes, 2015). In this context, competitive sports can work negatively as a biogenic stressor and cause injuries (Adirim & Cheng, 2003) and negative psychological impact such as over-training (Carfagno & Hendrix, 2014). On the other hand, some strategies were designed for exercise-induced pleasure.

Following the hedonic theory, pleasurable stimuli should be repeated while negative stimuli should be avoided. Exercises designed to activate the reward system and, consequently, induce a positive affective response can be an optimal tool for enhancing the number of people who are physically active. Currently, children and adolescents have many distractions such as video games and the internet, so finding pleasurable exercises for them is the first step in exercise promotion. Furthermore, exercise inducing pleasure can be a good strategy for stress management. Exercise can be a positive kind of stress, maybe because it can be perceived as a pleasurable stressor.

In this context, Annesi (2005) investigated the effects on mood of 12 weeks of an after-school exercise programme in 9–12-year-old preadolescents. A reduction in depression score and negative mood (total mood disturbance) was shown in the exercise group. Thus, possibly exercise can be a good strategy to manage stress by reducing negative mood.

Some studies investigated the acute effects of 15 minutes of exercise. Williamson, Dewey, and Steinberg (2001) compared the mood response of children aged 9 or 10 years old in two 'fun' exercise sessions (i.e. run round the school gymnasium and play with volley balls and space hoppers) compared to an educational film session without exercise. They showed that both exercise sessions improved positive mood and decreased negative mood, whereas the film session generated the opposite result.

Simple strategies designed to induce positive psychological effects in exercise were evaluated. Duncan et al. (2014) assessed age 14-year-olds in two cycling exercises in a moderate-intensity set in 50% heart rate reserve (HR_{Res}) for 15 minutes. In one exercise session the children cycled watching a film of cycling in a forest environment and in the other session they cycled viewing a black screen. With a very similar design, Wood, Angus, Pretty, Sandercock, and Barton (2013) did not find any difference between the exercise session with a film of the natural environment compared to another exercise session viewing the built environment. However, both exercise sessions induced a positive effect on mood. These 15-minute exercise sessions showed that watching a film during exercise does not impact the affective response significantly. Maybe the real-life situation of an exercise practice in a field or in the green environment could induce positive effects on affective response. Although the experiments failed to show differences between sessions, it was shown that 15 minutes of moderate exercise could be a good stimulus to improve mood.

Is the exercise a protective strategy against chronic stress?

Repetitive bouts of exercise also induce structural, physiological and psychological effects on mental health that help the body to manage the stress (Figure 7.3). Possibly exercise-induced resilience is one of the most valuable

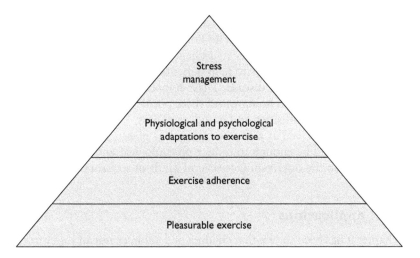

Figure 7.3 Exercise is a stressor, but it can be a strategy to manage the effects of other stressors.

effects in stress management (Deuster & Silverman, 2013). Following Deuster and Silverman (2013), resilience is defined as 'the ability to withstand, recover, and grow in the face of stressors and changing demands'. Childs and de Wit (2014) compared physically active individuals with sedentary individuals in an acute psychosocial stress test. After the stress test, sedentary individuals showed a decrease in positive affect, but physically active individuals did not. Following the authors, these modest results suggest that exercise can be related to resilience.

There are numerous papers on the long-term effects of exercise on the cardiovascular, immune, endocrine and nervous system on generating a low risk for several diseases in physically active individuals (Gordon-Larsen et al., 2009; Huai et al., 2013). Further, people who have diseases such as hypertension, diabetes and other diseases can significantly reduce their effects when they became physically active (Healy et al., 2008; Semlitsch et al., 2013).

More recent are scientific discoveries of the effects of exercise on mental health. As discussed, it is known that exercise can reduce the symptoms of some mental diseases (Matta Mello Portugal et al., 2013). In a meta-analysis of Silveira et al. (2013), positive effects of exercise on symptoms of depression were found in patients with major depression. Furthermore, another meta-analysis showed that people who suffer from anxiety disorder can benefit significantly from long-term exercise (Wegner et al., 2014).

The effects of exercise on mental health may operate by different routes. Growth factors such as brain-derived neurotrophic factors, vascular endothelial grow factor and insulin like growth factor are proteins that can stimulate cell survivor and plasticity (Dishman et al., 2006; Matta Mello Portugal et al., 2013). Regular exercise is a potent stimulus for the production and release of growth factors, as shown by different authors (Deslandes et al., 2009; Dishman et al., 2006; Matta Mello Portugal et al., 2013). It is possible to infer that these factors can induce neurogenesis (growth of new neurons), which may be a positive stimulus to help patients to build new memory circuits and reduce the effects of disease. These hypotheses seem to be reasonable, but need to be tested in humans. All these positive effects may improve other functions, such as affective and mood responses.

Exercise is not perceived as a stressor when it is pleasurable. Then, exercise adherence should be enough to induce physiological and psychological adaptations to help the organism face several kinds of stressors.

Practical applications

In this chapter it has been shown that children and adolescents can suffer from different kinds of stressors. Unfortunately, these stressors can generate negative impacts on the organism. Thus, teachers and parents must be careful to detect the signals of stress. Often children and adolescents have difficulty talking about their feelings, so analysing their behaviour is important. Psychologists can be important to help in stress management. Furthermore, exercise can be a useful strategy to improve the response to stress in different ways.

Exercise is a kind of stressor that be avoided by humans when it is perceived as unpleasant, boring or a threatening factor for body homeostasis. With that in mind, sports and exercise science professionals should aim to prescribe pleasurable exercises. Moreover, the exercise cannot be always too easy, because positive adaptations to exercise seem to be dose-dependent. Thus, exercises with dissociative stimuli such as balls, music and different aims for children and adolescents can be a useful strategy.

Young athletes can have reduce the impact of competitive sports following the strategies suggested by Adirim and Cheng (2003): '(i) the pre-season physical examination; (ii) medical coverage at sporting events; (iii) proper coaching; (iv) adequate hydration; (v) proper officiating; and (vi) proper equipment and field/surface playing conditions'.

Conclusion

Children and adolescents can suffer from negative stress caused by different stressors. Exercise can act by different routes to alleviate stress. It seems that exercise-induced stress management can be dependent on exercise programmes that are perceived as pleasurable. Thus, sports and exercise science professionals have to design exercise programmes that induce pleasure in children and adolescents.

References

Adirim, T. A., & Cheng, T. L. (2003). Overview of injuries in the young athlete. *Sports Med, 33*(1), 75–81.

American Psychological Association. (2009). *Identifying signs of stress in your children and teens.* Retrieved April 28, 2017 from: http://www.apa.org/helpcenter/stress-children.aspx.

Annesi, J. J. (2005). Correlations of depression and total mood disturbance with physical activity and self-concept in preadolescents enrolled in an after-school exercise program. *Psychol Rep, 96*(3 Pt 2), 891–898. doi: 10.2466/pr0.96.3c.891-898.

Arias-Carrion, O., Caraza-Santiago, X., Salgado-Licona, S., Salama, M., Machado, S., Nardi, A. E., . . . Murillo-Rodriguez, E. (2014). Orquestic regulation of neurotransmitters on reward-seeking behavior. *Int Arch Med, 7*, 29. doi: 10.1186/1755-7682-7-29.

Brillon, D. J., Zheng, B., Campbell, R. G., & Matthews, D. E. (1995). Effect of cortisol on energy expenditure and amino acid metabolism in humans. *Am J Physiol, 268*(3 Pt 1), E501–E513.

Carfagno, D. G., & Hendrix, J. C., 3rd. (2014). Overtraining syndrome in the athlete: Current clinical practice. *Curr Sports Med Rep, 13*(1), 45–51. doi: 10.1249/JSR.0000000000000027.

Childs, E., & de Wit, H. (2014). Regular exercise is associated with emotional resilience to acute stress in healthy adults. *Front Physiol, 5*, 161. doi: 10.3389/fphys.2014.00161.

Deslandes, A., Moraes, H., Ferreira, C., Veiga, H., Silveira, H., Mouta, R., . . . Laks, J. (2009). Exercise and mental health: many reasons to move. *Neuropsychobiology, 59*(4), 191–198. doi: 10.1159/000223730.

Deuster, P. A., & Silverman, M. N. (2013). Physical fitness: A pathway to health and resilience. *US Army Med Dep J*, 24–35.

Dishman, R. K., Berthoud, H. R., Booth, F. W., Cotman, C. W., Edgerton, V. R., Fleshner, M. R., . . . Zigmond, M. J. (2006). Neurobiology of exercise. *Obesity (Silver Spring), 14*(3), 345–356. doi: 10.1038/oby.2006.46.

Droste, S. K., Gesing, A., Ulbricht, S., Muller, M. B., Linthorst, A. C., & Reul, J. M. (2003). Effects of long-term voluntary exercise on the mouse hypothalamic–pituitary–adrenocortical axis. *Endocrinology, 144*(7), 3012–3023. doi: 10.1210/en.2003-0097.

Duncan, M. J., Clarke, N. D., Birch, S. L., Tallis, J., Hankey, J., Bryant, E., & Eyre, E. L. (2014). The effect of green exercise on blood pressure, heart rate and mood state in primary school children. *Int J Environ Res Public Health, 11*(4), 3678–3688. doi: 10.3390/ijerph110403678.

Ekkekakis, P., Hall, E. E., & Petruzzello, S. J. (2008). The relationship between exercise intensity and affective responses demystified: To crack the 40-year-old nut, replace the 40-year-old nutcracker! *Ann Behav Med, 35*(2), 136–149. doi: 10.1007/s12160-008-9025-z.

Everly, G. S., & Lating, J. M. (2013). *A clinical guide to the treatment of the human stress response* (3rd ed.). New York: Springer.

Faravelli, C., Lo Sauro, C., Godini, L., Lelli, L., Benni, L., Pietrini, F., . . . Ricca, V. (2012). Childhood stressful events, HPA axis and anxiety disorders. *World J Psychiatry, 2*(1), 13–25. doi: 10.5498/wjp.v2.i1.13.

Faravelli, C., Lo Sauro, C., Lelli, L., Pietrini, F., Lazzeretti, L., Godini, L., . . . Ricca, V. (2012). The role of life events and HPA axis in anxiety disorders: A review. *Curr Pharm Des, 18*(35), 5663–5674.

Goncharova, N. D. (2013). Stress responsiveness of the hypothalamic–pituitary–adrenal axis: Age-related features of the vasopressinergic regulation. *Front Endocrinol (Lausanne), 4*, 26. doi: 10.3389/fendo.2013.00026.

Gordon-Larsen, P., Boone-Heinonen, J., Sidney, S., Sternfeld, B., Jacobs, D. R., Jr, & Lewis, C. E. (2009). Active commuting and cardiovascular disease risk: The CARDIA study. *Arch Intern Med, 169*(13), 1216–1223. doi: 10.1001/archinternmed.2009.163.

Grant, K. E., Compas, B. E., Thurm, A. E., McMahon, S. D., Gipson, P. Y., Campbell, A. J., . . . Westerholm, R. I. (2006). Stressors and child and adolescent psychopathology: Evidence of moderating and mediating effects. *Clin Psychol Rev, 26*(3), 257–283. doi: 10.1016/j.cpr.2005.06.011.

Healy, G. N., Wijndaele, K., Dunstan, D. W., Shaw, J. E., Salmon, J., Zimmet, P. Z., & Owen, N. (2008). Objectively measured sedentary time, physical activity, and metabolic risk: The Australian Diabetes, Obesity and Lifestyle Study (AusDiab). *Diabetes Care, 31*(2), 369–371. doi: 10.2337/dc07-1795.

Herman, J. P., McKlveen, J. M., Ghosal, S., Kopp, B., Wulsin, A., Makinson, R., . . . Myers, B. (2016). Regulation of the hypothalamic–pituitary–adrenocortical stress response. *Compr Physiol, 6*(2), 603–621. doi: 10.1002/cphy.c150015.

Huai, P., Xun, H., Reilly, K. H., Wang, Y., Ma, W., & Xi, B. (2013). Physical activity and risk of hypertension: A meta-analysis of prospective cohort studies. *Hypertension, 62*(6), 1021–1026. doi: 10.1161/HYPERTENSIONAHA.113.01965.

Khani, S., & Tayek, J. A. (2001). Cortisol increases gluconeogenesis in humans: Its role in the metabolic syndrome. *Clin Sci (Lond), 101*(6), 739–747.

Lenze, E. J., Mantella, R. C., Shi, P., Goate, A. M., Nowotny, P., Butters, M. A., . . . Rollman, B. L. (2011). Elevated cortisol in older adults with generalized anxiety disorder is reduced by treatment: A placebo-controlled evaluation of escitalopram. *Am J Geriatr Psychiatry, 19*(5), 482–490. doi: 10.1097/JGP.0b013e3181ec806c.

Maier, S. F., Watkins, L. R., & Fleshner, M. (1994). Psychoneuroimmunology. The interface between behavior, brain, and immunity. *Am Psychol, 49*(12), 1004–1017.

Matta Mello Portugal, E., Cevada, T., Sobral Monteiro-Junior, R., Teixeira Guimaraes, T., da Cruz Rubini, E., Lattari, E., . . . Camaz Deslandes, A. (2013). Neuroscience of exercise: From neurobiology mechanisms to mental health. *Neuropsychobiology, 68*(1), 1–14. doi: 10.1159/000350946.

McNeely, C. A., & Blanchard, J. (2010). *The teen years explained: A guide to healthy adolescent development*. Baltimore, MD: Johns Hopkins University.

Merikangas, K. R., Nakamura, E. F., & Kessler, R. C. (2009). Epidemiology of mental disorders in children and adolescents. *Dialogues Clin Neurosci, 11*(1), 7–20.

Merkel, D. L. (2013). Youth sport: Positive and negative impact on young athletes. *Open Access J Sports Med, 4*, 151–160. doi: 10.2147/OAJSM.S33556.

Nestler, E. J., Barrot, M., DiLeone, R. J., Eisch, A. J., Gold, S. J., & Monteggia, L. M. (2002). Neurobiology of depression. *Neuron, 34*(1), 13–25.

Portugal, E. M., Lattari, E., Santos, T. M., & Deslandes, A. C. (2015). Affective responses to prescribed and self-selected strength training intensities. *Percept Mot Skills, 121*(2), 465–481. doi: 10.2466/29.PMS.121c17x3.

Schwabe, L., Dalm, S., Schachinger, H., & Oitzl, M. S. (2008). Chronic stress modulates the use of spatial and stimulus-response learning strategies in mice and man. *Neurobiol Learn Mem, 90*(3), 495–503. doi: 10.1016/j.nlm.2008.07.015.

Semlitsch, T., Jeitler, K., Hemkens, L. G., Horvath, K., Nagele, E., Schuermann, C., . . . Siebenhofer, A. (2013). Increasing physical activity for the treatment of hypertension: A systematic review and meta-analysis. *Sports Med, 43*(10), 1009–1023. doi: 10.1007/s40279-013-0065-6.

Silveira, H., Moraes, H., Oliveira, N., Coutinho, E. S., Laks, J., & Deslandes, A. (2013). Physical exercise and clinically depressed patients: A systematic review and meta-analysis. *Neuropsychobiology, 67*(2), 61–68. doi: 10.1159/000345160.

Stranahan, A. M., Lee, K., & Mattson, M. P. (2008). Central mechanisms of HPA axis regulation by voluntary exercise. *Neuromolecular Med, 10*(2), 118–127. doi: 10.1007/s12017-008-8027-0.

Vander, A. J., Sherman, J. H., & Luciano, D. S. (2001). *Human physiology: The mechanisms of the body function*. New York: McGraw-Hill.

Vogel, S., & Schwabe, L. (2016). Learning and memory under stress: Implications for the classroom. *Nature Partner J, 1*(1611), 1–10.

Wegner, M., Helmich, I., Machado, S., Nardi, A. E., Arias-Carrion, O., & Budde, H. (2014). Effects of exercise on anxiety and depression disorders: Review of meta-analyses and neurobiological mechanisms. *CNS Neurol Disord Drug Targets, 13*(6), 1002–1014.

Williamson, D., Dewey, A., & Steinberg, H. (2001). Mood change through physical exercise in nine- to ten-year-old children. *Percept Mot Skills, 93*(1), 311–316. doi: 10.2466/pms.2001.93.1.311.

Wood, C., Angus, C., Pretty, J., Sandercock, G., & Barton, J. (2013). A randomised control trial of physical activity in a perceived environment on self-esteem and mood in UK adolescents. *Int J Environ Health Res, 23*(4), 311–320. doi: 10.1080/09603123.2012.733935.

Zoref-Shani, E., Kessler-Icekson, G., Wasserman, L., & Sperling, O. (1984). Characterization of purine nucleotide metabolism in primary rat cardiomyocyte cultures. *Biochim Biophys Acta, 804*(2), 161–168.

Chapter 8

Structural and functional brain changes related to acute and chronic exercise effects in children, adolescents and young adults

*Claudia Voelcker-Rehage, Claudia Niemann
and Lena Hübner*

Introduction

In recent years, the influence of exercise and physical activity on cognitive performance in children and young adults has come into focus (e.g. Donnelly et al., 2016; Etnier, Nowell, Landers, & Sibley, 2006; Hillman, Erickson, & Kramer, 2008). In addition, studies examining the effects of exercise and physical activity on motor performance and motor learning processes (e.g. Roig, Skriver, Lundbye-Jensen, Kiens, & Nielsen, 2012) represent promising areas of research. Brain research methods such as electroencephalography (EEG) or functional and structural magnetic resonance imaging (MRI) provide valuable information on how exercise and physical activity affect brain structure and function and which possible mechanisms might underlie their relationship with cognition/motor performance.

One line of research focuses on the immediate effects of acute bouts of exercise. Studies that fall into this category can be further divided into approaches measuring cognitive or motor performance during or directly after exercising. These studies are often complemented by EEG measurements to investigate underlying neurophysiological mechanisms. Another line of research investigates chronic effects of physical activity. Investigations in this field examine either the association between an individual's overall physical fitness level with or the effect of a (long-term) exercise intervention on cognitive or motor performance. Only long-term intervention studies are assumed to lead to structural changes in the organism (e.g. increased vascularization or growth of synapses). For structural changes to occur, however, physiological changes must precede. Such physiological changes, which take place while the organism adapts to the physical demands of an activity, may already positively impact specific cognitive processes directly after an acute bout of exercise. Certain research questions so far have been thoroughly investigated only in certain target groups (e.g. chronic exercise effects mainly in older adults and acute exercise effects in younger adults). Further, research methods and paradigms differ immensely between studies.

In this chapter we will focus on studies performed with children, adolescents and young adults using neurophysiological methods, i.e. primarily EEG and MRI.

Physical activity incorporates bodily movements produced by skeletal muscles, including a variety of unspecified activities in daily life domains (e.g. work, household). In contrast, structured *exercise* is characterized as physical activity that is planned, repetitive and done with the purpose of improving physical fitness level. *Physical fitness level* (or *fitness level*) in turn refers to the status of someone's physical fitness, often measured by defining the maximal rate of oxygen consumption (Vo_{2max}) or the participant's energy expenditure using physical activity questionnaires.

Effects of acute bouts of exercise

Effects of acute bouts of exercise on cognitive performance

The relationship between acute exercise and cognition has been investigated with various physical intervention methods, sample characteristics, cognitive assessments and time points of measurement (e.g. McMorris, Sproule, Turner, & Hale, 2011). There is evidence that performance on complex cognitive tasks that tap into the executive control system, i.e. those cognitive functions that are related to attentional control, working memory and cognitive flexibility, suffers when performed *during* aerobic exercise (Pontifex & Hillman, 2007). These deficits, however, dissipate and even reverse when exercise is terminated, i.e. cognitive performance *following* exercise improves on average (see Chang, Pan, Chen, Tsai, & Huang, 2012, for a review).

Cardiovascular exercise

Most studies on acute exercise effects have been performed with young adults. A meta-analysis by McMorris et al. (2011) revealed significantly faster response times in tasks of executive function following moderate-intensity exercise. Only a few studies have investigated children. Drollette, Shishido, Pontifex, and Hillman (2012) as well as Hillman, Pontifex, Raine, and Kramer (2009) confirmed exercise-induced increases in response accuracy after acute bouts of moderate-intensity treadmill walking also in pre-adolescent children, indicating that acute exercise effects might be similar in children and young adults.

Key factors that add to the variation in findings on the exercise–cognition relationship are the *intensity* and *duration* of the exercise. A meta-analysis by McMorris and Hale (2012) supports the assumption of an inverted-U-shaped relationship between arousal and performance, referring to the Yerkes–Dodson Law (Yerkes & Dodson, 1908). Accordingly, the most beneficial and robust results for acute exercise on cognitive performance (particularly executive control) are achieved at submaximal, moderate intensities with durations between 20 and 60 minutes (McMorris et al., 2011; Tomporowski, 2003). High-intensity exercise, on the contrary, seems to be most beneficial in very fit subjects (Budde et al., 2012). For example, Budde and colleagues (2012) have shown that attention was improved after high-intensity exercise in young adults with a high participation rate in physical activity, whereas this was not the case in not very active individuals. This finding indicates that a higher participation rate in physical activity might lead to neurobiological adaptations that facilitate the effects of high-intensity exercise on cognitive processes (i.e. attention) (Budde et al., 2012; for further specification of the effects of high-intensity exercise, see the section 'Combination of acute and chronic exercise' later in this chapter).

Further, exercise effects differ with regard to the *time point of assessment* following exercising. Postexercise effects on executive functioning are evident immediately after exercise and last up to 30–40 minutes after exercise cessation (for a review, see Pontifex, Hillman, & Polich, 2009), but seem to be diminished after 2 hours (Hopkins, Davis, VanTieghem, Whalen, & Bucci, 2012). The finding that brief, moderate-intensity exercise can improve cognitive function has important implications for various target groups. For example, for adolescents in a school setting positive effects of single bouts of exercise on cognitive performance support the argument that physical activity could help to improve scholastic performance (Budde, Voelcker-Rehage, Pietrabyk-Kendziorra, Ribeiro, & Tidow, 2008), particularly for adolescents who are considered low cognitive performers (Budde et al., 2010).

Resistance exercise

Although most studies have been performed on cardiovascular exercise, recent research has revealed that in healthy young adults also an acute bout of resistance exercise facilitated cognitive functioning (Brush, Olson, Ehmann, Osovsky & Alderman, 2016). However, results differed in regard to the intensity of the acute bout, the time point of cognitive assessment and the cognitive task administered. At 15 minutes post exercise, high-intensity resistance exercise resulted in less interference and improved reaction time for the Stroop task, while 180 minutes of low- and moderate-intensity exercise resulted in improved performance on plus-minus and Simon tasks, respectively. Similarly, Chang and Etnier (2009) revealed a dose–response relationship between the intensity of resistance exercise and cognitive performance in healthy young adults such that high-intensity exercise benefits speed of processing, but moderate-intensity exercise is most beneficial for executive function. In contrast, in adolescents, a 30-minute single bout of resistance exercise resulted in similar cognitive benefits (Stroop test, Trail-Making Test) as cardiovascular exercise of the same length did (Harveson et al., 2016).

Neurophysiological studies

Several studies applied neurophysiological methods, predominantly EEG, during or after an acute bout of exercise to understand better underlying brain processes. In this vein it has been shown that acute bouts of exercise modulate event-related potentials (ERPs), short-lasting positive or negative voltage changes that are synchronized with certain internal or external events such as stimuli, tasks or responses. For example, there is some indication that acute bouts of moderate-intensity exercise lead to increased P3 amplitudes and earlier peak latencies alongside behavioural benefits (Drollette et al., 2014; Hillman, Pontifex, Raine, et al., 2009; Kamijo, Nishihira, Higashiura, & Kuroiwa, 2007; Magnie et al., 2000; Nakamura, Nishimoto, Akamatu, Takahashi, & Maruyama, 1999; Scudder, Drollette, Pontifex, & Hillman, 2012).

The P3 is a positive deflection peaking about 300–500 ms after stimulus onset and is related to the evaluation and classification of incoming information. The amplitude has been suggested to indicate processing intensity of the cognitive task at hand. An enlargement of the P3 amplitude due to exercise can be interpreted as an increase in attentional resources in the brain (see Kamijo, 2009, for an overview). Latency of the P3 is an index of the timing of respective cognitive processes. Own pilot data collected from younger adults immediately after cycling for 20 minutes at a moderate intensity (40–60% of individual Vo_2 peak values) reveal earlier P3 peaks and a trend for increased P3 amplitudes as compared to a rest condition (Winneke, Hübner, Godde, & Voelcker-Rehage, in preparation). Recent data in young adults by Pontifex, Parks, Henning, and Kamijo (2015) showed a maintenance of the P3 amplitude after a 20-minute bout of aerobic exercise, whereas resting for the same amount of time resulted in a decrease in P3 amplitude. For children (age 8–10 years), Drollette et al. (2014) showed earlier P3 latencies in a flanker task (a measure of selective attention and executive control that requires participants to inhibit irrelevant stimuli in order to respond to a relevant target stimulus) following moderate exercise, indicating a reduction in processing speed, i.e. faster processing. Interestingly, children classified as low performers showed particular behavioural gains in the more difficult incongruent flanker condition accompanied by P3 amplitude enlargements, suggesting a gain in selective attentional resource allocation (cf. Hillman, Buck, Themanson, Pontifex, & Castelli, 2009, for similar associations with cardiovascular fitness in the same age group).

A first study on resistance exercise investigated the effects of 30 minutes of acute resistance exercise on cognitive functioning (flanker task, Go/No-Go task) and ERPs (Tsai et al., 2014). The study revealed improved cognitive performance after exercise accompanied with increases in P3 amplitude.

Results regarding the effect of exercise on the N2 are scarce and mixed. The N2, the second negative deflection in the ERP, reaches its maximum amplitude around 200–300 ms after stimulus onset and reflects endogenous cognitive components associated with novelty detection (N2a), executive control (N2b) and classification (N2c). Themanson and Hillman (2006) did not find effects of acute exercise on the N2 in young adults, whereas Pontifex and Hillman (2007) in young adults as well as Drollette and colleagues (2014) in children reported a reduction in N2 amplitude while exercising, interpreted as an indication that fewer resources are required for attentional control while exercising.

Continuous EEG data

Continuous EEG data that are not time-locked to certain events can be regarded as the linear sum of various oscillatory components. Decomposing the data by, for example, Fourier transform reveals typical oscillations in different frequency bands that can be associated with certain cognitive or brain states. Alpha oscillations (~8–13 Hz) are associated with a relaxed brain state without active processing of external or internal stimuli.

Crabbe and Dishman (2004) did a quantitative synthesis of EEG studies investigating oscillations in the alpha frequency band (~8–12 Hz) after acute exercise, including participants ranging from young to older adults. The authors reported overall increased absolute alpha power (representing the strength of the respective oscillations) directly after exercise. For example, in 9–10-year-old children larger alpha activity was revealed in the precuneus after 15 minutes of moderate bike exercise (Schneider, Vogt, Frysch, Guardiera, & Strüder, 2009). This has been interpreted as a reflection of an overall state of physical relaxation which might improve the ability to concentrate and result in better cognitive performance following an acute exercise bout. Mierau and colleagues (2014) investigated cognitive performance and EEG in young children after 45 minutes of movement games. They found larger alpha activity in resting-state EEG, again a state of physical relaxation, but no changes in cognitive performance and task-related EEG measurements.

The phase consistency of oscillations between pairs of electrodes in each frequency band is called *coherence* and can be interpreted as functional interaction of corresponding brain areas. Decreased coherence in the lower alpha band (8–10 Hz) after acute exercise of moderate intensity as compared to rest condition was shown; this is regarded as an indicator for reduced cognitive effort after acute exercise (Hogan et al., 2013). Furthermore, individual alpha peak frequency (iAPF, the dominant EEG peak frequency within the individual alpha frequency band) was increased after exhaustive exercise but not after less intense exercise in young healthy adults (Gutmann et al., 2015). The increase in iAPF is interpreted as a marker of arousal and attention and is associated with increased information-processing speed (Gutmann et al., 2015).

To sum up the electrophysiological findings, research indicates enhanced attentional capacity related to acute exercise, as reflected in increased P3 amplitudes. Studies looking at EEG frequencies (alpha frequency in particular) suggest an increase in neural resources that can be devoted to the cognitive task at hand representing enhanced attention and better cognitive task performance. So far, no study has systematically compared effects for children, youth and young adults indicating differentiated results.

Effects of acute bouts of exercise on motor performance and motor learning

General findings

Effects of acute exercise on motor performance and motor learning have been studied for decades, with very heterogeneous findings.[1] Studies differ with respect to conducted exercise protocols (e.g. exercise intensity, termination criteria) and performed motor tasks (e.g. gross or fine motor skills) or whether the focus was on performance or learning.

When measuring effects of acute exercise on *motor performance*, the performance or adaptation of a motor task was measured directly after exercise (e.g. Thacker, Middleton, McIlroy, & Staines, 2014; Wegner, Koedijker, & Budde, 2014). Similarly to cognitive performance research, some findings partially supported the claim of an inverted-U-shape relationship between exercise intensity and motor performance (e.g. with the gross motor Bachman ladder task; Pack, Cotten, & Biasiotto, 1974). Others found improvements after intense exercise, e.g. in a task requiring fine motor control in very fit young subjects (e.g. Fitts' reciprocal tapping task; Dickinson, Medhurst, & Whittingham, 1979).

A recent meta-analysis on the effects of acute exercise on whole-body movements, i.e. sport-related skills like passing in soccer, by McMorris, Hale, Corbett, Robertson, and Hodgson (2015), not only disproved the inverted-U-shape relationship in healthy young adults, but also found no significant effect of moderate-intensity exercise on motor performance and a detrimental effect of intense exercise. So far, only the study by Wegner et al. (2014) investigated the effects of moderate-intensity exercise on manual dexterity performance in children (flower trail) and found no effect of acute exercise on fine motor performance.

When measuring the effects of acute exercise on *motor learning*, performance in the motor task was mostly measured on delayed retention tests (e.g. Mang, Snow, Campbell, Ross, & Boyd, 2014; Roig et al., 2012; Skriver et al., 2014) as motor memory needs time to be transformed into performance improvement (memory consolidation; Kantak & Winstein for a review, 2012). Findings regarding the effects of acute exercise on learning a motor skill are also inconsistent. Interestingly, in contrast to studies analysing exercise effects on cognitive or motor performance, these studies used bouts of exercise of high intensity (Mang et al., 2014; Roig et al., 2012; Skriver et al., 2014). High-intensity exercise (90% of maximal power output) led to better motor skill retention 24 hours and 7 days later than low-intensity exercise (45% of maximal power output) or a control condition in young adults with a force-tracking task (Thomas, Johnsen, Geertsen, et al., 2016). Accordingly, no effect on motor learning (24-hour retention, continuous force-tracking task) was reported after moderate-intensity exercise (Snow et al., 2016). A possible explanation is that a high level of lactate is a mediating mechanism, which is supposed to trigger the release of brain-derived neurotrophic factor (BDNF) (Skriver et al., 2014). BDNF is known to influence experience-dependent plasticity in the primary motor cortex (M1) (Kleim et al., 2006) and increased levels of BDNF were detected after motor skill training (Lu, 2003).

In samples of young adults, a high-intensity acute exercise protocol seemed to reveal positive effects on learning an implicit motor sequence task in terms of higher temporal precision but not spatial accuracy (force tracking) (Mang et al., 2014). It also revealed positive effects on retention performance (24 hours and 7 days after practice), but not immediately after exercise (Roig et al., 2012; Skriver et al., 2014) as compared to a resting control group. The latter finding reflects motor memory consolidation.

Roig and colleagues (2012) not only compared the amount of motor learning after an acute bout of exercise with the amount of learning after a rest condition in a sample of young males, but also varied the order of acute exercise and motor task. Interestingly, the experimental group practising the motor task before the acute bout of exercise revealed better performance 7 days after practice as compared to the group practising the motor task directly after a bout of intense exercise (Roig et al., 2012).

Furthermore, the timing between acute exercise and motor skill acquisition seems to be important, as (motor) memory seems to be facilitated only when a temporal proximity is given (for a recent review see Roig et al., 2016). Correspondingly, Thomas, Beck, Lind, and colleagues (2016) reported that exercise performed 20 minutes after acquisition showed higher effects on retention performance 1 and 7 days after acquisition than exercise performed 1 or 2 hours post motor acquisition in young adults.

These findings create the need to investigate further the optimal time point of acute exercise (before or after practising the motor task) to facilitate consolidation of motor learning processes. Some recent studies investigated the effects of acute exercise on *initial* or *short-term motor learning*, by measuring motor performance in tasks with focus performance speed directly after the acute exercise session (Perini, Bortoletto, Capogrosso, Fertonani, & Miniussi, 2016; Sage et al., 2016). For example, Perini and colleagues (2016) reported an immediate positive effect of moderate-intensity exercise in a thumb abduction task (as fast as possible). Further, Sage and colleagues (2016) found decreased error rates in a key-pressing task after moderate-intensity exercise, but no significant effect on response times. These findings might indicate that the specific demands of the motor task also play a role in the the exercise–performance relationship.

Neurophysiological studies

Recent studies have provided neural underpinnings for the positive impact of acute bouts of exercise on motor learning processes. First, it was revealed that acute bouts of exercise facilitate neuroplasticity in the (primary) motor cortex (M1) induced by repetitive transcranial magnetic stimulation (i.e. a non-invasive brain stimulation technique; see Coco, Perciavalle, Cavallari, & Perciavalle, 2016; Singh & Staines, 2015 for a review) as well as continuous theta burst stimulation (McDonnell, Buckley, Opie, Ridding, & Semmler, 2013). M1 is the most important source of ascending projections to the motor neurons, crucial for the voluntary control of movements and also involved in motor learning processes. This enhanced neuroplasticity might occur because acute exercise affects neurochemical processes that are in turn known to facilitate M1 excitability, like levels of the neurotransmitters dopamine, serotonin, noradrenaline (norepinephrine) and lactate (Coco et al., 2016; Singh, Neva, & Staines, 2014).

In accordance with that, Skriver and colleagues (2014) showed that the same neurochemical processes (plus increased levels of insulin-like growth factor, adrenaline (epinephrine) and vascular endothelial growth factor) are also involved in motor skill acquisition and retention. Furthermore, a bout of acute exercise enhanced resting-state functional connectivity in sensorimotor brain regions (Rajab et al., 2014), which might also indicate enhanced susceptibility of the motor system.

Interestingly, Coco and colleagues (2016) further reported decreased excitability of the supplementary motor area, which is known to be involved in linking cognition to action (Nachev, Kennard, & Husain, 2008). This finding might mean that the cognitive part of motor control is decreased right after exhaustive exercise, whereas the motor part is facilitated. Nevertheless, more studies are needed to examine the effects of acute exercise on motor functions and learning and motor areas, including physiological and neurochemical measures – also in children – and to understand the exact mechanisms and give recommendations about exercise intensity, duration and timing of exercise and motor paradigms (McMorris et al., 2015).

Long-term exercise or physical activity effects

Long-term exercise or physical activity effects on cognition

General findings

Meta-analyses and review articles (Donnelly et al., 2016; Prakash, Voss, Erickson, & Kramer, 2015; Voelcker-Rehage & Niemann, 2013) have shown that physical activity (cross-sectional data and intervention studies) is positively associated with cognitive functioning across the lifespan. For children, adolescents and young adults, positive associations of physical activity (mostly cross-sectional data) have been shown on executive functions (Buck, Hillman, & Castelli, 2008; Davis & Cooper, 2011; Pontifex et al., 2011; Scudder et al., 2014), perceptual speed (Mokgothu & Gallagher, 2010; Wu & Hillman, 2013) and memory performance (Chaddock, Hillman, Buck, & Cohen, 2011; Drollette et al., 2016, Mokgothu & Gallagher, 2010; Raine et al., 2013). Longitudinal studies found positive associations of baseline fitness levels with change in executive control performance after 9 months (Niederer et al., 2011; mean age 5 years) and 1 year (Chaddock, Hillman, Pontifex, et al., 2012; mean age 10 years). A study on 9–10-year old children using an interventional design revealed positive effects on working-memory performance after a 10-week additional afterschool exercise regime, which took place three times a week for 45 minutes (Koutsandréou, Niemann, Wegner, & Budde, 2016).

Most exercise paradigms utilized cardiovascular exercise, also referred to as aerobic or cardiorespiratory exercise, where highly automated movements like walking or cycling are performed. Fewer studies investigated other types of exercise, such as motor coordinative or resistance exercise (to our knowledge, so far, in children and young adults only studies using acute resistance exercise exist; cf. above). Similarly to cardiovascular fitness, resistance exercise (resistance training) affects metabolic and energetic processes and to some extent intramuscular coordination. Unlike metabolic exercise, motor coordination training comprises exercises for bilateral fine and gross motor body coordination, such as balance, eye–hand coordination and leg–arm coordination, as well as spatial orientation and reaction to moving objects/persons (Voelcker-Rehage, Godde, & Staudinger, 2011; Voelcker-Rehage, & Niemann, 2013). Coordination training induces less change in energy metabolism than cardiovascular and resistance exercise. Instead, coordinative movements require perceptual and higher-level cognitive processes, such as attention, that are essential for mapping sensation to action and ensuring anticipatory and adaptive aspects of coordination. Thus, changes induced by coordinative exercise are likely to be related to changes in information processing and cognitive tasks that demand, besides attention, the ability to handle visual and spatial information. By contrast, perceptual and higher-level cognitive processes are less relevant in highly automated movements like walking or cycling, as used in cardiovascular exercise. In this section, we will detail the differential effects of different types of exercise and fitness on brain and cognitive function.

Cardiovascular exercise

As for acute effects of exercise, there is increasing evidence for fitness-related modulations of cognitive ERPs. Higher physical activity levels were associated with shorter P3 latencies and/or larger amplitudes in children (Hillman et al., 2014) and younger adults (Kamijo & Takeda, 2010). Also a study with elementary school children revealed faster response times as well as shorter P3 latencies and increased P3 amplitudes on a flanker task and thereby underline the positive effect of physical activity intervention programmes on attentional processes in children (Hillman et al., 2014). Interestingly, benefits of physical exercise in children were reported not only for general cognitive tasks but also for specific aspects of arithmetic problem solving (Moore, Drollette, Scudder, Bharij, & Hillman, 2014). Similarly, larger P3 amplitudes have also been found by Hillman, Pontifex, Raine, et al. (2009) in very fit preadolescent children (flanker task; see Hillman, Buck, Themanson, et al., 2009, for similar results) and by our research group in young adults (working-memory task; Winneke et al., in preparation). Results are interpreted as a confirmation of the positive association between fitness and cognitive performance in an executive control task through increased cognitive control.

Themanson and Hillman (2006) reported that in young adults the fitness level was not associated with modulations of the N2, but very fit adults showed marked reductions in the amplitude of the error-related negativity (ERN; the ERN can be observed about 100 ms following an error even without the participant being aware of committing the error). Findings regarding the N2 and physical fitness in children and adolescents are also mixed with some studies reporting no association (Hillman, Pontifex, Raine, et al., 2009, in preadolescent children), others reporting smaller N2 amplitudes in highly fit children yet better cognitive control performance (see Pontifex et al., 2011, for preadolescent children; Stroth et al., 2009, for adolescents).

Given the diversity of experimental designs and testing parameters together with the small number of studies, the effects of exercise interventions on ERP components, as markers of cognitive functioning and attentional control, require further investigation. Also, differences in maturity of brain development have to be considered, particularly when comparing findings in children and young adults.

The first functional MRI study on the exercise–cognition relationship was conducted by Colcombe and colleagues (2004) with older adults. Results indicated that after cardiovascular training, older adults applied cognitive resources more effectively and cognition was improved. Brain activation of physically active and inactive older participants differed in prefrontal and parietal regions, and the anterior cingulate cortex. Only few studies investigated the possible association of physical activity and brain function in young adults and children. However, existing research in children confirmed findings from research with older adults. In cross-sectional and longitudinal studies highly fit children (or after exercise intervention) revealed better executive control performance (e.g. Chaddock, Erickson, Prakash et al., 2012; Raine, Scudder, Saliba, Kramer, & Hillman, 2016; Voss et al., 2011). Further, higher relational memory (Chaddock et al., 2010a) and learning benefits (Raine et al., 2013) were shown. These behavioural results from highly fit children were accompanied by more effective brain activation, as pronounced in either higher prefrontal cortex activity (Chaddock, Erickson, Prakash et al., 2012 for the early task blocks; Davis et al., 2011) or reduced frontal activity (Chaddock, Erickson, Prakash et al., 2012 for the later task blocks) and reduced parietal activity (Chaddock, Erickson, Prakash et al., 2012, for the later task blocks; Davis et al., 2011), presumably reflecting a reduction of resources required to complete the task. Findings indicate an important role of cardiovascular exercise/fitness in the facilitation of the cognitive control network.

Neural connectivity data bear the potential to reveal task-independent measures of brain function. For example, Kim, Cha, Kim, Kang, and Han (2015) found that resting-state functional connectivity from the cerebellum to the frontal and parietal cortex was enhanced in children from 10 to 13 years after 3 years of participation in a taekwondo training five times per week. Also hippocampal function as well as regions of the default mode network has been shown to be positively related to aerobic fitness in adolescents (Herting & Nagel, 2013).

On the level of brain anatomy, Colcombe and coworkers (2003) again were the first to examine the association between brain volume and cardiovascular fitness in older adults. They found that age-related decline in brain volume in frontal, parietal and temporal cortices was attenuated as a function of cardiovascular fitness (Colcombe et al., 2003). In young adults, one study related physical activity to brain structure, so far. Peters et al. (2009) revealed a positive association of aerobic capacity with volume of the right anterior insula, a brain region involved in cortical control of cardiovascular functions. No associations of aerobic capacity with memory performance could be revealed. Only a few studies have so far investigated the association between physical activity and brain structure in children. Higher levels of cardiovascular fitness or long-term exercise training have been related to larger volumes of the hippocampus accompanied by better relational memory performance (Chaddock et al., 2010a) and larger volumes of the basal ganglia accompanied by more efficient executive control performance (Chaddock et al., 2010b; see Chaddock, Hillman, Pontifex, et al., 2012, for an intervention analysis).

Even less research has been performed on physical activity and white-matter volume or integrity. However, associations of physical activity and white matter might be likely, as myelinization of white-matter fibers proceeds during adolescence. *Myelin* is a fatty layer surrounding the axons of neurons that enables fast information processing between neurons, and is responsible for the white colouring. *White-matter integrity* represents a measure of the quality of the white-matter microstructure, e.g. assessed by *fractional anisotropy* (value that refers to the coherence of the orientation of water diffusion). An 8-month intervention study by Krafft, Schaeffer, and Schwarz (2014) with 8–11-year-old children did not reveal any association between physical activity engagement and executive functioning nor general white-matter integrity measurement. Only frequency of attendance in the experimental group was positively related to change in white-matter integrity. Evaluation of the same study group, however, showed increased change of fractional anisotropy values of the uncinate fasciculus, a white-matter tract that connects parts of the limbic system such as the hippocampus and frontal brain areas, in the exercising group (Schaeffer, Krafft, & Schwarz, 2014). Research in healthy young adults on white-matter changes is scarce and, so far, has not revealed a relationship between white-matter volume and physical activity (Peters et al., 2009).

Motor coordination training

Motor coordination measured after an exercise intervention or via motor fitness level is also positively associated with cognitive function. This has been shown for different age groups. In elementary school-aged children, motor fitness levels have been positively related to complex executive control tasks (Luz, Rodrigues, & Cordivil, 2015) and academic achievement (Fernandes et al., 2016; Lopes, Santos, Pereira, & Lopes, 2013). After 3 months (Koutsandréou et al., 2016), 5-month (Gallotta et al., 2015) or 6 months (Crova et al., 2014) of motor-demanding and cognitively challenging interventions, executive control performance of 9–10-year old children was improved.

To the best of our knowledge, there is only one study that assessed the effect of coordination training on neurophysiological measures. Kindergarten children participating in an 8-week coordinative exercise programme revealed faster response times as well as shorter P3 latencies and increased P3 amplitudes on a flanker task at the end of the intervention relative to the beginning (Chang, Tsai, Chen, & Hung, 2013).

To sum up, current research indicates that not only cardiovascular demands contribute to cognitive benefits, since interventions without any cardiovascular impact also revealed positive effects on the behavioural and neurophysiological level. Therefore, coordination training including a variety of complex movements (for a discussion, see also Voelcker-Rehage & Niemann, 2013) might be essential for cognitive benefits as well.

*Effects of physical activity on motor performance and
motor learning*

As compared to cognitive skills, less is known about the relationship between
chronic engagement in physical activity and performance in motor tasks. No
controlled study so far has investigated the effects of chronic physical activity on motor learning processes in children or young adults. For example,
a study with older adults showed that an 8-week aerobic fitness intervention led to improved performance in a finger-tracking task, which might
be explained by enhanced information processing (Bakken et al., 2001).
Also animal studies showed that aerobic exercise interventions induced
changes in the motor cortex and other areas involved in motor function (cerebellum, basal ganglia, substantia nigra) expressed by enhanced oxidative
metabolism (McCloskey, Adamo, & Anderson, 2001; Vissing, Andersen,
& Diemer, 1996), hippocampal neurogenesis and synaptic plasticity (van
Praag, Shubert, Zhao, & Gage, 2005). These findings indicate that regular
exercise not only modulates brain areas involved in cognitive processing,
but also brain regions that are active during motor performance. Research
is needed to confirm these results in young humans as findings could have
a great impact for certain target groups, for example, in the school setting.

Combination of acute and chronic exercise

Few studies have investigated the interplay between the effects of acute and
chronic exercise on cognitive functioning. Such a relationship is assumed
because physiological changes, which take place while the organism adapts
to the demands of an acute bout of exercise, may lead to structural changes
in the long run. So far, these studies indicate that individual improvements in
physical fitness lead to larger cognitive benefits through acute bouts of exercise (e.g. Hopkins et al., 2012). For example, Zervas, Danis, and Klissouras
(1991) investigated in an acute–chronic mixed design the performance in
a visual discrimination task in preadolescent children. Twenty-five minutes
of treadmill running improved cognitive performance and was highest after
6 months of aerobic training. The fitness effect seems to be especially prominent in highly complex cognitive tasks (Weingarten, 1973). However, so far
intervention lengths have been limited (7 and 12 weeks) in studies, only children or young adults have been investigated and study designs were not well
controlled (Gutin, 1966; Weingarten, 1973). Roig, Nordbrandt, Geertsen,
and Nielsen (2013) concluded in their review that fitness level does not interact with acute exercise in tasks requiring short-term memory. In contrast,
in tasks requiring long-term memory, acute exercise seems to have a greater
effect in individuals with an average fitness level than with a low fitness level.

We assume that acute exercise effects sum up across an exercise intervention period and lead to pre-to-post test (chronic) changes in cognition and
(neuro-) physiological markers. High-intensity exercise seems to be most

beneficial for cognition in well-trained or highly fit subjects (Budde et al., 2012). This might indicate that long-term physical training may foster neurobiological adaptations that facilitate the effects of high-intensity exercise on cognitive processes. Findings regarding exercise intensity effects are, however, ambiguous as some studies revealed higher cognitive benefits for highly fit or very active participants in comparison to their less fit or inactive counterparts (Budde et al., 2012; Pesce, Cereatti, Forte, Crova, & Casella, 2011) and others did not show any differential effects regarding fitness levels (Magnie et al., 2000; Themanson & Hillman, 2006).

To sum up, these results underline the importance of assessing physical fitness status and a history of physical activity history (i.e. sport participation in the last 12 months) in studies examining effects of acute exercise to control for the interplay of acute and chronic exercise effects.

Outlook

In this chapter we have provided an overview about different research facets of the exercise–cognition interaction in children, adolescents and young adults. It turns out that research methods and paradigms differ immensely between studies. Systematic approaches that bring together the different research areas, methods and results are still missing. Especially the interaction of acute and chronic exercise effects on cognition needs to be examined in greater depth, because, as we outlined in this chapter, existing findings seem to be ambiguous. Moreover, studies are needed to investigate whether the effects of acute and chronic exercise on behaviour and neurophysiological processes are the same in children, adolescents and younger adults. More longitudinal studies and long-term follow-up measurements are desirable to expand our knowledge further of how the relationship develops over time. Also, research investigating the relationship between chronic physical activity or acute bouts of exercise and motor performance and motor learning in different age groups is needed. In this field of research studies measuring neurophysiological processes are missing. Furthermore, only very lab-oriented motor tasks have been used so far. Studies testing tasks more closely related to daily activities need to be conducted to estimate better the impact of physical activity and acute exercise on daily functioning and living.

Note

1 In some (earlier) studies acute bouts of exercise were named as physical fatigue (e.g. Pack, Cotten, & Biasiotto, 1974).

References

Bakken, R. C., Carey, J. R., Di Fabio, R. P., Erlandson, T. J., Hake, J. L., & Intihar, T. W. (2001). Effect of aerobic exercise on tracking performance in elderly people: A pilot study. *Physical Therapy*, 81(12), 1870–1879.

Brush, C. J., Olson, R. L., Ehmann. P. J., Osovsky, S., & Alderman, B. L. (2016). Dose–response and time course effects of acute resistance exercise on executive function. *Journal of Sports and Exercise Psychology, 29*, 1–35.

Buck, S. M., Hillman, C. H., & Castelli, D. M. (2008). The relation of aerobic fitness to Stroop task performance in preadolescent children. *Medicine and Science in Sports and Exercise, 40*(1), 166–172.

Budde, H., Brunelli, A., Machado, S., Velasques, B., Ribeiro, P., Arias-Carrion, O., & Voelcker-Rehage, C. (2012). Intermittent maximal exercise improves attentional performance only in physically active students. *Archives of Medical Research, 43*(2), 125–131.

Budde, H., Voelcker-Rehage, C., Pietrassyk-Kendziorra, S., Machado, S., Ribeiro, P., & Arafat, A. M. (2010). Steroid hormones in the saliva of adolescents after different exercise intensities and their influence on working memory in a school setting. *Psychoneuroendocrinology, 35*, 382–391.

Budde, H., Voelcker-Rehage, C., Pietrabyk-Kendziorra, S., Ribeiro, P., & Tidow, G. (2008). Acute coordinative exercise improves attentional performance in adolescents. *Neuroscience Letters, 441*(2), 219–223.

Chaddock, L., Erickson, K. I., Prakash, R. S., Kim, J. S., Voss, M. W., Vanpatter, M., . . . Kramer, A. F. (2010a). A neuroimaging investigation of the association between aerobic fitness, hippocampal volume, and memory performance in preadolescent children. *Brain Research, 1358*, 172–183.

Chaddock, L., Erickson, K. I., Prakash, R. S., VanPatter, M., Voss, M. W., Pontifex, M. B., . . . Kramer, A. F. (2010b). Basal ganglia volume is associated with aerobic fitness in preadolescent children. *Developmental Neuroscience, 32*(3), 249–256.

Chaddock, L., Erickson, K. I., Prakash, R. S., Voss, M. W., VanPatter, M., Pontifex, M. B., . . . Kramer, A. F. (2012). A functional MRI investigation of the association between childhood aerobic fitness and neurocognitive control. *Biological Psychology, 89*(1), 260–268.

Chaddock, L., Hillman, C. H., Buck, S. M., & Cohen, N. J. (2011). Aerobic fitness and executive control of relational memory in preadolescent children. *Medicine and Science in Sports and Exercise, 43*(2), 344–349.

Chaddock, L., Hillman, C. H., Pontifex, M. B., Johnson, C. R., Raine, L. B., & Kramer, A. F. (2012). Childhood aerobic fitness predicts cognitive performance one year later. *Journal of Sports Sciences, 30*(5), 421–430.

Chang, Y. K., & Etnier, J. (2009). Exploring the dose–response relationship between resistance exercise intensity and cognitive function. *Journal of Sports and Exercise Psychology, 31*(5), 640–656.

Chang, Y., Pan, C. Y., Chen, F. T., Tsai, C. L., & Huang, C. C. (2012). Effect of resistance-exercise training on cognitive function in healthy older adults: A review. *Journal of Aging and Physical Activity, 20*, 497–517.

Chang, Y., Tsai, Y., Chen, T., & Hung, T. (2013). The impacts of coordinative exercise on executive function in kindergarten children: An ERP study. *Experimental Brain Research, 225*(2), 187–196.

Coco, M., Perciavalle, V., Cavallari, P., & Perciavalle, V. (2016). Effects of an exhaustive exercise on motor skill learning and on the excitability of primary motor cortex and supplementary motor area. *Medicine, 95*(11).

Colcombe, S. J., Erickson, K. I., Raz, N., Webb, A. G., Cohen, N. J., McAuley, E., & Kramer, A. F. (2003). Aerobic fitness reduces brain tissue loss in aging humans.

The Journals of Gerontology. Series A, Biological Sciences and Medical Sciences, 58(2), 176–180.

Colcombe, S. J., Kramer, A. F., Erickson, K. I., Scalf, P., McAuley, E., Cohen, N. J., & Elavsky, S. (2004). Cardiovascular fitness, cortical plasticity, and aging. *Proceedings of the National Academy of Sciences of the United States of America, 101*(9), 3316–3321.

Crabbe, J. B., & Dishman, R. K. (2004). Brain electrocortical activity during and after exercise: A quantitative synthesis. *Psychophysiology, 41*(4), 563–574.

Crova, C., Struzzolino, I., Marchetti, R., Masci, I., Vannozzi, G., Forte, R., & Pesce, C. (2014). Cognitively challenging physical activity benefits executive function in overweight children. *Journal of Sports Sciences, 32*(3), 201–211.

Davis, C. L., & Cooper, S. (2011). Fitness, fatness, cognition, behavior, and academic achievement among overweight children: Do cross-sectional associations correspond to exercise trial outcomes? *Preventive Medicine, 52*, S65–S69.

Davis, C. L., Tomporowski, P. D., McDowell, J. E., Austin, B. P., Miller, P. H., Yanasak, N. E., . . . Naglieri, J. A. (2011). Exercise improves executive function and achievement and alters brain activation in overweight children: A randomized, controlled trial. *Health Psychology: Official Journal of the Division of Health Psychology, American Psychological Association, 30*(1), 91–98.

Dickinson, J., Medhurst, C., & Whittingham, N. (1979). Warm-up and fatigue in skill acquisition and performance. *Journal of Motor Behavior, 11*(1), 81–86.

Donnelly, J. E., Hillman, C. H., Castelli, D., Etnier, J., Lee, S., Tomporowski, P., Lambourne, K., & Szabo-Reed, A. (2016). Physical activity, fitness, cognitive function, and academic achievement in children: A systematic review. *Medicine and Science in Sports and Exercise, 48*(6), 1197–1222.

Drollette, E. S., Scudder, M. R., Raine, L. B., Davis, M. R., Pontifex, M. B., Erickson, K. I., & Hillman, C. H. (2016). The sexual dimorphic association of cardiorespiratory fitness to working memory in children. *Developmental Science, 19*(1), 90–108.

Drollette, E. S., Scudder, M. R., Raine, L. B., Moore, R. D., Saliba, B. J., Pontifex, M. B., & Hillman, C. H. (2014). Acute exercise facilitates brain function and cognition in children who need it most: An ERP study of individual differences in inhibitory control capacity. *Developmental Cognitive Neuroscience, 7*, 53–64.

Drollette, E. S., Shishido, T., Pontifex, M. B., & Hillman, C. H. (2012). Maintenance of cognitive control during and after walking in preadolescent children. *Medicine and Science in Sports and Exercise, 44*(10), 2017–2024.

Etnier, J. L., Nowell, P. M., Landers, D. M., & Sibley, B. A. (2006). A meta-regression to examine the relationship between aerobic fitness and cognitive performance. *Brain Research Reviews, 52*(1), 119–130.

Fernandes, V., Ribeiro, M. L., Melo, T., de Tarso Maciel-Pinheiro, P., Giumarães, T. T., Ribeiro, S., & Deslandes, A. C. (2016). Motor coordination correlates with academic achievement and cognitive function in children. *Frontiers in Psychology* 15(7), 318.

Gallotta, M. C., Emerenziani, G. P., Iazzoni, S., Meucci, M., Baldari, C., & Guidetti, L. (2015). Impacts of coordinative training on normal weight and overweight/obese children's attentional performance. *Front Human Neuroscience, 28*(9), 577.

Gutin, B. (1966). Effect of increase in physical fitness on mental ability following physical and mental stress. *Research Quarterly, 37*(2), 211–220.

Gutmann, B., Mierau, A., Hülsdünker, T., Hildebrand, C., Przyklenk, A., Hollmann, W., & Strüder, H. K. (2015). Effects of physical exercise on individual resting state EEG alpha peak frequency. *Neural Plasticity, 5*, 717312. doi: 10.1155/2015/717312.

Harveson, A. T., Hannon, J. C., Brusseau, T. A., Podlog, L., Papadopoulos, C., Durrant, L. H., Hall, M. S., & Kang, K. D. (2016). Acute effects of 30 minutes resistance and aerobic exercise on cognition in a high school sample. *Research Quarterly for Exercise and Sports, 87*(2), 214–220.

Herting, M. M., & Nagel, B. J. (2013). Differences in brain activity during a verbal associative memory encoding task in high- and low-fit adolescents. *Journal of Cognitive Neuroscience, 25*(4), 595–612.

Hillman, C. H., Buck, S. M., Themanson, J. R., Pontifex, M. B., & Castelli, D. M. (2009). Aerobic fitness and cognitive development: Event-related brain potential and task performance indices of executive control in preadolescent children. *Developmental Psychology, 45*(1), 114–129.

Hillman, C. H., Erickson, K. I., & Kramer, A. F. (2008). Be smart, exercise your heart: Exercise effects on brain and cognition. *Nature Reviews Neuroscience, 9*(1), 58–65.

Hillman, C. H., Pontifex, M. B., Castelli, D. M., Khan, N. A., Raine, L. B., Scudder, M. R., & Kamijo, K. (2014). Effects of the FITKids randomized controlled trial on executive control and brain function. *Pediatrics, 134*(4), e1063–e1071.

Hillman, C. H., Pontifex, M. B., Raine, L. B., & Kramer, A. F. (2009). The effect of acute treadmill walking on cognitive control and academic achievement in preadolescent children. *Neuroscience, 159*(3), 1044–1054.

Hogan, M., Kiefer, M., Kubesch, S., Collins, P., Kilmartin, L., & Brosnan, M. (2013). The interactive effects of physical fitness and acute aerobic exercise on electrophysiological coherence and cognitive performance in adolescents. *Experimental Brain Research, 229*(1), 85–96.

Hopkins, M. E., Davis, F. C., VanTieghem, M. R., Whalen, P. J., & Bucci, D. J. (2012). Differential effects of acute and regular physical exercise on cognition and affect. *Neuroscience, 215*, 59–68.

Kamijo, K. (2009). Effects of acute exercise on event-related brain potentials. In W. Chodzko-Zajko, A. F. Kramer, L. W. Poon, W. Chodzko-Zajko, A. F. Kramer, & L. W. Poon (Eds.), *Enhancing cognitive functioning and brain plasticity.* (pp. 111–132). Champaign, IL: Human Kinetics.

Kamijo, K., Nishihira, Y., Higashiura, T., & Kuroiwa, K. (2007). The interactive effect of exercise intensity and task difficulty on human cognitive processing. *International Journal of Psychophysiology: Official Journal of the International Organization of Psychophysiology, 65*(2), 114–121.

Kamijo, K., & Takeda, Y. (2010). Regular physical activity improves executive function during task switching in young adults. *International Journal of Psychophysiology, 75*(3), 304–311.

Kantak, S. S., & Winstein, C. J. (2012). Learning–performance distinction and memory processes for motor skills: A focused review and perspective. *Behavioural Brain Research, 228*(1), 219–231.

Kim, Y. J., Cha, E. J., Kim, S. M., Kang, K. D., & Han, D. H. (2015). The effects of taekwondo training on brain connectivity and body intelligence. *Psychiatry Investigation, 12*(3), 335–340.

Kleim, J. A., Chan, S., Pringle, E., Schallert, K., Procaccio, V., Jimenez, R., & Cramer, S. C. (2006). BDNF val66met polymorphism is associated with modified experience-dependent plasticity in human motor cortex. *Nature Neuroscience, 9*(6), 735–737.

Koutsandréou, F., Niemann, C., Wegner, M., & Budde, H. (2016). Effects of motor versus cardiovascular exercise training on children's working memory. *Medicine and Science in Sports and Exercise, 48*(6), 1144–1152.

Krafft, C. E., Schaeffer, D. J., & Schwarz, N. F. (2014). Improved frontoparietal white matter integrity in overweight children is associated with attendance at an after-school exercise program. *Developmental Neuroscience, 36*(1), 1–9.

Lopes, L., Santos, R., Pereira, B., & Lopes, V. P. (2013). Associations between gross motor coordination and academic achievement in elementary school children. *Human Movement Science, 32*(1), 9–20.

Lu, B. (2003). BDNF and activity-dependent synaptic modulation. *Learning and Memory, 10*(2), 86–98.

Luz, C., Rodrigues, L. P., & Cordovil, R. (2015). The relationship between motor coordination and executive functions in 4th grade children. *European Journal of Developmental Psychology, 12*(2), 129–141.

Magnie, M. N., Bermon, S., Martin, F., Madany-Lounis, M., Suisse, G., Muhammad, W., & Dolisi, C. (2000). P300, N400, aerobic fitness, and maximal aerobic exercise. *Psychophysiology, 37*(3), 369–377.

Mang, C. S., Snow, N. J., Campbell, K. L., Ross, C. J., & Boyd, L. A. (2014). A single bout of high-intensity aerobic exercise facilitates response to paired associative stimulation and promotes sequence-specific implicit motor learning. *Journal of Applied Physiology (Bethesda, Md.: 1985), 117*(11), 1325–1336.

McCloskey, D. P., Adamo, D. S., & Anderson, B. J. (2001). Exercise increases metabolic capacity in the motor cortex and striatum, but not in the hippocampus. *Brain Research, 891*(1), 168–175.

McDonnell, M. N., Buckley, J. D., Opie, G. M., Ridding, M. C., & Semmler, J. G. (2013). A single bout of aerobic exercise promotes motor cortical neuroplasticity. *Journal of Applied Physiology, 114*(9), 1174–1182.

McMorris, T., & Hale, B. J. (2012). Differential effects of differing intensities of acute exercise on speed and accuracy of cognition: A meta-analytical investigation. *Brain and Cognition, 80*(3), 338–351.

McMorris, T., Hale, B. J., Corbett, J., Robertson, K., & Hodgson, C. I. (2015). Does acute exercise affect the performance of whole-body, psychomotor skills in an inverted-U fashion? A meta-analytic investigation. *Physiology and Behavior, 141,* 180–189.

McMorris, T., Sproule, J., Turner, A., & Hale, B. J. (2011). Acute, intermediate intensity exercise, and speed and accuracy in working memory tasks: A meta-analytical comparison of effects. *Physiology and Behavior, 102*(3–4), 421–428.

Mierau, A., Hülsdünker, T., Mierau, J., Hense, A., Hense, J., & Strüder, H. K. (2014). Acute exercise induces cortical inhibition and reduces arousal in response to visual stimulation in young children. *International Journal of Developmental Neuroscience, 34,* 1–8.

Mokgothu, C. J., & Gallagher, J. D. (2010). Effects of aerobic fitness on attention, memory and decision-making in children. *International Journal of Body Composition Research Impact, 8,* 37–44.

Moore, R. D., Drollette, E. S., Scudder, M. R., Bharij, A., & Hillman, C. H. (2014). The influence of cardiorespiratory fitness on strategic, behavioral, and electrophysiological indices of arithmetic cognition in preadolescent children. *Frontiers in Human Neuroscience, 8,* 258.

Nachev, P., Kennard, C., & Husain, M. (2008). Functional role of the supplementary and pre-supplementary motor areas. *Nature Reviews in Neuroscience, 9*(11), 856–869.

Nakamura, Y., Nishimoto, K., Akamatu, M., Takahashi, M., & Maruyama, A. (1999). The effect of jogging on P300 event related potentials. *Electromyography and Clinical Neurophysiology, 39*(2), 71–74.

Niederer, I., Kriemler, S., Gut, J., Schindler, C., Barral, J., & Puder, J. J. (2011). Relationship of aerobic fitness and motor skills with memory and attention in preschoolers (Ballabeina): A cross-sectional and longitudinal study. *BMC Pediatrics, 11,* 34.

Pack, M. D., Cotten, D. J., & Biasiotto, J. (1974). Effect of four fatigue levels on performance and learning of a novel dynamic balance skill. *Journal of Motor Behavior, 6*(3), 191–197.

Perini, R., Bortoletto, M., Capogrosso, M., Fertonani, A., & Miniussi, C. (2016). Acute effects of aerobic exercise promote learning. *Scientific Reports, 6,* 25440.

Pesce, C., Cereatti, L., Forte, R., Crova, C., & Casella, R. (2011). Acute and chronic exercise effects on attentional control in older road cyclists. *Gerontology, 57*(2), 121–128.

Peters, J., Dauvermann, M., Mette, C., Platen, P., Franke, J., Hinrichs, T., & Daum, I. (2009). Voxel-based morphometry reveals an association between aerobic capacity and grey matter density in the right anterior insula. *Neuroscience, 163*(4), 1102–1108.

Pontifex, M. B., & Hillman, C. H. (2007). Neuroelectric and behavioral indices of interference control during acute cycling. *Clinical Neurophysiology, 118*(3), 570–580.

Pontifex, M. B., Hillman, C. H., & Polich, J. (2009). Age, physical fitness, and attention: P3a and P3b. *Psychophysiology, 46*(2), 379–387.

Pontifex, M. B., Parks, A. C., Henning, D. A., & Kamijo, K. (2015). Single bouts of exercise selectively sustain attentional processes. *Psychophysiology, 52*(5), 618–625.

Pontifex, M. B., Raine, L. B., Johnson, C. R., Chaddock, L., Voss, M. W., Cohen, N. J., . . . Hillman, C. H. (2011). Cardiorespiratory fitness and the flexible modulation of cognitive control in preadolescent children. *Journal of Cognitive Neuroscience, 23*(6), 1332–1345.

Prakash, R. S., Voss, M. W., Erickson, K. I., & Kramer, A. F. (2015). Physical activity and cognitive vitality. *Annual Review of Psycholgy, 3*(66), 769–797.

Raine, L. B., Lee, H. K., Saliba, B. J., Chaddock-Heyman, L., Hillman, C. H., & Kramer, A. F. (2013). The influence of childhood aerobic fitness on learning and memory. *PloS One, 8*(9), e72666.

Raine, L. B., Scudder, M. R., Saliba, B. J., Kramer, A. F., & Hillman, C. (2016). Aerobic fitness and context processing in preadolescent children. *Journal of Physical Activity and Health, 13*(1), 94–101.

Rajab, A. S., Crane, D. E., Middleton, L. E., Robertson, A. D., Hampson, M., & MacIntosh, B. J. (2014). A single session of exercise increases connectivity in sensorimotor-related brain networks: A resting-state fMRI study in young healthy adults. *Frontiers in Human Neuroscience, 8*, 625.

Roig, M., Nordbrandt, S., Geertsen, S. S., & Nielsen, J. B. (2013). The effects of cardiovascular exercise on human memory: A review with meta-analysis. *Neuroscience and Biobehavioral Reviews, 37*(8), 1645–1666.

Roig, M., Skriver, K., Lundbye-Jensen, J., Kiens, B., & Nielsen, J. B. (2012). A single bout of exercise improves motor memory. *PloS One, 7*(9), e44594.

Roig, M., Thomas, R., Mang, C. S., Snow, N. J., Ostadan, F., Boyd, L. A., & Lundbye-Jensen, J. (2016). Time-dependent effects of cardiovascular exercise on memory. *Exercise and Sport Sciences Reviews, 44*(2), 81–88.

Sage, M. D., Beyer, K. B., Laylor, M., Liang, C., Roy, E. A., & McIlroy, W. E. (2016). A single session of exercise as a modulator of short-term learning in healthy individuals. *Neuroscience Letters, 629*, 92–98.

Schaeffer, D. J., Krafft, C. E., & Schwarz, N. F. (2014). An 8-month exercise intervention alters frontotemporal white matter integrity in overweight children. *Psychophysiology, 51*(8), 728–733.

Schneider, S., Vogt, T., Frysch, J., Guardiera, P., & Strüder, H. K. (2009). School sport – a neurophysiological approach. *Neuroscience Letters, 467*(2), 131–134.

Scudder, M. R., Drollette, E. S., Pontifex, M. B., & Hillman, C. H. (2012). Neuroelectric indices of goal maintenance following a single bout of physical activity. *Biological Psychology, 89*(2), 528–531.

Scudder, M. R., Lambourne, K., Drollette, E. S., Herrmann, S. D., Washburn, R. A., Donnelly, J. E., & Hillman C. H. (2014). Aerobic capacity and cognitive control in elementary school-age children. *Medicine and Science in Sports and Exercise, 46*(5), 1025–1035.

Singh, A. M., Neva, J. L., & Staines, W. R. (2014). Acute exercise enhances the response to paired associative stimulation-induced plasticity in the primary motor cortex. *Experimental Brain Research, 232*(11), 3675–3685.

Singh, A. M., & Staines, W. R. (2015). The effects of acute aerobic exercise on the primary motor cortex. *Journal of Motor Behavior, 47*(4), 328–339.

Skriver, K., Roig, M., Lundbye-Jensen, J., Pingel, J., Helge, J. W., Kiens, B., & Nielsen, J. B. (2014). Acute exercise improves motor memory: Exploring potential biomarkers. *Neurobiology of Learning and Memory, 116*, 46–58.

Snow, N. J., Mang, C. S., Roig, M., McDonnell, M. N., Campbell, K. L., & Boyd, L. A. (2016). The effect of an acute bout of moderate-intensity aerobic exercise on motor learning of a continuous tracking task. *PloS One, 11*(2), e0150039.

Stroth, S., Kubesch, S., Dieterle, K., Ruchsow, M., Heim, R., & Kiefer, M. (2009). Physical fitness, but not acute exercise modulates event-related potential indices for executive control in healthy adolescents. *Brain Research, 1269*, 114–124.

Thacker, J. S., Middleton, L. E., McIlroy, W. E., & Staines, W. R. (2014). The influence of an acute bout of aerobic exercise on cortical contributions to motor preparation and execution. *Physiological Reports, 2*(10), 10.14814/phy2.12178.

Themanson, J. R., & Hillman, C. H. (2006). Cardiorespiratory fitness and acute aerobic exercise effects on neuroelectric and behavioral measures of action monitoring. *Neuroscience, 141*(2), 757–767.

Thomas, R., Beck, M. M., Lind, R. R., Korsgaard Johnsen, L., Geertsen, S. S., Christiansen, L., . . . Lundbye-Jensen, J. (2016a). Acute exercise and motor memory consolidation: The role of exercise timing. *Neural Plasticity, 2016*, 6205452.

Thomas, R., Johnsen, L. K., Geertsen, S. S., Christiansen, L., Ritz, C., Roig, M., & Lundbye-Jensen, J. (2016b). Acute exercise and motor memory consolidation: The role of exercise intensity. *PloS One, 11*(7), e0159589.

Tomporowski, P. D. (2003). Effects of acute bouts of exercise on cognition. *Acta Psychologica, 112*(3), 297–324.

Tsai, C. L., Wang, C. H., Pan, C. Y., Chen, F. C, Huang, T. H., & Chou, F. Y. (2014). Executive function and endocrinological responses to acute resistance exercise. *Frontiers in Behavioral Neuroscience, 1*(8), 262.

van Praag, H., Shubert, T., Zhao, C., & Gage, F. H. (2005). Exercise enhances learning and hippocampal neurogenesis in aged mice. *The Journal of Neuroscience: The Official Journal of the Society for Neuroscience, 25*(38), 8680–8685.

Vissing, J., Andersen, M., & Diemer, N. H. (1996). Exercise-induced changes in local cerebral glucose utilization in the rat. *Journal of Cerebral Blood Flow and Metabolism, 16*(4), 729–736.

Voelcker-Rehage, C., Godde, B., & Staudinger, U. M. (2011). Cardiovascular and coordination training differentially improve cognitive performance and neural processing in older adults. *Frontiers in Human Neuroscience, 5*, 26. doi: 10.3389/fnhum.2011.00026.

Voelcker-Rehage, C., & Niemann, C. (2013). Structural and functional brain changes related to different types of physical activity across the life span. *Neuroscience and Biobehavioral Reviews, 37*(9 Pt B), 2268–2295.

Voss, M. W., Chaddock, J. S., Kim, M., Vanpatter, M. B., Pontifex, L. B., Raine, N. J., Cohen, C. H., Hillman, C. H., & Kramer, A. F. (2011). Aerobic fitness is associated with greater efficiency of the network underlying cognitive control in preadolescent children. *Neuroscience, 199*, 166–176.

Wegner, M., Koedijker, J. M., & Budde, H. (2014). The effect of acute exercise and psychosocial stress on fine motor skills and testosterone concentration in the saliva of high school students. *PloS One, 9*(3), e92953.

Weingarten, G. (1973). Mental performance during physical exertion: The benefits of being phyiscally fit. *International Journal of Sport Psychology, 4*, 16–26.

Winneke, A. H., Hübner, L., Godde, B., Voelcker-Rehage, C. (in preparation). Brief bout of exercise boosts neurophysiological marker of attentional control.

Wu, C. T., & Hillman, C. H. (2013). Aerobic fitness and the attentional blink in preadolescent children. *Neuropsychology, 27*(6), 642–653.

Yerkes, R. M., & Dodson, J. (1908). The relation of strength of stimulus to rapidity of habit-formation. *Journal of Comparative Neurology and Psychology, 18*, 459–482.

Zervas, Y., Danis, A., & Klissouras, V. (1991). Influence of physical exertion on mental performance with reference to training. *Perceptual and Motor Skills, 72*(3), 1215–1221.

Chapter 9

The impact of physical activities on age-related brain function and structure and the underlying neural mechanisms

Patrick Müller, Anita Hökelmann and Notger G. Müller

Introduction

Western societies are currently experiencing a tremendous demographic change with an unprecedented increase in absolute and relative numbers of senior citizens. This change is a consequence of two processes: falling birth rates on the one hand, and continuously increasing life expectancies on the other hand. The demographic change entails a plethora of challenges for the healthcare system and for democratic society in general. As the incidence of many diseases correlates with age, the number of persons affected by age-related diseases will rise; at the same time the complexity and quantity (multimorbidity) of impairments will increase. In that respect, neurodegenerative diseases with their severe cognitive deficits and eventual loss of self-dependence, i.e. dementia, constitute a major problem and represent one of the largest health issues.

According to recent predictions, the global number of people affected by dementia will rise from currently 40 million to 115 million by 2050, whereby Alzheimer's disease as the most common cause of dementia accounts for up to 75% of cases. Hope for the imminent development of disease-modifying drug therapies has faded after more than 130 clinical trials with new drugs having failed in the recent past (Rubinstein et al., 2015). In this context, concepts of healthy ageing are becoming increasingly important. Several studies indicate that physical exercise could play a key role in healthy ageing and prevention of cognitive decline and neurodegenerative diseases.

Normal ageing, mild cognitive impairment (MCI) and Alzheimer's disease

The ageing process varies widely between individuals; nevertheless, it is apparent that many physical, cognitive and motoric parameters degrade in old age. Impairments of memory and other cognitive functions are attributed to structural and functional alterations of the ageing brain (Gregory, Parker & Thompson, 2012). Among them reduced cerebrovascular blood circulation along with metabolite and beta-amyloid plaque deposits are of special importance (Jernigan et al., 2001). Intact cognitive functions are crucial for successful ageing and self-dependence of seniors. Therefore, much research in neuroscience is currently directed towards the understanding of the underlying neural mechanisms for decreased cognitive functions, especially fluid intelligence, with age.

The 'normal' process of ageing

Age-related structural involution processes occur in almost all cortical and subcortical regions, whereby the manifestation varies greatly between different regions (Good et al., 2001; Gregory, Parker & Thompson, 2012). The most significant age-related alterations are reported for prefrontal and temporal areas (Raz et al., 2005). These areas are of particular importance for executive functions and memory. Just as the neural changes during the 'normal' ageing process differ across the brain, specific cognitive domains are also differently affected by ageing. In particular, executive functions, episodic memory, working memory and alertness regress with age. On the other hand, cognitive functions such as autobiographical memory are hardly affected by the normal ageing process (Hedden & Gabrieli, 2004).

Mild cognitive impairment

The transition between normal and pathological ageing, namely dementia, is smooth and clinically often difficult to detect. The most common model for this transitional phase is that of MCI (Petersen et al., 1999). MCI is defined as a subjective deterioration in intellectual performance, which can be objectified by below-average cognitive test results. Unlike in dementia, daily living abilities are preserved. MCI is associated with an increased risk for later Alzheimer's disease, especially when memory functions are affected in the first place (amnestic MCI: Mitchell & Shiri-Feshki, 2009).

Alzheimer's disease

First described by Alois Alzheimer in 1906, and later named after him, probable Alzheimer's disease is diagnosed according to the tenth edition of *International Classification of Diseases* (ICD-10: World Health Organization, 2015) when signs of dementia are present and other potential causes for the observed cognitive deficits have been excluded (e.g. vascular encephalopathy, vitamin deficiency, alcohol abuse). In order to diagnose Alzheimer's disease unambiguously, histological postmortem examinations of the brain are required. These will reveal the typical neuropathological changes, already described by Alzheimer, namely intracellular tau tangles and extracellular beta-amyloid plaques. These are accompanied by neuronal loss and, consequently, brain atrophy (Förstl, Short, & Hartmann, 2011). Only two types of drugs are currently approved for the treatment of Alzheimer's disease: the non-competitive N-methyl-D-aspartate (NMDA) antagonist memantine and the acetylcholinesterase inhibitors donepezil, galantamine and rivastigmine (Deuschl et al., 2009). These drugs relieve symptoms to some extent but have no influence on the progress of the neurodegenerative processes itself. Whether such disease-modifying drugs, e.g. immunotherapies, will be developed at some time in the future is an open question (Cummings et al., 2014). In the meantime the focus of research is directed to so-called modifiable risk factors. Norton et al. (2014) postulate that one-third of global Alzheimer's disease is related to modifiable risk factors. The following factors have been identified (Barnes & Yaffe, 2011):

- Low educational attainment
- Physical inactivity
- Depression
- Overweight
- Midlife hypertension
- Smoking
- Diabetes mellitus.

These factors open an opportunity for various preventive strategies. According to a computational model, a 10% reduction of risk factors per decade could lead to an 8.3% decrease in the global Alzheimer's prevalence by 2050 (Barnes & Yaffe, 2011).

Prevention approaches

Despite the age-related degradation processes, the brain is able to adapt dynamically to changing requirements throughout life, both functionally and structurally. This adaptive process is called neuroplasticity. Sporting activities (Gregory, Parker & Thompson, 2012), healthy diets (Murphy, Dias & Thuret, 2014), and social contacts (Fratiglioni, Paillard-Borg & Winblad, 2004) have all been shown to have positive outcomes on brain function. Therefore, these measures have a potential in the prevention of neurodegenerative diseases.

Neurodegenerative diseases, such as Alzheimer's disease, are multifactorial and characterized by a long preclinical or prodromal phase, in which neuropathological changes have already started but have not yet resulted in detectable clinical symptoms as initially these changes can be compensated for (Sperling et al., 2011). During this preclinical phase it is impossible to rule out that a person who appears cognitively unimpaired already suffers from Alzheimer's pathology. On the other hand, this long preclinical phase opens the opportunity for a targeted intervention in terms of neuroprotection. In this respect, it is noteworthy that because neurodegenerative dementias are usually found in advanced age, even a small delay of the neurodegenerative process can have a substantial clinical impact on the quality of life of an affected person. When delayed, an aged person may die before the disease has progressed to an advanced stage where the most feared symptom, the loss of self-reliance, manifests (Figure 9.1).

The starting point for preventive measures is the reduction of cardiovascular risk factors (high blood pressure, obesity, diabetes mellitus), adaptation of lifestyle factors (nutrition, exercise, alcohol and drug consumption, smoking) as well as other modifiable aspects, for example, sleep (Steiner, Witte & Flöel, 2011). All these measures can be assumed to convey neuroprotective effects, whereby neuroprotection not only includes all measures taken to reduce the risk factors but also those that enhance neuroplastic processes (Figure 9.2). Neuroplasticity is based on the ability of the human

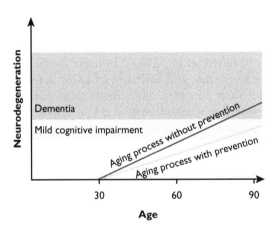

Figure 9.1 Schematic account of the effect of prevention on neurodegeneration and clinical symptoms. A slight delay in the neurodegenerative process can have a relevant impact on clinical symptoms and quality of life in old age.

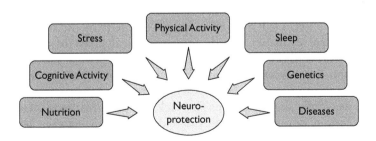

Figure 9.2 Factors that contribute to neuroprotection.

brain continuously and dynamically to adapt to ever-changing requirements, both structurally and functionally.

In the following, the impact of diverse lifestyle factors on neuroplasticity and the prevention of dementia will be illustrated. The main focus is on the influence of physical exercise, as lack of physical activity presumably represents the most important modifiable risk factor in Western industrial nations (Barnes & Yaffe, 2011).

Neuroprotection by physical activities

Epidemiological studies

Several epidemiological studies have examined how lifestyle factors correlate with cognitive performance or the incidence of dementia in old age. Evidence for positive impact of physical activity on neuroplasticity in the elderly was reported both in observational and interventional studies (Bamadis et al., 2014). For example, it was stated that older individuals who had indicated that they had adhered to a physically active lifestyle had a lower risk of developing dementia later in life than less active persons (Larson et al., 2006; Verghese et al., 2003). In more detail, Larson et al. (2006) captured the frequency and intensity of sport activities in 1,740 healthy seniors older than 65 years. Individuals who were physically active at least three times a week showed a 34% smaller risk of dementia after a mean observation period of 6.2 years. A meta-analysis including 16 prospective studies reported a 28–45% reduction in risk of dementia related to physical activity (Hamer & Chida, 2009). However, correlation and causality cannot be distinguished in observational studies. Therefore, an inverse causality between physical activity and dementia risk is also conceivable: Persons in a preclinical phase of dementia may refrain from sporting activities as they may be already less fit or motivated compared to really healthy persons. In retrospective observational studies, this might result in overestimating the protective impact of physical activity. Indeed, in the study of Verghese et al. (2003), the authors could not confirm the protective effect of recreational activities when persons who developed a manifest dementia over the first 9 years of the observation period were excluded from the analysis. These persons, at the time of inclusion, were probably already in a preclinical phase of dementia. Additionally, the authors did not find a correlation between the amount of activity and the incidence of dementia; that is, the impact on the risk of dementia was not lower for persons who were very active compared to those who were only slightly active. This lack of a dose–response relationship casts certain doubts on the postulated correlation between leisure activities and dementia risk.

Stronger conclusions can be derived from longitudinal intervention trials in which subjects are randomized to either an experimental or a control group. Such randomized clinical trials usually assess surrogate markers for the risk of dementia, i.e. cognitive performance or neuroimaging of the participants' brains, as otherwise the study duration would be too long. In general, these studies propose a positive effect of sport on brain function and structure (reviewed in Bamadis et al., 2014). For example, Erickson et al. (2011) showed that seniors who took part in a 12-month aerobic fitness training programme had larger hippocampal volumes than their control counterparts who engaged in stretching exercises. Indeed, aerobic endurance sport is the best-studied intervention, as detailed below.

Impact of aerobic endurance training

The World Health Organization general sport-for-health training recommendations (2010) favour traditional endurance sports like bicycling and walking for the elderly because these types are characterized by repetitive movements which strengthen the cardiovascular system and simultaneously involve only a minimal risk of injury.

In 2003, Colcombe et al. examined for the first time the relationship between aerobic fitness measured by means of maximal oxygen uptake (Vo_{2max}) and brain volume. This cross-sectional study revealed typical age-related volume reductions of the grey matter in frontal, temporal and parietal regions, and in the anterior white matter. Compared to individuals with low aerobic fitness, individuals with high aerobic fitness showed larger volumes, especially in brain regions, which are most affected by the ageing process. In a cross-sectional study comprising 165 participants, Erickson et al. (2009) found cardiorespiratory fitness, also determined by Vo_{2max}, as a predictor for left and right hippocampus volume. Furthermore, the authors postulate that the hippocampus serves as a mediator between aerobic fitness and memory performance.

In contrast to cross-sectional studies, interventional longitudinal studies enable one to deduce causalities. Most of these studies feature a positive impact of endurance training on cognitive function and brain plasticity in the elderly (Bamadis et al., 2014). However, it must be pointed out that these studies are often beset with methodological problems (Miller et al., 2012). For example, although the experimental group of the interventional study of Erickson et al. (2011) showed a stronger increase in certain brain volumes than the control group, no significant improvement of memory performance was observed. Moreover, there was no significant correlation between the improvement of fitness and memory, nor did the changes in brain-derived neurotrophic factor (BDNF) level (see below) correlate with memory performances.

Impact of strength training

The current research situation regarding the impact of strength training on neuroplasticity and dementia prevention is deficient. Some studies report positive effects of strength training on cognitive functions in healthy seniors (Cassilhas et al., 2007; Liu-Ambrose et al., 2010). However, the achieved improvements were not dependent on training frequency (once or twice a week) or exercise intensity (from moderately to highly intensive). This lack of a dose–response interaction diminishes the interpretability of the results. By contrast, Kimura et al. (2010) did not find any significant improvements of executive functions after a 12-week strength training programme with three weekly training units. These contradictory results underline the necessity for further investigations regarding the impact of strength training in the context of dementia prevention.

Impact of sensorimotor coordination training

The lderly still have the ability to learn new and complex motion patterns. For instance, Boyke et al. (2008) studied 93 healthy seniors who learned to juggle over 3 months. Using voxel-based morphometry of magnetic resonance brain images, the researchers found volume increases in the visual cortex, the left hippocampus and bilaterally in the nucleus accumbens. The volume increases in the hippocampus and nucleus accumbens, however, were not stable and vanished after another 3 months without further training. Sehm et al. (2014) could also demonstrate volume increases in the left hippocampus of healthy seniors after 6-week balance training with a 45-minute exercise unit per week.

Is dancing an optimum measure for neuroprotection?

Results from animal studies suggest that a combination of physical and cognitive activity is superior to one-dimensional intervention training in inducing long-lasting neuroplasticity (Kempermann et al., 2010). According to this view, exercising (treadmill running) would stimulate neurogenesis in the hippocampus of mice. In order for the newborn cells to be integrated into the brain permanently, however, additional sensory enrichment, i.e. equipping the animals' cage with toys, would be required; otherwise the newly formed nerve cells would not survive. Dancing has been suggested as a human homologue of this combined challenge as it involves both physical exercise and cognitive performance, such as memory of the choreography and spatial orientation (Kattenstroth et al., 2013). This combination, in the context of evolutionary and epigenetic factors, is the basis of neuroplastic processes. During dancing much afferent (perception of melody and rhythm in context of time pressure) and efferent (transformation into complex

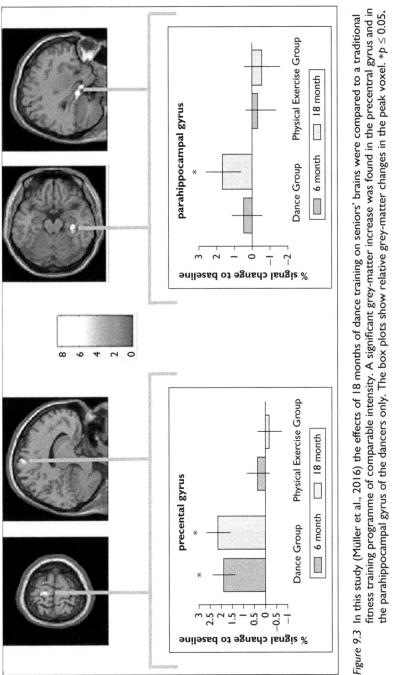

Figure 9.3 In this study (Müller et al., 2016) the effects of 18 months of dance training on seniors' brains were compared to a traditional fitness training programme of comparable intensity. A significant grey-matter increase was found in the precentral gyrus and in the parahippocampal gyrus of the dancers only. The box plots show relative grey-matter changes in the peak voxel. *$p \leq 0.05$.

movements, which involved different body parts) information must be processed in the brain. Moreover dancing involves different balance situations (one-leg standing position, single-leg turns, and bipedal leg turns) which require the integration of input from vestibular, visual und sensory systems.

Based on these considerations we recently performed a study with 26 healthy seniors who took part either in an 18-month dance or a traditional sport fitness programme. The dance programme was especially designed to boost constant learning by presenting participants with new choreography all the time. Compared to participants in the sports group, dancers showed volume increases in brain grey matter in parahippocampal and precentral regions (Müller et al., 2016; Figure 9.3).

The results suggest that dance training is particularly suitable for dementia prevention since volume decreases in parahippocampal regions are an early finding in Alzheimer's disease (Echávarri et al., 2011). Indeed, the above-mentioned study by Verghese et al. (2003) revealed that regular dancing, in comparison to all other recreational activities examined, was associated with the largest (76%) reduction of risk of later dementia. As mentioned above, the lack of a dose–response relationship and the potential inclusion of preclinical patients somehow diminish the validity of this observation. Moreover, and regarding our own study, it should be critically stated that the stronger neuroplastic effects in the dancers did not result in better cognitive function than in the sportsmen.

Mechanisms of neuroplasticity in response to physical activity

Several theories try to explain the neuroprotective and neuroplastic effects of physical activity. However, the exact neurobiological mechanisms are still largely unknown (Kempermann, 2015). Kirk-Sanchez and McGough (2014) assume that exercise affects neuroplasticity of the brain via two mechanisms of action. They suggest that endurance sports cause both generally improved cardiovascular health and an increased level of neurotrophic factors. These two factors would stimulate neurogenesis, synaptogenesis and further neuroplastic processes, resulting in improved cognitive performance. Since cardiovascular diseases (hypertension, dyslipidaemia and diabetes) are known to be a risk factor for all-type dementias, cardiovascular effects could provide a universal explanatory approach for the neuroprotective impact of physical activity. Regarding the significance of neurotrophic growth factors such as BDNF, insulin-like growth factor (IGF-1) and vascular endothelial growth factor (VEGF), research results are inconsistent (Cotman et al., 2007).

BDNF plays a key role in early brain development and later in life in adaptive changes and survival of neurons. The BDNF level is modulated by many factors, among them stress, physical activity or dietary restriction (Laske & Eschweiler, 2007). Several studies reported an increase of

BDNF levels following sporting interventions (Erickson et al., 2012; Müller et al., 2016). Others, however, failed to observe changes in any neurotrophic factor assessed (Maass et al., 2015). Research in animals draws a more consistent picture; here increases in BDNF, IGF-1, VEGF, neurotrophic growth factor and antioxidants as a result of exercise are routinely reported (e.g. Constans et al., 2016). BDNF, in particular, is therefore assumed as a significant mediator of sports-induced neuroplasticity.

Besides neurotrophic growth factors many other molecular mediators of brain plasticity have been proposed (Figure 9.4). Physical activity has acute and chronic effects on stress, metabolism, transcription factors, inflammation and epigenetic factors. These factors strongly interact and induce complex biochemical cascades that underlie brain plasticity (Erickson et al., 2012; Thomas et al., 2012).

Possible cellular mechanisms of grey-matter plasticity are neurogenesis, angiogenesis, synaptogenesis, glial changes and axon sprouting. Candidate mechanisms of white-matter plasticity are volume increases based on angiogenesis and glial adaptations and increases in fractional anisotropy based on myelin changes and fibre organization (Zatorre et al., 2012). Results from animal research suggest different time courses for the different components of brain plasticity. Processes of neurogenesis and angiogenesis develop faster than volume increases in astrocytes and neuropil. Additionally, animal studies show different components of structural brain changes when only aerobic activity is promoted than when it is combined with sensory and social enrichment. While aerobic activity alone only induces angiogenesis and neurogenesis, aerobic activity together with enrichment leads to additional changes in neuropil and astrocytes.

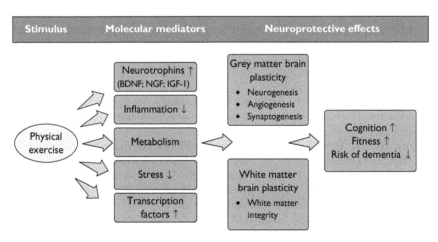

Figure 9.4 Theoretical model of physical exercise-induced neuroplasticity and the underlying neurobiological mechanisms. BDNF, brain-derived neurotrophic factor; NGF, neurotrophic growth factor; IGF-1, insulin-like growth factor.

Conclusion and practical recommendations

In summary, prevention of age-associated diseases such as Alzheimer's dementia by the modification of lifestyle factors seems possible – albeit to a limited extent. Numerous epidemiological, cross-sectional and interventional studies suggest that particularly long-term physical in combination with cognitive activity can enhance brain structure and function and has the potential to reduce the risk of dementia. It is therefore recommended to adhere to an active lifestyle from early in life. This lifestyle should comprise cognitive, physical and social components. Even slight modifications in lifestyle seem to be reasonable, such as learning a new musical instrument, using a bicycle as vehicle for short distances, using the stairs instead of an elevator, eating a Mediterranean diet and maintaining social relationships.

In summary, there are still considerable gaps in knowledge, especially regarding the underlying neuronal mechanisms of activity-induced brain changes, which need to be filled. Further, randomized clinical long-term intervention trials are needed that assess not only surrogate markers (e.g. brain volumes) for the risk of dementia but the real incidence of neurodegenerative diseases in the experimental and control group. Fortunately, such studies are under way (e.g. FINGER, Kivipelto et al., 2013). These trials fulfil the stringent criteria of pharmacological and clinical studies (representative sample, double-blinded, predetermined outcomes). Future research should also assess which type of sport, which duration and which intensity are most effective in terms of neuroprotection and which combination of various measures (exercise, nutrition, mental activity, etc.) could be particularly reasonable. Furthermore, individual differences and preferences in terms of an individualized (specified) prevention should be considered to determine the most effective individual form of intervention and, moreover, to strengthen motivation and compliance. For one thing is clear: the best preventive measure is worth nothing unless it is kept going.

References

Bamadis, P.D., Vivas, A.B., Styliadis, C. et al. (2014). A review of physical and cognitive interventions in. *Neuroscience and Biobehavioral Reviews, 44,* 206–220.

Barnes, D.E., & Yaffe, K. (2011). The projected impact of risk factor reduction on Alzheimer's disease prevalence. *Lancet Neurology, 10,* 819–828.

Boyke, J., Driemeyer, J., Gaser, C. et al. (2008). Training-induced brain structure changes in the elderly. *The Journal of Neuroscience, 28,* 7031–7035.

Cassilhas, R.C., Viana, V.A., Grassmann, V. et al. (2007). The impact of resistance exercise on the cognitive function of the elderly. *Medicine and Science in Sports and Exercise, 39*(8), 1401–1407.

Colcombe, S.J., Erickson, K.I., Raz, N. et al. (2003). Aerobic fitness reduces brain tissue loss in aging humans. *Journal of Gerontology: Medical Sciences, 58A*(2), 176–180.

Constans, A., Pin-Barre, C., Temprado, J.-J., Decherchi, P., & Laurin, J. (2016). Influence of aerobic training and combinations of interventions on cognition and neuroplasticity after stroke. *Frontiers in Aging Neuroscience, 8*, 164. doi: 10.3389/fnagi.2016.00164.

Cotman, C.W., Berchtold, N.C., & Christie, L.A. (2007). Exercise builds brain health: Key roles of growth factor cascades and inflammation. *Trends in Neurosciences, 30*, 464–472.

Cummings, J.L., Morstoff, T., & Zhong, K. (2014). Alzheimer's disease drug-development pipeline: Few candidates, frequent failures. *Alzheimer's Research and Therapy, 6*, 37–42.

Deuschl, G., Maier, W., Jessen, F. et al. (2009). *S3 Leitlinie Demenzen In: Diagnose- und Behandlungsleitlinie Demenz*. Deutsche Gesellschaft für Neurologie. Heidelberg: Springer.

Echávarri, C., Aalten, P., Uyling, H.B.M. et al. (2011). Atrophy in the parahippocampal gyrus as an early biomarker of Alzheimer's disease. *Brain Structure and Function, 215*(3–4), 265–271.

Erickson, K.I., Miller, D.I., & Roecklein, K.A. (2012). The aging hippocampus: Interactions between exercise, depression and BDNF. *Neuroscientist, 18*, 82–97.

Erickson, K.I., Prakash, R.S., Voss, M.W. et al. (2009). Aerobic fitness is associated with hippocampal volume in elderly humans. *Hippokampus, 19*(10), 1030–1039.

Erickson, K.I., Voss, M.W., Prakash, R.S. et al. (2011). Exercise training increases size of hippocampus and improves memory. *Proceedings of the National Academy of Sciences of the U.S.A., 108*(7), 3017–3022.

Förstl, H., Short, A., & Hartmann, T. (2011). Alzheimer-Demenz. In: Förstl, H. (Eds.), *Demenzen in Theorie und Praxis*. Heidelberg: Springer.

Fratiglioni, L., Paillard-Borg, S., & Winblad B (2004). An active and socially integrated lifestyle in late life might protect against dementia. *Lancet Neurology, 3*(6), 343–353.

Good, C.D., Johnsrude, I.S., Ashburner, J. et al. (2001). A voxel-based morphometric study of ageing in 465 normal adult human brains. *Neuroimage, 14*, 21–36.

Gregory, S.M., Parker, B., & Thompson, P.D. (2012). Physical activity, cognitive function, and brain health: What is the role of exercise training in the prevention of dementia? *Brain Sciences, 2*(4), 684–708.

Hamer, M., & Chida, Y. (2009). Physical activity and risk of neurodegenerative disease: A systematic review of prospective evidence. *Psychological Medicine, 39*(1), 3–11.

Hedden, T., & Gabrieli, J.D. (2004). Insights into the ageing mind: A view from cognitive neuroscience. *Nature Reviews Neuroscience, 5*(2), 87–96.

Jernigan, T.L., Archibald, S.L., Fennema-Notestine, C. et al. (2001). Effects of age on tissues and regions of the cerebrum and cerebellum. *Neurobiology of Aging, 22*(4), 581–594.

Kattenstroth, J.C., Kalisch, T., Holt, S. et al. (2013). Six months of dance intervention enhances postural, sensorimotor, and cognitive performance in elderly without affecting cardiorespiratory functions. *Frontiers in Aging Neuroscience, 5*, 1–16.

Kempermann, G. (2015). Neurodegenerative Erkrankungen und zelluläre Plastizität als sportmedizinische Herausforderung. *Deutsche Zeitschrift für Sportmedizin, 66*, 31–35, doi: 10.5960/dzsm.2015.163.

Kempermann, G., Fabel, K., Ehninger, D. et al. (2010). Why and how physical activity promotes experience-induced brain plasticity. *Frontiers in Neuroscience, 4*, 189.

Kimura, K., Obuchi, S., Arai, T. et al. (2010). The influence of short-term strength training on health-related quality of life and executive cognitive function. *Journal of Physiological Anthropology, 29*(3), 95–101.

Kirk-Sanchez, N., & McGough E. (2014). Physical exercise and cognitive performance in the elderly: Current perspectives. *Clinical Interventions in Aging, 9*, 51–62.

Kivipelto, M., Solomon, A., Ahtiluoto, S. et al. (2013). The Finnish Geriatric intervention study to prevent cognitive impairment and disability (FINGER): Study design and progress. *Alzheimers Dementia, 9*, 657–665.

Laske, C., & Eschweiler, G.W. (2007) Brain-derived neurotrophic factor. *Nervenarzt, 77*, 523. doi: 10.1007/s00115-005-1971-0.

Larson, E.B., Wang, L., Bowen, J.D. et al. (2006). Exercise is associated with reduced risk for incident dementia among persons 65 years and older. *Annals of Internal Medicine, 144*(2), 73–81.

Liu-Ambrose, T., Nagamatsu, L.S., Graf, P. et al. (2010). Resistance training and executive functions: A 12-month randomized controlled trial. *Archives of Internal Medicine, 170*(2), 170–178.

Maass, A., Duzel, S., Goerke, M. et al. (2015). Relationship between peripheral IGF-1, VEGF and BDNF levels and exercise-related changes in memory, hippocampal perfusion and volumes in older adults. *Neuroimage, 131*, 142–154. doi: 10.1016/j.neuroimage.2015.10.084.

Miller, D.I., Taler, V., Davidson, P.S., & Messier, C. (2012). Measuring the impact of exercise on cognitive aging: Methodological issues. *Neurobiology Aging, 33*(3), 622–643.

Mitchell, A.J., & Shiri-Feshki M. (2009). Rate of progression of mild cognitive impairment to dementia meta-analysis of 41 robust inception cohort studies. *Acta Psychiatriatrica Scandinavica, 119*, 252–265.

Müller, P., Rehfeld, K., Lüders, A. et al. (2016). Effekte eines Tanz- und eines Gesundheitssporttrainings auf die graue Hirnsubstanz gesunder Senioren. *Sportwissenschaft, 46*(3), 213–222. doi: 10.1007/s12662-016-0411-6.

Murphy, T., Dias, G., & Thuret, S. (2014). Effects of diet on brain plasticity in animal and human studies: Mind the gap. *Neural Plasticity, 563160*.

Norton, S., Matthews, F.E., Barnes, D.E., Yaffe, K., & Brayne, C. (2014). Potential for primary prevention of Alzheimer's disease: An analysis of population-based data. *Lancet Neurology, 13*, 788–794.

Petersen, R.C., Smith, G.E., Waring, S.C. et al. (1999). Mild cognitive impairment: Clinical characterization and outcome. *Archives of Neurology, 56*(3), 303–308.

Raz, N., Lindenberger, U., Rodrigue, K.M. et al. (2005). Regional brain changes in aging healthy adults: General trends, individual differences and modifiers. *Cerebral Cortex, 15*(11), 1676–1689.

Rubinstein, E., Duggan, C., Landingham, B. et al. (2015). A call to action: The global response to dementia through policy innovation. Report of the WISH Dementia Forum 2015. Available online at: http://mhinnovation.net/sites/default/files/downloads/resource/WISH_Dementia_Forum_Report_08.01.15_WEB.pdf.

Sehm, B., Taubert, M., Conde, V. et al. (2014). Structural brain plasticity in Parkinson's disease induced by balance training. *Neurobiology of Aging, 35*, 232–239.

Sperling, R.A., Aisen, P.S., Beckett, L.A. et al. (2011). Toward defining the preclinical stages of Alzheimer's disease: Recommendations from the National Institute on Aging-Alzheimer's Association workgroups on diagnostic guidelines for Alzheimer's disease. *Alzheimers Dement*, 7, 280–292.

Steiner, B., Witte, V., & Flöel A. (2011). Lebensstil und Kognition. *Der Nervenarzt*, 82, 1566–1577.

Thomas, A.G., Dennis, A., Bandettini, P.A., & Johansen-Berg, H. (2012). The effects of aerobic activity on brain structure. *Frontiers in Psychology*, 3, 86. doi: 10.3389/fpsyg.2012.00086.

Verghese, J., Lipton, R.B., & Katz, M.J. (2003). Leisure activities and the risk of dementia in the elderly. *New England Journal of Medicine*, 348(25), 2508–2016.

World Health Organization (WHO). (2010). *World health report 2010: Global recommendations on physical activity for health*. Geneva: WHO.

World Health Organization. (2015). *International classification of diseases* (10th ed.). Geneva: World Health Organization.

Zatorre, R.J., Fields, R.D., & Johansen-Berg, H. (2012). Plasticity in gray and white: Neuroimaging changes in brain structure during learning. *Nature Neuroscience*, 15(4), 528–536, doi: 10.1038/nn.3045.

Chapter 10

A review of laboratory studies on the acute effects of movement and exercise on cognition in children

Nadja Walter and Sabine Schaefer

Teachers in kindergarten and elementary school often report that classroom behaviour of children tends to be better after a break. They argue that children can focus more effectively on the to-be-learned material, and are less distracted. Many children use the breaks in school for physical activity (PA) (e.g. playing soccer in the school yard, rope skipping or climbing), so parts of the effect are possibly caused by exercise. But in order to give valuable recommendations to practitioners, it is necessary to investigate these effects in detail. How much exercise is needed to achieve positive outcomes, do all children profit to the same extent, what is the time course of such effects, and which types of cognitive activities profit the most?

In a different vein, in the early kindergarten years, acquiring knowledge about the physical world seems to rely on children's own physical experiences. There are studies showing that young children's early understanding of abstract concepts, like numbers, can be fostered by providing opportunities to move through space (Fischer, Moeller, Bientzle, Cress, & Nuerk, 2011; Link, Moeller, Huber, Fischer, & Nuerk, 2013).

This chapter has two main parts. The first part presents findings on the acute effects of exercise in children, and the second part introduces recent empirical evidence that movement is important for young children when acquiring abstract concepts.

Laboratory studies on the acute effects of exercise on school-aged children

The chapter presents a selection of lab studies on the acute effects of exercise. Selected studies are presented in some detail, such that important design issues can be discussed. Our review is not exhaustive, and the interested reader is referred to Best (2010), Chang, Labban, Gapin, and Etnier (2012), Janssen, Toussaint, van Mechelen, and Verhagen (2014b) and Tomporowski (2003) for more systematic reviews of the topic.

Most studies on the acute effects of exercise on cognition have used aerobic exercises, such as jogging, fast walking or cycling on bicycle ergometers.

These exercises lead to an increase in heart rate, which can influence arousal levels (Lambourne & Tomporowski, 2010). The positive effect on cognition may also be caused by changes in specific neurotransmitters. Exercise affects the central dopaminergic, noradrenergic and serotonergic system (Meeusen & De Meirleir, 1995), and leads to increased synthesis of amino acid neurotransmitters, especially glutamate and gamma-aminobutyric acid (Maddock, Casazza, Fernandez, & Maddock, 2016).

Laboratory studies allow for a manipulation of crucial variables, such that hypotheses about the underlying mechanisms of the observed effects can be tested. There are several design features that researchers should take into consideration.

Within- or between-subjects design?

In a within-subjects design, all participants perform all conditions of a task. For example, cognition can be tested after a period of seated rest, after a low-intensity exercise bout or after a high-intensity exercise bout. Since the same person is tested in each condition, performance changes are (in part) caused by the changes in condition. However, practice effects or fatigue can also influence cognition. These influences can be controlled for by randomly distributing participants across different testing schemes. For example, some participants start with the seated rest condition and do the high-intensity exercise in the last session, while others start with the high-intensity exercise and do the seated rest in the last session. Experimental psychology textbooks offer a variety of designs that can be used in this respect (e.g. Goodwin & Goodwin, 2012; Shadish, Cook, & Campbell, 2001).

In a between-subjects design, participants only perform one condition. One person performs the cognitive test after a period of seated rest, another person after low-intensity exercise, and yet another after high-intensity exercise. While influences of practice and/or fatigue are not relevant, results can be influenced by pre-existing differences between people. For example, people with a higher working-memory capacity will perform better in such tasks. It is therefore crucial to assign participants randomly across conditions. If certain characteristics that influence task performance have been assessed, another option is to distribute participants with similar background characteristics equally across the different conditions.

Assessment of performance before and after exercise, practice effects

In order to assess a reliable baseline, cognition should be tested before the bout of exercise, and during and/or after the exercise episode. If the cognitive task is very likely to improve with practice, providing participants with sufficient practice before the exercise starts can be helpful. Although this requires more time and effort, the advantage is that one gets a 'purer' and more reliable cognitive measure, and potential exercise-induced changes in cognition are less likely to be confounded by other factors (see also literature on 'testing-the-limits' effects in developmental psychology: Kliegl, Smith, & Baltes, 1989).

Floor and ceiling effects in cognition

Researchers should make sure that participants are not exposed to tasks that are too easy (ceiling effects) or too difficult (floor effects). If difficulty of the cognitive task does not correspond to the ability levels of participants, effects of exercise will not be detectable. It might be worth individually adjusting task difficulties if performances differ a lot across people (see Brehmer, Li, Müller, von Oertzen, & Lindenberger, 2007; Schaefer, Krampe, Lindenberger, & Baltes, 2008, for examples).

Adherence to exercise protocol

It is important that participants actively take part in the exercise protocol. This issue is easier to control in laboratory studies, where exercise intensity can be closely monitored and individually adjusted. In a school setting, however, it can be more difficult to assure that everybody is exercising at the predefined intensity level. Devices like heart rate monitors or accelerometry can be used to control for exercise intensities and time-on-task.

Expertise effects concerning exercise

Experiences with specific sports can influence the effects of exercise on cognition. Some effects can only be shown in trained athletes (Cereatti, Casella, Manganelli, & Pesce, 2009), while other effects can be even more pronounced in less active individuals. Not all studies assess and report whether children take part in regular PA, but this information should be provided.

The following section presents studies on the acute effects of exercise in children.

A study by Schaefer, Lövdén, Wieckhorst, and Lindenberger (2010) asked 9-year-old children and young adults to walk on a treadmill in two conditions: either at their preferred speed, or at a fixed speed of 2.5 km/h, which was slower than preferred. Participants were also asked to perform a working-memory task, n-back, under different difficulty conditions. For the n-back task, participants are presented with a series of numbers over loudspeakers. They had to indicate whether the current number is identical to the number presented n positions earlier in the sequence. The easiest condition was n-back 1 (comparing the number to the previous number), and the most difficult condition was n-back 4 (comparing the number to the number that was presented four positions earlier). Since the task requires a constant updating of memory, it is rather demanding. When performing the task while walking at their preferred speed as opposed to sitting, participants were more successful in the cognitive task, and this effect was more pronounced in the children (Figure 10.1). However, when the treadmill speed was fixed, performances in n-back did not differ between walking and sitting. The authors argue that preferred-speed walking might have optimized arousal levels, whereas walking at a slower than preferred speed requires some attention, such that the cognitive task does not profit from this task condition.

Treadmill walking has been used in several studies on the effects of exercise on children's cognition. Drollette, Shishido, Pontifex, and Hillman (2012) extended the finding from Schaefer et al. (2010) by testing 9–11-year-olds in two different cognitive tasks: a modified flanker task that requires inhibitory control, and a spatial version of n-back, for which participants had to compare the position of stimuli to previous positions (1-back or 2-back). For the flanker task, participants were instructed to attend to the centre target stimulus amid four identical flanking stimuli that are either congruent (i.e. facing the same direction) or incongruent

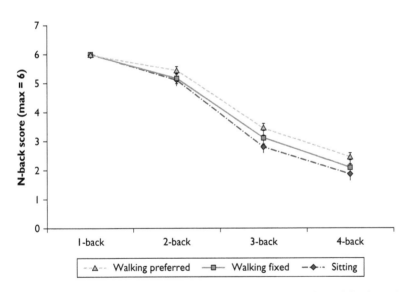

Figure 10.1 Working-memory score in children as a function of task difficulty and sitting or treadmill walking at fixed or preferred speed in the study by Schaefer et al. (2010). Children showed the highest cognitive performances while walking at their preferred speed (error bars = SE mean).

(i.e. facing the opposite direction). Performance in incongruent trials tends to be slower and more error-prone, since participants have to inhibit the distraction caused by the flanking stimuli. The authors also tested each participant's fitness level with a Vo_{2max} test. One experimental session took place during seated rest, and the other one included a bout of walking at 60% of each individual's maximum heart rate. The order of these sessions was counterbalanced across participants. In each session, cognition was assessed three times: before walking/seated rest, during walking/ seated rest or after walking/seating rest. Task performances for the flanker and the n-back task did not differ during exercise as compared to during rest, indicating that exercising does not have negative effects on cognition. Decrements in flanker accuracy occurred over the course of the seated rest session, whereas flanker accuracies did not deteriorate in the walking session. There were no such changes for the n-back task. The authors state that 'physical activity does not interfere with working memory and may facilitate maintenance of attention over time in cognitively demanding settings, which has public health implications for the educational environment and the context of learning' (Drollette et al., 2012, p. 2022).

Hillman et al. (2009) also used treadmill walking as a motor task to assess potential effects on cognition. Study participants were 9 years old, and each participant's cardiovascular fitness was measured by a graded exercise test. On two separate days, participants performed a flanker test either after a period of seated rest, or after 20 minutes of treadmill walking at 60% of their estimated maximum heart rate. Participants started working on the cognitive tasks when their heart rate had returned to within 10% of their pre-exercise levels. The flanker test was followed by a test on academic achievement, measuring reading comprehension, arithmetic and spelling. The order of sessions (seated rest and treadmill walking) was counterbalanced across participants. Electroencephalogram (EEG) was also measured during the performance of the cognitive tasks. Results indicated an improvement in response accuracy, larger P3 amplitude and better performance on the academic achievement test following aerobic exercise relative to the resting session. The authors conclude that single bouts of exercise can be helpful in enhancing children's cognitive performances.

Findings by Drollette et al. (2014) indicate that the extent to which cognition profits from exercise can be influenced by cognitive ability level. They tested a sample of 40 preadolescent children who performed a flanker task after a resting period or after a 20-minute bout of treadmill walking at 60–70% of their maximum heart rate. The authors also recorded EEG to assess event-related potentials (ERPs) during task performance. Children were classified as either high-performers or low-performers in the cognitive task, based on their performances in the seated rest condition. While high-performers showed similar performance levels after rest and after treadmill walking, the performances of low-performers were improved after walking: They reacted with a higher accuracy to the target stimuli. ERP changes in the two groups supported this pattern of findings: The amplitude of the P3 component, which reflects attentional resource allocation during stimulus engagement, is unchanged in high-performers, but increased in low-performers when comparing the walking to the seated rest condition. Both groups displayed smaller N2 amplitude and shorter P3 latency following exercise, suggesting an overall facilitation in response conflict and the speed of stimulus classification.

A study by Best (2012) compared the influence of different activities on an executive control task in elementary school children. The crucial manipulation consisted of the amount of PA and cognitive engagement (CE) in each activity. In separate sessions, each child watched an instructional video (low PA, low CE), played a sedentary video game (low PA, high CE), played an exergame which only involved jogging in place on a response mat (high PA, low CE), or played an exergame that was physically and cognitively demanding, because children had to jump and change their position to overcome obstacles while jogging on the mat (high PA, high CE). Immediately following each activity, children performed a computerized cognitive task that required high levels of executive control, a modified flanker task.

CE had no effect on task performance, but PA enhanced children's speed to resolve interference from conflicting visuospatial material in the flanker task. This indicates that a bout of PA helps children in subsequent mental tasks, but in this particular study, adding cognitive challenges to the exercise did not have additional positive effects on cognition.

It is conceivable that expert athletes profit even more from exercise when performing a cognitive task, since they are confronted with such types of situations during practice. A study by Cereatti et al. (2009) asked adolescents who were experienced orienteers and a group of physically active adolescents not practising orienteering to perform a visual attention task at rest and under acute submaximal exercise. Both groups reacted faster during exercise as compared to rest, but the effect was larger in the orienteers than in the non-practisers. This might be due to the fact that orienteers are skilled in directing the available resources to task demands. The paper also reports several aspects of the cognitive task in which orienteers were better than their non-practising peers (behaving more adult-like), which indicates that long-term training of a certain sport can influence cognitive performances and can accelerate the maturation of cognitive abilities.

This review focuses on controlled laboratory studies, but there are numerous studies conducted in school settings showing that acute bouts of exercise can enhance children's cognitive and/or academic performances (Altenburg, Chinapaw, & Singh, 2016; Budde et al., 2010; Budde, Voelcker-Rehage,

Pietraßyk-Kendziorra, Ribeiro, & Tidow, 2008; Gallotta et al., 2015; Jäger, Schmidt, Conzelmann, & Roebers, 2014; Janssen et al., 2014a; Niemann et al., 2013; Pesce, Crova, Cereatti, Casella, & Bellucci, 2009). There are also findings that children suffering from attention deficit-hyperactivity disorder can profit from exercise (Pontifex, Saliba, Raine, Picchietti, & Hillman, 2013). In addition, there are interesting recent findings in young and older adults (for a review, see Roig, Nordbrandt, Geertsen, & Nielsen, 2013; and Roig et al., 2016) that indicate that acute bouts of exercise are particularly supportive for the formation of new memory traces. If these findings can be replicated in school-aged children, active school breaks should be helpful for priming the molecular processes involved in the encoding and consolidation of newly acquired information.

Embodiment: physically moving through space can help to acquire abstract concepts

The effects of acute exercise on cognition are probably caused by the optimization of arousal levels or by changes in neurotransmitter secretion. Exercise in the studies described above challenged the cardiovascular system, often by asking participants to walk or run on a treadmill at a certain intensity level. There are currently too few studies that systematically investigate other types of movements, such as coordination, in a laboratory setting. The findings by Budde et al. (2008) indicate that coordinative exercises might be helpful as well.

In a different vein, physical movements can be helpful in solving cognitive tasks. This effect can occur when bodily experiences are used to form abstract cognitive representations. Research on these effects has been conducted under the term 'embodied cognition' (Andres, Olivier, & Badets, 2008; Körner, Topolinski, & Strack, 2015; Wilson, 2002) or 'grounded cognition' (Barsalou, 2008, 2010; Gentsch, Weber, Synofzik, Vosgerau, & Schütz-Bosbach, 2016). Early childhood is a developmental period in which physical experiences are particularly important for cognitive development (Boncoddo, Dixon, & Kelley, 2010; Kontra, Goldin-Meadow, & Beilock, 2012; Loeffler, Raab, & Canal-Bruland, 2016). The studies that are described in this section are interventions, addressing the question whether performances can be improved if specific underlying abilities are trained.

Based on the assumption that children's early basic numerical competencies predict their future arithmetic abilities, a study by Fischer et al. (2011) tried to improve theses early abilities by sensorimotor spatial training. In the embodied condition, kindergarten children were placed on a dance mat and shown an Arabic digit (e.g. 8) and a hypothetical number line on the floor in front of them. They had to compare the magnitude of the digit to that of simultaneously presented standard (e.g. 5). The standard was presented together with its position on the number line. If the target digit was larger than the standard, children were asked to take a step to the right; if it was smaller, they were asked to take a step to the left. The same task was also administered with arrays of dots instead of digits. In this case, children indicated whether the target included more or less dots than the standard. The control condition consisted of the same task, but children worked on a tablet PC instead of the dance mat, so the full-body movement was not required. Each child received three training sessions per condition, and half of the sample started with the embodied training, while the other half started with PC training. The embodied training was more effective than the control training in enhancing children's performances on a paper-and-pencil number line estimation task and on a standardized maths test (counting principles; e.g. counting in steps of two, counting backwards). However, there were no significant differential improvements in other subtests of the maths test. It is assumed that the effects were caused by an improvement of children's mental number line representations, and that they are not merely a result of changes in motivation or attention.

To investigate further whether numerical representations profit from an embodied training, the paradigm was extended to elementary school-aged subjects in a subsequent study (Link et al., 2013). The authors asked first-graders to work on two different training regimes. In the embodied condition, children were shown a number between 0 and 100 (e.g. 78) and asked to walk to the estimated location of that number on a number line on the floor. In the non-embodied training condition, children performed the same task on a computer screen. They always received feedback about the exact location after each trial, and all children underwent both training regimes. Children showed more pronounced training effects after the embodied training as compared to the control training on a paper-and-pencil version of the number line task. There was also a more pronounced transfer effect of the embodied training to another numerical task, namely single-digit sums (e.g. 4 + 3 = 7). Moreover, children with lower measures on a covariate test of general cognitive ability profited more from the embodied training condition than children with higher cognitive ability scores. The authors conclude that there are 'beneficial effects of embodied processes for the training of seemingly abstract cognitive representations in general and for the amelioration of basic numerical representations in particular' (Link et al., 2013, p. 74).

Many young children initially use their fingers when counting or solving easy mathematical problems. Gracia-Baffaluy and Noel (2008) investigated whether training in finger differentiation would increase finger gnosis and numerical performance. 'Finger gnosis' refers to the ability to differentiate one's own fingers when they are touched without any visual cue. Finger gnosis in early childhood is a powerful predictor of numerical abilities several years later. The authors argue that some children may not be able to use their fingers efficiently to count, calculate or show numerosities and this might prevent them from developing good numerical skills. For the study, they tested 112 first-graders for their finger gnosis and recruited the 33 children with the lowest scores and the 14 children with the highest scores for the study. Children with poor scores were randomly divided into a finger representation training group and a story comprehension training group, which served as the control group. The high-scoring group did not receive any training.

The finger representation training used a color scheme, such that children learned an association between each finger and a specific colour (i.e. thumb–white, index–green, middle–blue . . .). They were then trained on a labyrinth task, a pointing task, a piano task, and a grip task, all of which relied on the colour-coded fingers. Both training regimes lasted for 8 weeks, with two sessions a week. Before any intervention, children with good finger gnosis outperformed the two groups with poor finger gnosis in two numerical tasks, one tapping the level of elaboration of the verbal numerical chain and the other involving counting collections. After the intervention, children in the finger representation training group outperformed those of the control training group in finger gnosis, and even those of the high-performing group who had not received any training. They had improved their scores on a 'draw a hand' test, could react faster in a task that required them to say how many fingers were raised in pictures, and reacted faster in a subitizing task compared to the story comprehension training group. The authors argue that improving finger gnosis in young children is possible and that it can provide a useful support to learning mathematics.

Conclusions and suggestions for learning environments

The first part of the chapter presented empirical evidence indicating that bouts of exercise can help children on subsequent cognitive tasks. The review has focused on laboratory studies, but evidence for the positive influences of exercise on cognition and academic performance is currently also accumulating in school settings. Based on these findings, teachers should assure that there are enough breaks throughout the school day, and that children are encouraged to use these breaks for exercise. Wherever possible, the number of physical education classes should be increased, and school subjects that are known to be cognitively challenging might profit from taking place after physical education lessons. Additional research is needed to find out how memory consolidation can be optimized by a clever timing of exercise bouts, and on the exact nature of helpful physical activities (e.g. aerobic exercise versus coordination).

Findings that currently emerge from the embodied cognition approach indicate that actively moving through space or training children how to use their fingers when counting can be helpful for the acquisition of basic numerical concepts. Kindergarten and elementary school teachers should be encouraged to come up with creative ways to address not only the mind, but also the body when teaching this type of material. The empirical evidence suggests that this can be particularly helpful for children of lower ability levels.

In order to progress on these issues, practitioners and scientists should exchange their experiences whenever possible. It is nice to know about the outcomes of studies, but it is as least as important to know what actually works 'in the real world'.

References

Altenburg, T. M., Chinapaw, M. J. M., & Singh, A. S. (2016). Effects of one versus two bouts of moderate intensity physical activity on selective attention during a school morning in Dutch primary school children: A randomized controlled trial. *Journal of Science and Medicine in Sport, 19*(10), 820–824. doi: 10.1016/j.jsams.2015.12.003.

Andres, M., Olivier, E., & Badets, A. (2008). Actions, words, and numbers: A motor contribution to semantic processing? *Current Directions in Psychological Science, 17*, 313–317.

Barsalou, L. W. (2008). Grounded cognition. *Annual Review of Psychology, 59*, 617–645. doi: 10.1146/annurev.psych.59.103006.093639.

Barsalou, L. W. (2010). Grounded cognition: Past, present, and future. *Topics in Cognitive Sciences, 2*, 716–724. doi: 10.1111/j.1756-8765.2010.01115.x.

Best, J. R. (2010). Effects of physical activity on children's executive function: Contributions of experimental research on aerobic exercise. *Developmental Review, 30*, 331–351. doi: 10.1016/j.dr.2010.08.001.

Best, J. R. (2012). Exergaming immediately enhances children's executive function. *Developmental Psychology, 48*, 1501–1510. doi: 10.1037/a0026648.

Boncoddo, R., Dixon, J. A., & Kelley, E. (2010). The emergence of a novel representation from action: Evidence from preschoolers. *Developmental Science, 13*, 370–377. doi: 10.1111/j.1467-7687.2009.00905.x.

Brehmer, Y., Li, S.-C., Müller, V., von Oertzen, T., & Lindenberger, U. (2007). Memory plasticity across the lifespan: Uncovering children's latent potential. *Developmental Psychology, 43*, 465–478. doi: 10.1037/0012-1649.43.2.465.

Budde, H., Voelcker-Rehage, C., Pietraßyk-Kendziorra, S., Machado, S., Ribeiro, P., & Arafat, A. M. (2010). Steroid hormones in the saliva of adolescents after different exercise intensities and their influence on working memory in a school setting. *Psychoneuroendocrinology, 35*, 382–391. doi: 10.1016/j.psyneuen.2009.07.015.

Budde, H., Voelcker-Rehage, C., Pietraßyk-Kendziorra, S., Ribeiro, P., & Tidow, G. (2008). Acute coordinative exercise improves attentional performance in adolescents. *Neuroscience Letters, 441*, 219–223.

Cereatti, L., Casella, R., Manganelli, M., & Pesce, C. (2009). Visual attention in adolescents: Facilitating effects of sport expertise and acute physical exercise. *Psychology of Sport and Exercise, 10*, 136–145. doi: 10.1016/j.psychsport.2008.05.002.

Chang, Y. K., Labban, J. D., Gapin, J. I., & Etnier, J. L. (2012). The effects of acute exercise on cognitive performance: A meta-analysis. *Brain Research, 1453*, 87–101. doi: 10.1016/j.brainres.2012.02.068.

Drollette, E. S., Scudder, M. R., Raine, L. B., Moore, R. D., Saliba, B. J., Pontifex, M. B., & Hillman, C. (2014). Acute exercise facilitates brain function and cognition in children who need it most: An ERP study of individual differences in inhibitory control capacity. *Developmental Cognitive Neuroscience, 7*, 53–64. doi: 10.1016/j.dcn.2013.11.001.

Drollette, E. S., Shishido, T., Pontifex, M. B., & Hillman, C. (2012). Maintenance of cognitive control during and after walking in preadolescent children. *Medicine and Science in Sports and Exercise, 44*, 2017–2024. doi: 10.1249/MSS.0b013e318258bcd5.

Fischer, U., Moeller, K., Bientzle, M., Cress, U., & Nuerk, H.-C. (2011). Sensorimotor spatial training of number magnitude representation. *Psychonomic Bulletin and Review, 18*, 177–183. doi: 10.3758/s13423-010-0031-3.

Gallotta, M. C., Emerenziani, G. P., Franciosi, E., Meucci, M., Guidetti, L., & Baldari, C. (2015). Acute physical activity and delayed attention in primary school students. *Scandinavian Journal of Medicine and Science in Sports, 25*, e3331–3338. doi: 10.1111/sms.12310.

Gentsch, A., Weber, A., Synofzik, M., Vosgerau, G., & Schütz-Bosbach, S. (2016). Towards a common framework of grounded action cognition: Relating motor control, perception and cognition. *Cognition, 146*, 81–89. doi: 10.1016/j.cognition.2015.09.010.

Goodwin, C. J., & Goodwin, K. A. (2012). *Research in psychology: Methods and design* (7th ed.). New York: Wiley.

Gracia-Baffaluy, M., & Noel, M.-P. (2008). Does finger training increase young children's numerical performance? *Cortex, 4*, 368–375. doi: 10.1016/j.cortex.2007.08.020.

Hillman, C. H., Pontifex, M. B., Raine, L. B., Castelli, D. M., Hall, E. E., & Kramer, A. F. (2009). The effect of acute treadmill walking on cognitive control and academic achievement in preadolescent children. *Neuroscience, 159*, 1044–1054.

Jäger, K., Schmidt, M., Conzelmann, A., & Roebers, C. (2014). Cognitive and physiological effects of an acute physical activity intervention in elementary school children. *Frontiers in Psychology, 5*, 1–11. doi: 10.3389/fpsyg.2014.01473.

Janssen, M., Chinapaw, M. J. M., Rauh, S. P., Toussaint, H. M., van Mechelen, W., & Verhagen, E. (2014a). A short physical activity break from cognitive tasks increases selective attention in primary school children aged 10–11. *Mental Health and Physical Activity, 7*, 129–134. doi: 10.1016/j.mhpa.2014.07.001.

Janssen, M., Toussaint, H. M., van Mechelen, W., & Verhagen, E. (2014b). Effects of acute bouts of physical activity on children's attention: A systematic review of the literature. *SpringerPlus, 3*, 410–420. doi: 10.1186/2193-1801-3-410.

Kliegl, R., Smith, J., & Baltes, P. B. (1989). Testing-the-limits and the study of adult age differences in cognitive plasticity of a mnemonic skill. *Developmental Psychology, 25*, 247–256.

Kontra, C., Goldin-Meadow, S., & Beilock, S. L. (2012). Embodied learning across the lifespan. *Topics in Cognitive Science, x*, 1–9. doi: 10.1111/j.1756-8765.2012.01221.x.

Körner, A., Topolinski, S., & Strack, F. (2015). Routes to embodiment. *Frontiers in Psychology, 6*, 1–10. doi: 10.3389/fpsyg.2015.00940.

Lambourne, K., & Tomporowski, P. D. (2010). The effect of exercise-induced arousal on cognitive task performance: A meta-regression analysis. *Brain Research, 1341*, 12–24. doi: 10.1016/j.brainres.2010.03.091.

Link, T., Moeller, K., Huber, S., Fischer, U., & Nuerk, H.-C. (2013). Walk the number line – An embodied training of numerical concepts. *Trends in Neurosciences and Education, 2*, 74–84. doi: 10.1016/j.tine.2013.06.005.

Loeffler, J., Raab, M., & Canal-Bruland, R. (2016). A lifespan perspective on embodied cognition. *Frontiers in Psychology, 7*, 845. doi: 10.3389/fpsyg.2016.00845.

Maddock, R. J., Casazza, G. A., Fernandez, D. H., & Maddock, M. I. (2016). Acute modulation of cortical glutamate and GABA content by physical activity. *The Journal of Neuroscience, 36*, 2449–2457. doi: 10.1523/JNEUROSCI.3455-15.2016.

Meeusen, R., & De Meirleir, K. (1995). Exercise and brain neurotransmitters. *Sports Medicine, 20*, 160–188.

Niemann, C., Wegner, M., Voelcker-Rehage, C., Holzweg, M., Arafat, A. M., & Budde, H. (2013). Influence of acute and chronic physical activity on cognitive performance and saliva testosterone in preadolescent school children. *Mental Health and Physical Activity, 6*, 197–204. doi: 10.1016/j.mhpa.2013.08.002.

Pesce, C., Crova, C., Cereatti, L., Casella, R., & Bellucci, M. (2009). Physical activity and mental performance in preadolescents: Effects of acute exercise on free-recall memory. *Mental Health and Physical Activity, 2*, 16–22. doi: 10.1016/j.mhpa.2009.02.001.

Pontifex, M. B., Saliba, B. J., Raine, L. B., Picchietti, D. L., & Hillman, C. H. (2013). Exercise improves behavioral, neurocognitive, and scholastic performance in children with attention-deficit/hyperactivity disorder. *The Journal of Pediatrics, 162*, 543–551. doi: 10.1016/j.peds.2012.08.036.

Roig, M., Nordbrandt, S., Geertsen, S. S., & Nielsen, J. B. (2013). The effects of cardiovascular exercise on human memory: A review with meta-analysis. *Neuroscience and Biobehavioral Reviews, 37*, 1645–1666. doi: 10.1016/j.neubiorev.2013.06.012.

Roig, M., Thomas, A. G., Mang, C. S., Snow, N. J., Ostadan, F., Boyd, L. A., & Lundbye-Jensen, J. (2016). Time-dependent effects of cardiovascular exercise on memory. *Exercise and Sport Science Reviews, 44*, 81–88. doi: 10.1249/JES.0000000000000078.

Schaefer, S., Krampe, R. T., Lindenberger, U., & Baltes, P. B. (2008). Age differences between children and young adults in the dynamics of dual-task prioritization: Body (balance) versus mind (memory). *Developmental Psychology, 44*, 747–757. doi: 10.1037/0012-1649.44.3.747.

Schaefer, S., Lövdén, M., Wieckhorst, B., & Lindenberger, U. (2010). Cognitive performance is improved while walking: Differences in cognitive-sensorimotor couplings between children and young adults. *European Journal of Developmental Psychology, 7*, 371–389. doi: 10.1037/0012-1649.44.3.747.

Shadish, W. R., Cook, T. D., & Campbell, D. T. (2001). *Experimental and quasi-experimental designs for generalized causal inference* (2nd ed.). Boston: Cengage Learning.

Tomporowski, P. D. (2003). Effects of acute bouts of exercise on cognition. *Acta Psychologica, 112*, 297–324. doi: 10.1016/S0001-6918(02)00134.

Wilson, M. (2002). Six views of embodied cognition. *Psychonomic Bulletin and Review, 9*, 625–636. doi: 10.3758/BF03196322.

Chapter 11

Exercise as neuroenhancer in children with ADHD

Cognitive and behavioural effects

Sebastian Ludyga, Serge Brand,
Markus Gerber and Uwe Pühse

Introduction

With a global prevalence rate of around 6%, attention deficit-hyperactivity disorder (ADHD) is considered to be the most common neurodevelopmental disorder affecting children (Polanczyk, Willcutt, Salum, Kieling, & Rohde, 2014). Epidemiological data show that gender has a significant influence on prevalence rate, so that boys are diagnosed with ADHD more often than girls (Polanczyk, Lima, Horta, Biederman, & La Rohde, 2007). The behavioural symptoms of this neuropsychiatric disorder include a developmentally inappropriate pattern of inattention and impulsiveness/hyperactivity with an initial manifestation before children have reached 12 years of age (American Psychiatric Association, 2013; World Health Organization, 2004). Those symptoms are persistent and impairments therefore severely affect ADHD sufferers at different stages throughout life. In children, the disorder is associated with poor school performance, low academic achievement as well as school suspensions and expulsions (Loe & Feldman, 2007).

As the children grow older, problems with peers and poor family relations become more pronounced. Additionally, adolescents with ADHD are more vulnerable to substance abuse/dependence than their healthy peers (Lee, Humphreys, Flory, Liu, & Glass, 2011). In 65% of all cases, ADHD persists into adulthood and continues to cause a variety of behavioural problems. Higher rates of marital dissatisfaction and discord, higher divorce rates and parenting difficulties are only some examples of how social dysfunction affects relationships in adults with ADHD (Barkley & Fischer, 2010). Moreover, a developmentally inappropriate state of impulsivity has also been associated with problems with vehicle handling (Kieling et al., 2011) and increases the likeliness of involvement in other criminal activities (Fletcher & Wolfe, 2009).

The trajectory of the disorder is further complicated by a number of comorbidities, which are often associated with ADHD. Common comorbid psychiatric disorders include oppositional defiant disorder, conduct disorder, learning disabilities, substance use disorder as well as mood and anxiety disorders (Wilens et al., 2002). Based on the wide range of impairments and comorbidities, it is not surprising that ADHD appears to increase the risk of suicide significantly (James, Lai, & Dahl, 2004).

Considering this prognosis, an early treatment seems to be necessary to influence the trajectory of ADHD positively. Regarding evidence-based medicine, pharmacological interventions and behavioural therapies target-ing psychosocial dimensions have been reported to improve inattention and hyperactivity/impulsivity and their behavioural consequences (Charach et al., 2013; Tamminga, Reneman, Huizenga, & Geurts, 2016). Although those therapies seem to be efficient during active treatment, results from prospective studies leave open the question of long-term benefits for the trajectory of ADHD (van Lieshout et al., 2016; Vitiello et al., 2015). Moreover, the currently employed treatments might be able to reduce the impact of the disorder on life functioning, but children with ADHD under-going treatment still show a variety of behavioural deficits compared to their healthy peers (Shaw et al., 2012). To investigate the potential of new treatment approaches, such as regular exercise included in a multimodal concept, it is important to consider the aetiology of ADHD first.

Pathophysiology of ADHD

Brain function and structure

Despite the multidimensional character of ADHD, researchers have made attempts to understand the mechanisms underlying the behavioural symp-toms. Investigations of brain structure and function in particular have advanced our understanding of the neurobiological underpinnings of the disorder, so that abnormalities in frontostriatal and frontoparietal networks as well as other regions are considered to be central to ADHD dysfunc-tions (Cherkasova & Hechtman, 2009). The frontoparietal network is also described as the executive control circuit, which guides goal-directed execu-tive processes and configures information processing in response to variable task demands (Menon, 2011; Vincent, Kahn, Snyder, Raichle, & Buckner, 2008). In several prefrontal brain regions involved in the frontoparietal net-work children with ADHD showed volume reductions compared to healthy controls (Valera, Faraone, Murray, & Seidman, 2007). This cortical thin-ning is possibly due to a 2–3-year delay in structural maturation (Shaw et al., 2007). Moreover, children with ADHD show disruptions in unci-nate fasciculus (Hamilton et al., 2008), a white-matter fibre tract connecting frontal and temporal lobes.

Those morphological changes within the brain are accompanied by abnormal activation patterns, such as hypoactivation in the dorsal and ven-trolateral prefrontal cortex (PFC) during cognitive tasks requiring sustained attention, inhibitory control and temporal processing (Cubillo, Halari,

Smith, Taylor, & Rubia, 2012). Additionally, children with ADHD show reduced activation of ventromedial regions in the PFC during tasks relating to reward processing (Rubia, 2011). This is suggested to reflect motivational control deficits and poor emotion regulation, which largely correspond to the behavioural symptoms of ADHD. Apart from the frontoparietal circuit, the disorder appears to affect the default mode network as well. This network of interacting brain regions typically becomes active during rest and mind wandering, but it is deactivated during external goal-oriented tasks. There is evidence to suggest that people with ADHD fail to suppress the activity of the default mode network during such tasks, resulting in attentional lapses (Rubia, Alegria, & Brinson, 2014). Consequently, hypoactivation of task-relevant structures concomitant with a failure to suppress the default mode network might cause poor top-down control over inhibition, attention and timing functions.

Catecholamines

From a neuroendocrinological perspective, ADHD-related deficits of higher-order cognitive function might also be attributed to disturbances of catecholamine neurotransmission (Prince, 2008; Tripp & Wickens, 2008). Noradrenaline (norepinephrine) released from the PFC activates different intracellular signalling pathways and modulates arousal, vigilance and executive functions, such as working memory, behavioural inhibition and planning (Ramos & Arnsten, 2007). In contrast, dopamine receptor stimulation suppresses the transduction of task-irrelevant signals and influences locomotion, cognition, affect and neuroendocrine secretion (Tripp & Wickens, 2008). Interestingly, the effects of dopamine and noradrenaline on PFC functioning depend on their concentration or availability to receptors. By increasing the signal-to-noise ratio during processing of information, moderate catecholamine release from the PFC enhances higher-order cognitive functions (Ramos & Arnsten, 2007). In turn, small and high concentrations of noradrenaline and dopamine impair the ability of the PFC to guide behaviour.

Based on a summary of findings from experimental studies, ADHD is characterized by a dysfunction of both the dopaminergic and noradrenergic systems, leading to a hypocatecholaminergic state within the PFC (Prince, 2008). In this state, processes relating to the suppression of distractors and the inhibition of inappropriate behaviours are affected. Additionally, this might explain why children and adolescents with ADHD have difficulties in sustaining focus on important information that is not intrinsically interesting. Based on the association of the hypocatecholaminergic state with behavioural symptoms of the disorder, it is not surprising that effective pharmacological treatments augment the neurotransmission of dopamine and noradrenaline in the PFC (Del Campo, Chamberlain, Sahakian, & Robbins, 2011).

Executive function

As outlined above, cortical thinning, reduced activation of the PFC and the hypocatecholaminergic state play a role in the pathophysiology of ADHD. Those mechanisms are considered to be responsible for an impairment of cognitive functioning and executive control in particular. This cognitive domain encompasses processes responsible for organizing and controlling goal-directed behaviour (Banich, 2009). Although the subcomponents of executive control are still a subject of controversial debate, inhibition, working memory and task switching are included in most definitions (Diamond, 2013). In a review of neuroimaging studies, Royall et al. (2002) conclude that specific functions of the executive system are mediated by the frontal cortices and projections to other brain regions. In this respect, the authors found the dorsolateral prefrontal circuit to be linked with planning abilities, goal selection, task switching and working memory. Moreover, the lateral orbitofrontal region is considered to be involved in risk assessment and the inhibition of feelings and inappropriate behaviour. Recalling the morphological and functional abnormalities of those structures in ADHD, it follows that sufferers are characterized by deficits of executive control. Based on a meta-analytical examination of studies comparing children and adolescents with and without ADHD, Willcutt, Doyle, Nigg, Faraone, and Pennington (2005) found impairments to be most pronounced on response inhibition, vigilance, working memory and planning. Castellanos, Sonuga-Barke, Milham, and Tannock (2006) further suggest that ADHD also affects another important domain of executive control, which is termed 'hot executive functioning' and relates to emotional problem solving. In this respect, the authors note that children with ADHD perform poorly on tasks characterized by a high affective involvement and tasks demanding flexible appraisals of the significance of emotion-laden stimuli.

Previous studies have consistently shown that this lack of skills in emotional problem solving predicts behavioural problems, whereas poor abilities in cognitive problem solving are associated with low academic performance (Brock, Rimm-Kaufman, Nathanson, & Grimm, 2009; Kim, Nordling, Yoon, Boldt, & Kochanska, 2013; Willoughby, Kupersmidt, Voegler-Lee, & Bryant, 2011). In a review of the ADHD literature, Daley and Birchwood (2010) suggest that both behavioural symptoms and deficits in executive functioning are at the heart of ADHD-related academic underperformance. The discrepancies between academic outcomes in children with ADHD relative to healthy controls have been well documented and appear to be independent of the intelligence quotient (Arnold, Hodgkins, Kahle, Madhoo, & Kewley, 2015).

However, the risk of academic failure is not the only adverse consequence of poor executive control. Children with ADHD also encounter social impairments within the family and with peers (Wehmeier, Schacht, & Barkley, 2010). Reviewing peer functioning, Hoza (2007) found that sufferers display poorer scores on social preference, lack friendships and their relationships to others are characterized by a high number of conflicts. Furthermore, children and adolescents affected by the disorder face emotional difficulties, including poor self-regulation, excessive emotional expression and problems in coping with frustrating experiences (Wehmeier et al., 2010). There is compelling evidence that this emotional dysregulation is a risk factor for suicidal behaviour (Anestis, Bagge, Tull, & Joiner, 2011) and depressive disorders (Yap, Allen, & Sheeber, 2007), which are often comorbid with ADHD. Based on a review of longitudinal studies, Riggs, Jahromi, Razza, Dillworth-Bart, and Mueller (2006) have found the development of both social and emotional competences to be closely linked with executive functioning. As ADHD-related deficits of the executive system are suggested to be at the root of academic, social and emotional impairments, this specific cognitive domain is an important target for interventions.

Role of exercise in ADHD

The behavioural problems and cognitive deficits associated with ADHD as well as their long-term consequences highlight the need for effective treatment approaches. So far, evidence-based treatments result in significant short-term improvements of ADHD-related symptoms (Charach et al., 2013; Tamminga et al., 2016), but fail to normalize affected children in the long term (Shaw et al., 2012). Additionally, a review by Graham and Coghill (2008) indicates that adverse effects, such as insomnia and anorexia, are relatively common in pharmacological therapy. The authors also note that the likeliness of severe side effects decades after the onset of treatment cannot be predicted from the current literature. Therefore, the limited efficiency of evidence-based methods and some safety issues with pharmacotherapy highlight the need for additional complementary or alternative interventions in ADHD. Targeting the poor executive control and the cortical hypoactivation of people with ADHD, neurofeedback and cognitive training are now discussed as complementary treatments. Unfortunately, evidence for the positive effects of neurofeedback on the symptomatology of the disorder is still limited (Lofthouse, Arnold, Hersch, Hurt, & Debeus, 2012) and cognitive training has been shown to produce selective rather than general improvements in executive function (Melby-Lervåg & Hulme, 2013).

Furthermore, physical exercise is thought to possess great potential as complementary treatment for ADHD, because previous studies with healthy children and adults have consistently reported exercise-induced improvements of cognitive performance. In a recent meta-analytical examination, Ludyga, Gerber, Brand, Holsboer-Trachsler, and Pühse (2016) found acute benefits of moderate aerobic exercise on cognitive flexibility, working memory and task switching. These improvements in executive functioning were moderated by age, so that preadolescent children and older adults experienced the greatest benefits from exercise. Based on a review of the current literature, Tomporowski, McCullick, Pendleton, and Pesce (2015) support both acute and long-term effects of aerobic exercise on children's cognitive performance. However, the authors further suggest that other exercise programmes, which are intended to be physically and cognitively challenging, might well have a capacity to enhance cognition.

Although there is growing evidence for both acute and chronic benefits for cognition in healthy children, it does not necessarily mean that children with ADHD can expect similar improvements from exercise. Despite first preliminary evidence for the usefulness of exercise programmes in ADHD (Grassmann, Alves, Santos-Galduroz, & Galduroz, 2017), previous reviews have concluded that data are insufficient to recommend an implementation of such interventions in this population (Berwid & Halperin, 2012; Gapin, Labban, & Etnier, 2011). As the number of studies in this field has increased within the last years, a thorough review of the extant literature is necessary to clarify whether or not the potential neuroenhancing effect of exercise also applies to children and adolescents diagnosed with ADHD.

Acute exercise and cognition

Exercise benefits for cognition are considered to be dose-dependent, so that acute and long-term effects of exercise on cognition have to be differentiated. As changes of cognitive performance in response to a single exercise session are temporary and transient in nature, they are not expected to contribute to a facilitation of the trajectory of ADHD. Nonetheless, temporary benefits for cognitive performance are still of practical relevance, because they might allow preparation for a situation demanding high cognitive control, e.g. school examinations and competitions requiring tactical planning. Recalling that ADHD-related impairments are known to cause problems in such situations, researchers have targeted acute effects of exercise on different cognitive domains in children with ADHD.

Chang, Liu, Yu, and Lee (2012) randomly assigned children with ADHD to 30 minutes of moderately intense running on a treadmill or watching a video while seated. Compared with the physically inactive condition, improvements on tasks assessing inhibitory control and set shifting were found immediately after exercise cessation. Using a cross-over design, Piepmeier et al. (2015) also investigated different aspects of executive function in children with and without ADHD after 30 minutes of cycling at moderate intensity and after watching a documentary. Affected children and healthy controls showed increased inhibitory control following exercise, whereas planning and set shifting were not influenced by the intervention.

This finding is further supported by the results of Pontifex, Saliba, Raine, Picchietti, and Hillman (2013), who reported greater inhibitory control after 20 minutes of running on a treadmill than after seated reading in children with and without ADHD. Assessing neuroelectric indices of cognitive control, the authors were able to relate exercise-induced benefits to an increased allocation of attentional resources toward the task as well as a selective enhancement in stimulus classification and processing speed. Consequently, exercise seems to reduce ADHD-related deficits in executive functioning, which are linked with hypoactivation of the PFC.

Targeting the neuroendocrinologic response to exercise, Gapin, Labban, Bohall, Wooten, and Chang (2015) investigated the role of brain-derived neurotrophic factor (BDNF), which has an influence on plasticity of synapses and neurons, for exercise-induced benefits for cognitive control. Whereas healthy controls improved inhibition, working memory and task switching after 30 minutes of moderately intense running on a treadmill, exercise-induced benefits in children with ADHD were limited to measures on inhibition. However, improvements of cognitive performance were independent from BDNF levels.

As most findings on the acute benefits of exercise were conducted in laboratories, Hill, Williams, Aucott, Thomson, and Mon-Williams (2011) examined whether or not the positive influence of a single exercise session on executive function can be replicated in a school setting. Using a cross-over design, a large sample of 552 children performed cognitive testing after an active break, including 15 minutes of moderately intense aerobic activities (e.g. jumping and running on the spot) and after enjoyable curricular activities. The authors found that exercise enhanced children's performance on tracking tasks, which involved dividing or shifting attention, independent of ADHD symptoms. Consequently, the positive effects of moderate exercise on aspects of higher-order cognition reported from laboratory studies can also be observed in the school setting.

Compared to the effects of moderately intense exercise on cognitive performance, possible acute benefits of exercise at low or high intensities have been less well studied. However, there is some evidence that high-intensity exercise might also elicit temporary improvements in cognitive performance. Using a randomized controlled trial, Gawrilow, Stadler, Langguth, Naumann, and Boeck (2016) assigned children with ADHD either to jumping on a trampoline for 5 minutes or to colouring pictures depicting activities. Following the short exercise bout at high intensity, the authors found greater performance on an inhibition task than after the control condition.

Similarly, Medina et al. (2010) reported higher vigilance and sustained attention on the continuous performance test after 30 minutes of high-intensity interval training compared to 30 minutes of stretching. As the authors found that exercise-related improvements were not different between methylphenidate users and non-users, this further supports the role of high-intensity exercise as potential complementary treatment in ADHD.

Apart from intensity, the environment in which exercise is performed should also be considered an influencing factor for acute benefits for cognitive outcomes in children diagnosed with ADHD. In this respect, Taylor and Kuo (2008) showed that a 20-minute individually guided walk in the park was sufficient to improve working memory relative to the same amount of time in other settings, such as a neighbourhood and town centre. Consequently, mild exercise can also elicit favourable changes in executive function, when the appropriate surroundings are available.

In summary, the findings of the reviewed studies consistently support a positive effect of acute moderate aerobic exercise on cognitive performance. However, a few studies have shown that aerobic activities at mild and high intensity may also elicit improvements in cognitive outcomes. Due to the limited number of studies in this field, it remains unclear whether intensity and duration of the exercise session influence the magnitude of such benefits. Regarding qualitative aspects of exercise, there is compelling evidence for a neuroenhancing effect of aerobic activities in ADHD. At the same time, it should be noted that possible cognitive benefits elicited by other exercise modalities have not been investigated yet. Using a single aerobic exercise session, most studies have targeted aspects of executive function in ADHD. Whereas results were heterogeneous for working memory and set shifting, exercise-induced improvements of the inhibition component were mostly consistent. As impaired inhibitory control is one core deficit in children and adolescents with ADHD, exercise might be used to normalize this aspect of executive function temporarily.

Chronic exercise, cognition and behaviour

In contrast to acute benefits of exercise, changes in behavioural and cognitive outcomes elicited by regular engagement in exercise are considered to be long-lasting. This continuous approach is suggested to be a prerequisite for the facilitation of the trajectory of ADHD. The initial indications of a potential role of exercise in the treatment of ADHD and related symptoms were provided by cross-sectional studies. In this respect, Kiluk, Weden, and Culotta (2009) found that children with ADHD, who regularly participated in three or more sports, displayed fewer anxiety and depression symptoms than their less active peers. Additionally, engagement in moderate-to-vigorous physical activity (MVPA) has been shown to predict planning ability in boys with ADHD (Gapin & Etnier, 2010). Thus, the risk of comorbidities and impairments in specific executive functions seems to be reduced in ADHD sufferers with high MVPA levels compared to peers with low MVPA levels.

Further evidence for the positive influence of chronic exercise on ADHD-related symptoms is provided by longitudinal studies, which implemented a training intervention involving aerobic activities combined with other exercise modalities. Smith et al. (2013) investigated possible behavioural and cognitive benefits of such an exercise programme (5 × 26 minutes of MVPA per week) in children with ADHD. Each session was administered prior to school and involved activities that required children to employ different motor skills. Following the 8-week intervention period, the authors found improved performance on tasks demanding inhibitory control as well as a reduction in inappropriate behaviour that was evident from teacher, staff and parental ratings.

Verret, Guay, Berthiaume, Gardiner, and Beliveau (2012) also investigated the effects of an exercise programme which was designed to foster MVPA. Using a randomized controlled trial design, children with ADHD were assigned to mixed aerobic activities (3 × 45 minutes weekly), such as tag and ball games, or a control group. After the 10-week intervention period, children in the experimental group showed a higher level of information processing compared to controls, attributed to improved selective hearing and sustained attention. Additionally, mixed aerobic activities led to a reduction in impulsive behaviour.

Similarly, Bustamante et al. (2016) reported cognitive and behavioural improvements after a 10-week exercise programme, in which children with ADHD engaged either in 60 minutes of cooperative and competitive active games five times a week or participated in an art project. Whereas the control group improved visuospatial working memory and oppositional defiant symptoms, the 10-week exercise programme led to greater reductions in impulsive behaviour and increased verbal working memory.

Some researchers have examined whether or not such benefits for ADHD-related symptoms can also be elicited when aerobic activities are performed in shallow water. Pursuing this line of research, Chang, Hung, Huang, Hatfield, and Hung (2014) assigned children diagnosed with ADHD to an 8-week programme of moderately intense aquatic exercise consisting of two 90-minute sessions per week or a wait-list control group. The posttests revealed that the exercise group compared to controls improved the inhibition component of executive functioning.

Using an identical intervention protocol, Huang et al. (2014) investigated the effect of aquatic exercise on cortical activity at rest in children with ADHD. Following the intervention period, the exercise group showed decreased frontal and central theta–beta ratio compared to controls. High theta–beta ratio is an abnormal electroencephalogram characteristic evident in ADHD, which is associated with impaired inhibitory control and cortical hypoarousal. Thus, the aquatic exercise programme induced a favourable change of the cortical activation pattern in children diagnosed with ADHD.

Although the majority of studies focused on possible benefits of some kind of aerobic activities, coordinative exercise and skill training have also received some attention in ADHD research. For example, Pan et al. (2015) randomly assigned children with ADHD to 12 weeks of table tennis training with two 70-minute sessions weekly or no training. The exercise intervention, which was supposed to promote motor skills, led to improvements on all cognitive measures, including inhibitory control and task switching.

Focusing on the efficacy of different exercise programmes, Ziereis and Jansen (2015) compared the effects of motor skill training with a sports programme including a variety of activities, such as swimming, climbing and track and field. Children with ADHD were assigned to one of the 12-week training interventions, which consisted of one 60-minute session weekly, or a control group. Irrespective of the exercise type, participants in the exercise groups improved performance on all measures of working memory, whereas cognitive outcomes remained unchanged in controls.

Regarding exercise modality, tai chi and yoga have also been considered candidates for eliciting a beneficial effect on ADHD-related symptoms as they link physical exercise with meditation/concentration training. However, the results of Jensen and Kenny (2004) do not support this assumption, as children assigned to a 20-week yoga programme (one 60-minute session per week) did not show improvements in ADHD symptom severity and sustained attention. In contrast, a control group, which engaged in communication training, significantly reduced hyperactivity, anxiety and social problems. Increasing the frequency of yoga classes to two sessions per week, Harrison, Manocha, and Rubia (2004) found improvements in ADHD-related symptoms after 6 weeks. Along with these benefits, children with ADHD performing yoga also reported fewer conflicts and increased attention in school. Following a 5-week tai chi intervention with two 30-minute sessions per week, Hernandez-Reif, Field, and Thimas (2001) found similar improvements in children's ADHD behaviour, including the suppression of hyperactivity and inappropriate emotions.

Rather than using sports therapy alone, some researchers have systematically combined pharmacotherapy and exercise training to assess its value as a complementary treatment method. In the study by Kang, Choi, Kang, and Han (2011), children with ADHD received methylphenidate and education on behavioural control or engaged in 90 minutes of mixed aerobic activities twice a week. The authors were able to show that exercise combined with pharmacotherapy reduced parent and teacher ratings of inattention and improved various aspects of executive function, such as working memory and task switching.

These findings are supported by Choi, Han, Kang, Jung, and Renshaw (2015), who also examined the impact of adding mixed aerobic activities or an educational programme to methylphenidate treatment on ADHD-related symptoms. Compared to the group receiving behavioural education, adolescents completing three 90-minute sessions of mixed aerobic activities per week showed improved behavioural symptoms of ADHD and performance on a set-shifting task. This favourable change was related to an increase in cortical activity in the right PFC during the task. Therefore, it is reasonable to suggest that exercise-induced benefits in ADHD are partly due to a normalization of the task-related hypoactivation of the PFC.

As a combination of evidence-based treatment methods and exercise training seems to be promising, some researchers have also implemented elements of behavioural approaches in exercise therapy. In a study by Lufi and Parish-Plass (2011), children diagnosed with ADHD and children with other behavioural problems participated in weekly group therapy sessions over 1 year. Those sessions always involved a 30-minute group discussion led by psychologists, 30 minutes of aerobic activities and 30 minutes of team sports (e.g. basketball and soccer). As evident from self and parental ratings, treatment led to improvements in multiple behaviour domains, such as aggression, anxiety and attention.

In contrast, Smith et al. (2016) could not observe a reduction of ADHD-related symptoms after an integrative treatment approach consisting of coordinative exercise, cognitive training and behavioural education. Moreover, 15 weeks of integrative therapy with 60 sessions did not improve working memory in comparison to treatment-as-usual.

Summarizing the findings from experimental trials, it becomes evident that regular exercise has a beneficial impact on cognitive performance and ADHD-related behaviour. This finding is supported by a recent meta-analysis by Cerrillo-Urbina et al. (2015). Combining effect sizes from eight studies, the authors reported moderate to large effects of aerobic exercise on core symptoms, including attention, hyperactivity, social behaviour and executive function in children with ADHD. The reviewed studies further show that improvements in cognitive performance after 8–10 weeks of mixed aerobic activities were most pronounced for working memory and inhibitory control. In contrast, other exercise modalities have been less well studied in children with ADHD. However, there is some evidence for improved executive functioning after skill training and a favourable change in ADHD-related behaviour following tai chi and yoga. More promising is the combination of pharmaceutical or behavioural therapy with aerobic activities. Using this exercise modality in complementary treatment, experimental studies reported significant reductions of behavioural symptoms and executive function deficits in children with ADHD. The experimental studies therefore suggest that exercise is an efficient complement to medication, but exercise without systematic pharmacological treatment may also reduce core symptoms of ADHD. However, due to scarcity of relevant knowledge, it remains to be elucidated how exercise dose and characteristics influence the efficiency of training interventions in ADHD.

Underlying mechanisms for exercise-induced benefits in ADHD

Whereas intensive research has been conducted into the neurobiological underpinnings of ADHD, the mechanisms by which exercise reduces cognitive and behavioural impairments are still largely unknown. In an attempt to gain a deeper understanding of the effects of exercise on brain function and structure, many researchers have focused on healthy young and older adults. In contrast, possible underlying mechanisms of exercise-induced improvements in children with and without ADHD have rarely been studied. Consequently, it remains unclear whether or not the link between cognitive performance, brain function and morphology found in healthy adults (Erickson, Hillman, & Kramer, 2015) also exists in children and adolescents. Moreover, the time course of cognitive benefits in response to acute and chronic exercise suggests that there are different mechanisms driving the change. Due to the scarcity of relevant knowledge, findings from various target groups are combined to provide possible explanations for the neuroenhancing effect of exercise in ADHD.

Catecholamines and cerebral blood flow

Based on the arousal–performance interaction theory (Yerkes & Dodson, 1908), exercise intensity is suggested to influence cognitive performance in healthy samples in an inverted-U effect (Brisswalter, Collardeau, & René, 2002). Although there is a lack of knowledge on this dose–response relationship in ADHD, experimental studies consistently found improvements of executive function after aerobic exercise at moderate intensity. Similar to cognitive performance, cerebral blood flow and oxygenation are increased at moderate intensity and decrease when the load becomes more demanding (Ide & Secher, 2000; Mekari et al., 2015). These observations from healthy adults suggest that moderate aerobic exercise creates a nutritive environment by increasing the availability and supply of energetic substances to the brain. Children with ADHD might also benefit from this mechanism, as Gustafsson, Thernlund, Ryding, Rosén, and Cederblad (2000) have found that cerebral blood flow in the PFC is correlated with the degree of behavioural symptoms. A single exercise session might therefore elicit a temporary normalization of the hypoactivation and hypoperfusion of the PFC that is evident in children with ADHD.

Moreover, this disorder is also characterized by a hypocatecholaminergic state affecting regions of the frontal lobe (Prince, 2008). Interestingly, exercise has been shown to increase the expression of catecholamines, with an exponential increase in concentration occurring when the individual trains above the anaerobic threshold (Zouhal, Jacob, Delamarche, & Gratas-Delamarche, 2008). Whereas a low to moderate release of dopamine and noradrenaline is related to improvements of working memory, inhibition and attention regulation, a higher expression of these neurotransmitters impairs executive control due to severe neural traffic (Arnsten & Li, 2005; Cai & Arnsten, 1997). If moderate aerobic exercise triggers a similar release of dopamine and noradrenaline in children with ADHD, a facilitation of the hypocatecholaminergic state might partly explain exercise-induced benefits for cognition. In this case, the physiological effect of exercise would be similar to the effect of pharmacological treatments in ADHD, which positively influence information processing by augmenting the neurotransmission of dopamine and noradrenaline in the PFC (Del Campo et al., 2011).

BDNF, brain function and structure

Whereas acute exercise is suggested to facilitate the neurotransmission of catecholamines and brain function, a period of regular exercise is required to evoke morphological changes (Thomas, Dennis, Bandettini, & Johansen-Berg, 2012). Experimental studies have shown increases of grey matter in PFC and other regions concurrent with cognitive benefits in older adults after 6 months of aerobic training (Colcombe et al., 2006; Ruscheweyh et al., 2011). In contrast, possible benefits of aerobic exercise on grey mass have not yet been examined in children. However, Chaddock et al. (2010) found greater volumes in dorsal striatum in highly fit children compared to their not very fit peers. This is a first indication that regular exercise designed to increase cardiovascular fitness might also improve brain structure in children. Recalling that children with ADHD are characterized by volume reductions in several prefrontal brain regions (Valera et al., 2007), exercise might have a beneficial effect for the delayed structural maturation.

Regarding white-matter integrity, Schaeffer et al. (2014) found that 8 months of aerobic training had a positive influence on uncinated fasciculus in overweight children. Similar to ADHD, this group is characterized by uncinate perturbation (Yau, Castro, Tagani, Tsui, & Convit, 2012), which causes impairments in decision making and social-emotional problems (Heide, Skipper, Klobusicky, & Olson, 2013). Conversely, increased white-matter tract integrity might contribute to exercise-induced improvements on executive function and ADHD-related behaviour.

Regarding functional properties of the brain, there is compelling evidence for hypoactivation of the PFC in ADHD. Fortunately, exercise interventions including aerobic activities have been shown to increase task-related activation of the PFC (Choi et al., 2015) and to normalize cortical activity in the resting state (Huang et al., 2014). As insufficient activation of the PFC is related to impairments in goal-oriented behaviour, the tendency of aerobic exercise to facilitate this hypoaroused state of the central nervous system might partly explain how regular exercise benefits executive function in ADHD.

Furthermore, the expression of growth factors in response to exercise is considered a potential mechanism for favourable changes in the trajectory of ADHD. Especially BDNF has received much attention in brain research, because it plays a key role in neurogenesis, promotes synaptic plasticity and increases neuronal cell survival (Cotman & Berchtold, 2002). In turn, structural abnormalities and functional impairments are linked with a reduced expression of BDNF (Brunoni, Lopes, & Fregni, 2008).

In a recent meta-analysis, Szuhany, Bugatti, and Otto (2015) showed that both acute and chronic exercise have an impact on the regulation of this growth factor. Interestingly, regular exercise increases resting BDNF levels as well as the responsivity of BDNF to a single exercise session, so that the magnitude of acute effects is intensified after a training period. As the response of growth factors to exercise has been studied in adults only, it remains unclear whether or not exercise similarly increases BDNF levels in children with and without ADHD. However, Lou, Liu, Chang, and Chen (2008) found enhanced neurogenesis along with an increased expression of BDNF after aerobic exercise in juvenile rats. Kim et al. (2011) provide further support for the link between this growth factor and exercise-related benefits in an animal model of ADHD. Rats receiving methylphenidate and rats participating in treadmill exercise similarly increased BDNF levels, improved cognitive performance and reduced symptoms of hyperactivity. Taken together, these findings suggest that the BDNF response contributes to chronic effects of exercise on cognition and ADHD-related behaviour.

Exercise recommendations

A growing body of evidence shows that exercise reduces cognitive impairments and developmentally inappropriate behaviour in children and adolescents with ADHD. Regarding the acute effects of exercise, controlled studies have consistently found improvements in executive functioning, which were most pronounced in inhibitory control. Such cognitive enhancements were reported after children with ADHD engaged in aerobic activities with durations ranging from 5 to 30 minutes. So far, there is no indication of any moderating effect of exercise intensity and duration on the magnitude of cognitive benefits. Consequently, there is currently no need to formulate specific exercise prescriptions, apart from the fact that children with ADHD should be encouraged to perform aerobic exercise for a temporary enhancement of capabilities in executive functioning. However, it should be noted that most studies investigated moderate aerobic exercise, so that it remains unclear whether or not children with ADHD can expect similar or even greater benefits from other exercise modalities. Although the positive effects of a single exercise session on executive function are transient, they have a high practical relevance. Children and adolescents with ADHD may use a short aerobic exercise bout to prepare for situations demanding high executive control, such as oral tests and final examinations in school.

In contrast to acute effects of exercise, regular exercise is considered to elicit long-term benefits for cognitive performance and behaviour in children and adolescents with ADHD. Findings from experimental studies strongly indicate that mixed aerobic activities over a period of 8–10 weeks improve core deficits in ADHD, including inattention, hyperactivity, antisocial behaviour and decrements in executive function. Moreover, some evidence suggests that other exercise modalities, such as yoga, tai chi and skill training, also reduce symptoms of the disorder. As quantitative aspects of the exercise programmes varied between the reviewed studies, it is difficult to derive recommendations on intensity, frequency and duration of exercise for children and adolescents with ADHD. However, it is apparent that one or two sessions of skill training, yoga or tai chi per week elicited similar benefits for executive function and behaviour as three to five weekly sessions of mixed aerobic activities. This does not necessarily mean that aerobic activities are less efficient, because so far the effect of an aerobic exercise programme with lower frequency of sessions has only been investigated in combination with systematic methylphenidate treatment.

Such complementary approaches are promising as pharmacological treatment combined with regular exercise has consistently been found to reduce impairments in executive control and behavioural deficits. Consequently, ADHD research has reached a point where regular engagement in physical exercise can safely be recommended as complementary treatment for children and adolescents affected by the disease. Due to a lack of long-term studies and follow-up assessments, the current evidence does not indicate that exercise can actually replace pharmacological or behavioural therapy. Future studies should therefore address the question of if and how a manipulation of qualitative and quantitative aspects of exercise can increase the long-term effectiveness of exercise interventions in ADHD.

References

American Psychiatric Association. (2013). *Diagnostic and statistical manual of mental disorders: DSM-5* (5th ed.). Washington, D.C.: American Psychiatric Association.

Anestis, M. D., Bagge, C. L., Tull, M. T., & Joiner, T. E. (2011). Clarifying the role of emotion dysregulation in the interpersonal-psychological theory of suicidal behavior in an undergraduate sample. *Journal of Psychiatric Research*, 45(5), 603–611. doi: 10.1016/j.jpsychires.2010.10.013.

Arnold, L. E., Hodgkins, P., Kahle, J., Madhoo, M., & Kewley, G. (2015). Long-term outcomes of ADHD academic achievement and performance. *Journal of Attention Disorders*, 1087054714566076. doi: 10.1177/1087054714566076.

Arnsten, A. F. T., & Li, B.-M. (2005). Neurobiology of executive functions: Catecholamine influences on prefrontal cortical functions. *Biological Psychiatry*, 57(11), 1377–1384. doi: 10.1016/j.biopsych.2004.08.019.

Banich, M. T. (2009). Executive function: The search for an integrated account. *Current Directions in Psychological Science*, 18(2), 89–94. doi: 10.1111/j.1467-8721.2009.01615.x.

Barkley, R. A., & Fischer, M. (2010). The unique contribution of emotional impulsiveness to impairment in major life activities in hyperactive children as adults. *Journal of the American Academy of Child and Adolescent Psychiatry*, 49(5), 503–513.

Berwid, O. G., & Halperin, J. M. (2012). Emerging support for a role of exercise in attention-deficit/hyperactivity disorder intervention planning. *Current Psychiatry Reports*, 14(5), 543–551. doi: 10.1007/s11920-012-0297-4.

Brisswalter, J., Collardeau, M., & René, A. (2002). Effects of acute physical exercise characteristics on cognitive performance. *Sports Medicine, 32*(9), 555–566. doi: 10.2165/00007256-200232090-00002.

Brock, L. L., Rimm-Kaufman, S. E., Nathanson, L., & Grimm, K. J. (2009). The contributions of 'hot' and 'cool' executive function to children's academic achievement, learning-related behaviors, and engagement in kindergarten. *Early Childhood Research Quarterly, 24*(3), 337–349. doi: 10.1016/j.ecresq.2009.06.001.

Brunoni, A. R., Lopes, M., & Fregni, F. (2008). A systematic review and meta-analysis of clinical studies on major depression and BDNF levels: Implications for the role of neuroplasticity in depression. *International Journal of Neuropsychopharmacology, 11*(8), 1169–1180. doi: 10.1017/S1461145708009309.

Bustamante, E. E., Davis, C. L., Frazier, S. L., Rusch, D., Fogg, L. F., Atkins, M. S., & Marquez, D. X. (2016). Randomized controlled trial of exercise for ADHD and disruptive behavior disorders. *Medicine and Science in Sports and Exercise, 48*(7), 1397–1407. doi: 10.1249/MSS.0000000000000891.

Cai, J. X., & Arnsten, A. F. (1997). Dose-dependent effects of the dopamine D1 receptor agonists A77636 or SKF81297 on spatial working memory in aged monkeys. *The Journal of Pharmacology and Experimental Therapeutics, 283*(1), 183–189.

Castellanos, F. X., Sonuga-Barke, E. J., Milham, M. P., & Tannock, R. (2006). Characterizing cognition in ADHD: Beyond executive dysfunction. *Trends in Cognitive Sciences, 10*(3), 117–123. doi: 10.1016/j.tics.2006.01.011.

Cerrillo-Urbina, A. J., Garcia-Hermoso, A., Sanchez-Lopez, M., Pardo-Guijarro, M. J., Santos Gomez, J. L., & Martinez-Vizcaino, V. (2015). The effects of physical exercise in children with attention deficit hyperactivity disorder: A systematic review and meta-analysis of randomized control trials. *Child: Care, Health and Development, 41*(6), 779–788. doi: 10.1111/cch.12255.

Chaddock, L., Erickson, K. I., Prakash, R. S., VanPatter, M., Voss, M. W., Pontifex, M. B., . . . Kramer, A. F. (2010). Basal ganglia volume is associated with aerobic fitness in preadolescent children. *Developmental Neuroscience, 32*(3), 249–256. doi: 10.1159/000316648.

Chang, Y. K., Hung, C. L., Huang, C. J., Hatfield, B. D., & Hung, T. M. (2014). Effects of an aquatic exercise program on inhibitory control in children with ADHD: A preliminary study. *Archives of Clinical Neuropsychology: The Official Journal of the National Academy of Neuropsychologists, 29*(3), 217–223. doi: 10.1093/arclin/acu003.

Chang, Y. K., Liu, S., Yu, H. H., & Lee, Y. H. (2012). Effect of acute exercise on executive function in children with attention deficit hyperactivity disorder. *Archives of Clinical Neuropsychology: The Official Journal of the National Academy of Neuropsychologists, 27*(2), 225–237. doi: 10.1093/arclin/acr094.

Charach, A., Carson, P., Fox, S., Ali, M. U., Beckett, J., & Lim, C. G. (2013). Interventions for preschool children at high risk for ADHD: A comparative effectiveness review. *Pediatrics*, peds.2012-0974. doi: 10.1542/peds.2012-0974.

Cherkasova, M. V., & Hechtman, L. (2009). Neuroimaging in attention-deficit hyperactivity disorder: Beyond the frontostriatal circuitry. *The Canadian Journal of Psychiatry, 54*(10), 651–664. doi: 10.1177/070674370905401002.

Choi, J. W., Han, D. H., Kang, K. D., Jung, H. Y., & Renshaw, P. F. (2015). Aerobic exercise and attention deficit hyperactivity disorder: Brain research.

Medicine and Science in Sports and Exercise, 47(1), 33–39. doi: 10.1249/MSS.0000000000000373.

Colcombe, S. J., Erickson, K. I., Scalf, P. E., Kim, J. S., Prakash, R., McAuley, E., . . . Kramer, A. F. (2006). Aerobic exercise training increases brain volume in aging humans. *The Journals of Gerontology. Series A, Biological Sciences and Medical Sciences, 61*(11), 1166–1170.

Cotman, C. W., & Berchtold, N. C. (2002). Exercise: A behavioral intervention to enhance brain health and plasticity. *Trends in Neurosciences, 25*(6), 295–301. doi: 10.1016/S0166-2236(02)02143-4.

Cubillo, A., Halari, R., Smith, A., Taylor, E., & Rubia, K. (2012). A review of fronto-striatal and fronto-cortical brain abnormalities in children and adults with attention deficit hyperactivity disorder (ADHD) and new evidence for dysfunction in adults with ADHD during motivation and attention. *Frontal Lobes, 48*(2), 194–215. doi: 10.1016/j.cortex.2011.04.007.

Daley, D., & Birchwood, J. (2010). ADHD and academic performance: Why does ADHD impact on academic performance and what can be done to support ADHD children in the classroom? *Child: Care, Health and Development, 36*(4), 455–464. doi: 10.1111/j.1365-2214.2009.01046.x.

Del Campo, N., Chamberlain, S. R., Sahakian, B. J., & Robbins, T. W. (2011). The roles of dopamine and noradrenaline in the pathophysiology and treatment of attention-deficit/hyperactivity disorder. *Prefrontal Cortical Circuits Regulating Attention, Behavior and Emotion, 69*(12), e145–e157. doi: 10.1016/j.biopsych.2011.02.036.

Diamond, A. (2013). Executive functions. *Annual Review of Psychology, 64*, 135–168. doi: 10.1146/annurev-psych-113011-143750.

Erickson, K. I., Hillman, C. H., & Kramer, A. F. (2015). Physical activity, brain, and cognition. *Current Opinion in Behavioral Sciences, 4*, 27–32. doi: 10.1016/j.cobeha.2015.01.005.

Fletcher, J., & Wolfe, B. (2009). Long-term consequences of childhood ADHD on criminal activities. *The Journal of Mental Health Policy and Economics, 12*(3), 119–138.

Gapin, J. I., & Etnier, J. L. (2010). The relationship between physical activity and executive function performance in children with attention-deficit hyperactivity disorder. *Journal of Sport and Exercise Psychology, 32*(6), 753–763.

Gapin, J. I., Labban, J. D., Bohall, S. C., Wooten, J. S., & Chang, Y.-K. (2015). Acute exercise is associated with specific executive functions in college students with ADHD: A preliminary study. *Journal of Sport and Health Science, 4*(1), 89–96. doi: 10.1016/j.jshs.2014.11.003.

Gapin, J. I., Labban, J. D., & Etnier, J. L. (2011). The effects of physical activity on attention deficit hyperactivity disorder symptoms: The evidence. *Preventive Medicine, 52*(Suppl), S70–S74. doi: 10.1016/j.ypmed.2011.01.022.

Gawrilow, C., Stadler, G., Langguth, N., Naumann, A., & Boeck, A. (2016). Physical activity, affect, and cognition in children with symptoms of ADHD. *Journal of Attention Disorders, 20*(2), 151–162. doi: 10.1177/1087054713493318.

Graham, J., & Coghill, D. (2008). Adverse effects of pharmacotherapies for attention-deficit hyperactivity disorder: Epidemiology, prevention and management. *CNS Drugs, 22*(3), 213–237.

Grassmann, V., Alves, M. V., Santos-Galduroz, R. F., & Galduroz, J. C. F. (2017). Possible cognitive benefits of acute physical exercise in children with

ADHD: A systematic review. *Journal of Attention Disorders, 21*(5), 367–371. doi: 10.1177/1087054714526041.

Gustafsson, P., Thernlund, G., Ryding, E., Rosén, I., & Cederblad, M. (2000). Associations between cerebral blood-flow measured by single photon emission computed tomography (SPECT), electro-encephalogram (EEG), behaviour symptoms, cognition and neurological soft signs in children with attention-deficit hyperactivity disorder (ADHD). *Acta Paediatrica, 89*(7), 830–835. doi: 10.1111/j.1651-2227.2000.tb00391.x.

Hamilton, L. S., Levitt, J. G., O'Neill, J., Alger, J. R., Luders, E., Phillips, O. R., . . . Narr, K. L. (2008). Reduced white matter integrity in attention-deficit hyperactivity disorder. *Neuroreport, 19*(17), 1705. doi: 10.1097/WNR.0b013e3283174415.

Harrison, L. J., Manocha, R., & Rubia, K. (2004). Sahaja yoga meditation as a family treatment programme for children with attention deficit-hyperactivity disorder. *Clinical Child Psychology and Psychiatry, 9*(4), 479–497. doi: 10.1177/1359104504046155.

Heide, R. J., von der, Skipper, L. M., Klobusicky, E., & Olson, I. R. (2013). Dissecting the uncinate fasciculus: Disorders, controversies and a hypothesis. *Brain, 136*(6), 1692–1707. doi: 10.1093/brain/awt094.

Hernandez-Reif, M., Field, T. M., & Thimas, E. (2001). Attention deficit hyperactivity disorder: Benefits from tai chi. *Journal of Bodywork and Movement Therapies, 5*(2), 120–123. doi: 10.1054/jbmt.2000.0219.

Hill, L. J., Williams, J. H., Aucott, L., Thomson, J., & Mon-Williams, M. (2011). How does exercise benefit performance on cognitive tests in primary-school pupils? *Developmental Medicine and Child Neurology, 53*(7), 630–635. doi: 10.1111/j.1469-8749.2011.03954.x.

Hoza, B. (2007). Peer functioning in children with ADHD. *Ambulatory Pediatrics: The Official Journal of the Ambulatory Pediatric Association, 7*(1 Suppl), 101–106. doi: 10.1016/j.ambp.2006.04.011.

Huang, C.-J., Huang, C.-W., Tsai, Y.-J., Tsai, C.-L., Chang, Y.-K., & Hung, T.-M. (2014). A preliminary examination of aerobic exercise effects on resting EEG in children with ADHD. *Journal of Attention Disorders.* doi: 10.1177/1087054714554611.

Ide, K., & Secher, N. H. (2000). Cerebral blood flow and metabolism during exercise. *Progress in Neurobiology, 61*(4), 397–414.

James, A., Lai, F. H., & Dahl, C. (2004). Attention deficit hyperactivity disorder and suicide: A review of possible associations. *Acta Psychiatrica Scandinavica, 110*(6), 408–415. doi: 10.1111/j.1600-0447.2004.00384.x.

Jensen, P. S., & Kenny, D. T. (2004). The effects of yoga on the attention and behavior of boys with attention-deficit/hyperactivity disorder (ADHD). *Journal of Attention Disorders, 7*(4), 205–216.

Kang, K. D., Choi, J. W., Kang, S. G., & Han, D. H. (2011). Sports therapy for attention, cognitions and sociality. *International Journal of Sports Medicine, 32*(12), 953–959. doi: 10.1055/s-0031-1283175.

Kieling, R. R., Szobot, C. M., Matte, B., Coelho, R. S., Kieling, C., Pechansky, F., & La Rohde. (2011). Mental disorders and delivery motorcycle drivers (motoboys): A dangerous association. *European Psychiatry: The Journal of the Association of European Psychiatrists, 26*(1), 23–27. doi: 10.1016/j.eurpsy.2010.03.004.

Kiluk, B. D., Weden, S., & Culotta, V. P. (2009). Sport participation and anxiety in children with ADHD. *Journal of Attention Disorders, 12*(6), 499–506. doi: 10.1177/1087054708320400.

Kim, H., Heo, H.-I., Kim, D.-H., Ko, I.-G., Lee, S.-S., Kim, S.-E., . . . Kim, C.-J. (2011). Treadmill exercise and methylphenidate ameliorate symptoms of attention deficit/hyperactivity disorder through enhancing dopamine synthesis and brain-derived neurotrophic factor expression in spontaneous hypertensive rats. *Neuroscience Letters, 504*(1), 35–39. doi: 10.1016/j.neulet.2011.08.052.

Kim, S., Nordling, J. K., Yoon, J. E., Boldt, L. J., & Kochanska, G. (2013). Effortful control in "hot" and "cool" tasks differentially predicts children's behavior problems and academic performance. *Journal of Abnormal Child Psychology, 41*(1), 43–56. doi: 10.1007/s10802-012-9661-4.

Lee, S. S., Humphreys, K. L., Flory, K., Liu, R., & Glass, K. (2011). Prospective association of childhood attention-deficit/hyperactivity disorder (ADHD) and substance use and abuse/dependence: A meta-analytic review. *Clinical Psychology Review, 31*(3), 328–341. doi: 10.1016/j.cpr.2011.01.006.

Loe, I. M., & Feldman, H. M. (2007). Academic and educational outcomes of children with ADHD. *Journal of Pediatric Psychology, 32*(6), 643–654. doi: 10.1093/jpepsy/jsl054.

Lofthouse, N., Arnold, L. E., Hersch, S., Hurt, E., & Debeus, R. (2012). A review of neurofeedback treatment for pediatric ADHD. *Journal of Attention Disorders, 16*(5), 351–372. doi: 10.1177/1087054711427530.

Lou, S.-J., Liu, J.-Y., Chang, H., & Chen, P.-J. (2008). Hippocampal neurogenesis and gene expression depend on exercise intensity in juvenile rats. *Brain Research, 1210*, 48–55. doi: 10.1016/j.brainres.2008.02.080.

Ludyga, S., Gerber, M., Brand, S., Holsboer-Trachsler, E., & Pühse, U. (2016). The acute effects of moderate aerobic exercise on specific aspects of executive function in different age and fitness groups: A meta-analysis. *Psychophysiology, 53*(11), 1611–1626. doi: 10.1111/psyp.12736.

Lufi, D., & Parish-Plass, J. (2011). Sport-based group therapy program for boys with ADHD or with other behavioral disorders. *Child and Family Behavior Therapy, 33*(3), 217–230. doi: 10.1080/07317107.2011.596000.

Medina, J. A., Netto, T. L., Muszkat, M., Medina, A. C., Botter, D., Orbetelli, R., . . . Miranda, M. C. (2010). Exercise impact on sustained attention of ADHD children, methylphenidate effects. *Attention Deficit and Hyperactivity Disorders, 2*(1), 49–58. doi: 10.1007/s12402-009-0018-y.

Mekari, S., Fraser, S., Bosquet, L., Bonnery, C., Labelle, V., Pouliot, P., . . . Bherer, L. (2015). The relationship between exercise intensity, cerebral oxygenation and cognitive performance in young adults. *European Journal of Applied Physiology, 115*(10), 2189–2197. doi: 10.1007/s00421-015-3199-4.

Melby-Lervåg, M., & Hulme, C. (2013). Is working memory training effective? A meta-analytic review. *Developmental Psychology, 49*(2), 270. doi: 10.1037/a0028228.

Menon, V. (2011). Large-scale brain networks and psychopathology: A unifying triple network model. *Trends in Cognitive Sciences, 15*(10), 483–506. doi: 10.1016/j.tics.2011.08.003.

Pan, C.-Y., Tsai, C.-L., Chu, C.-H., Sung, M.-C., Huang, C.-Y., & Ma, W.-Y. (2015). Effects of physical exercise intervention on motor skills and executive functions in children with ADHD: A pilot study. *Journal of Attention Disorders*, *31*, 149–157. doi: 10.1177/1087054715569282.

Piepmeier, A. T., Shih, C.-H., Whedon, M., Williams, L. M., Davis, M. E., Henning, D. A., . . . Etnier, J. L. (2015). The effect of acute exercise on cognitive performance in children with and without ADHD. *Journal of Sport and Health Science*, *4*(1), 97–104. doi: 10.1016/j.jshs.2014.11.004.

Polanczyk, G. V., Lima, M. S. de, Horta, B. L., Biederman, J., & La Rohde. (2007). The worldwide prevalence of ADHD: A systematic review and metaregression analysis. *The American Journal of Psychiatry*, *164*(6), 942–948. doi: 10.1176/ajp.2007.164.6.942.

Polanczyk, G. V., Willcutt, E. G., Salum, G. A., Kieling, C., & Rohde, L. A. (2014). ADHD prevalence estimates across three decades: An updated systematic review and meta-regression analysis. *International Journal of Epidemiology*, *43*(2), 434–442. doi: 10.1093/ije/dyt261.

Pontifex, M. B., Saliba, B. J., Raine, L. B., Picchietti, D. L., & Hillman, C. H. (2013). Exercise improves behavioral, neurocognitive, and scholastic performance in children with ADHD. *The Journal of Pediatrics*, *162*(3), 543–551. doi: 10.1016/j.jpeds.2012.08.036.

Prince, J. (2008). Catecholamine dysfunction in attention-deficit/hyperactivity disorder: An update. *Journal of Clinical Psychopharmacology*, *28*(3 Suppl 2), 45. doi: 10.1097/JCP.0b013e318174f92a.

Ramos, B. P., & Arnsten, A. F. (2007). Adrenergic pharmacology and cognition: Focus on the prefrontal cortex. *Pharmacology and Therapeutics*, *113*(3), 523–536. doi: 10.1016/j.pharmthera.2006.11.006.

Riggs, N. R., Jahromi, L. B., Razza, R. P., Dillworth-Bart, J. E., & Mueller, U. (2006). Executive function and the promotion of social–emotional competence. *Journal of Applied Developmental Psychology*, *27*(4), 300–309. doi: 10.1016/j.appdev.2006.04.002.

Royall, D. R., Lauterbach, E. C., Cummings, J. L., Reeve, A., Rummans, T. A., Di Kaufer, . . . Coffey, C. E. (2002). Executive control function: A review of its promise and challenges for clinical research. A report from the Committee on Research of the American Neuropsychiatric Association. *The Journal of Neuropsychiatry and Clinical Neurosciences*, *14*(4), 377–405. doi: 10.1176/jnp.14.4.377.

Rubia, K. (2011). "Cool" inferior frontostriatal dysfunction in attention-deficit/hyperactivity disorder versus "hot" ventromedial orbitofrontal-limbic dysfunction in conduct disorder: A review. *Prefrontal Cortical Circuits Regulating Attention, Behavior and Emotion*, *69*(12), e69–e87. doi: 10.1016/j.biopsych.2010.09.023.

Rubia, K., Alegria, A. A., & Brinson, H. (2014). Brain abnormalities in attention-deficit hyperactivity disorder: A review. *Revista de Neurologia*, *58*(Suppl 1), 16.

Ruscheweyh, R., Willemer, C., Krüger, K., Duning, T., Warnecke, T., Sommer, J., . . . Flöel, A. (2011). Physical activity and memory functions: An interventional study. *Neurobiology of Aging*, *32*(7), 1304–1319. doi: 10.1016/j.neurobiolaging.2009.08.001.

Schaeffer, D. J., Krafft, C. E., Schwarz, N. F., Chi, L., Rodrigue, A. L., Pierce, J. E., . . . McDowell, J. E. (2014). An 8-month exercise intervention alters frontotemporal white matter integrity in overweight children. *Psychophysiology*, *51*(8). doi: 10.1111/psyp.12227.

Shaw, M., Hodgkins, P., Caci, H., Young, S., Kahle, J., Woods, A. G., & Arnold, L. E. (2012). A systematic review and analysis of long-term outcomes in attention deficit hyperactivity disorder: Effects of treatment and non-treatment. *BMC Medicine*, 10(1), 1. doi: 10.1186/1741-7015-10-99.

Shaw, P., Eckstrand, K., Sharp, W., Blumenthal, J., Lerch, J. P., Greenstein, D., . . . Rapoport, J. L. (2007). Attention-deficit/hyperactivity disorder is characterized by a delay in cortical maturation. *Proceedings of the National Academy of Sciences of the United States of America*, 104(49), 19649–19654. doi: 10.1073/pnas.0707741104.

Smith, A. L., Hoza, B., Linnea, K., McQuade, J. D., Tomb, M., Vaughn, A. J., . . . Hook, H. (2013). Pilot physical activity intervention reduces severity of ADHD symptoms in young children. *Journal of Attention Disorders*, 17(1), 70–82. doi: 10.1177/1087054711417395.

Smith, S. D., Vitulano, L. A., Katsovich, L., Li, S., Moore, C., Li, F., . . . Leckman, J. F. (2016). A randomized controlled trial of an integrated brain, body, and social intervention for children with ADHD. *Journal of Attention Disorders*, 20, 1–15. doi: 10.1177/1087054716647490.

Szuhany, K. L., Bugatti, M., & Otto, M. W. (2015). A meta-analytic review of the effects of exercise on brain-derived neurotrophic factor. *Journal of Psychiatric Research*, 60, 56–64. doi: 10.1016/j.jpsychires.2014.10.003.

Tamminga, H. G., Reneman, L., Huizenga, H. M., & Geurts, H. M. (2016). Effects of methylphenidate on executive functioning in attention-deficit/hyperactivity disorder across the lifespan: A meta-regression analysis. *Psychological Medicine*, 46(9), 1791–1807. doi: 10.1017/S0033291716000350.

Taylor, A. F., & Kuo, F. E. (2008). Children with attention deficits concentrate better after walk in the park. *Journal of Attention Disorders*, 12(5), 402–409. doi: 10.1177/1087054708323000.

Thomas, A. G., Dennis, A., Bandettini, P. A., & Johansen-Berg, H. (2012). The effects of aerobic activity on brain structure. *Frontiers in Psychology*, 3. doi: 10.3389/fpsyg.2012.00086.

Tomporowski, P. D., McCullick, B., Pendleton, D. M., & Pesce, C. (2015). Exercise and children's cognition: The role of exercise characteristics and a place for metacognition. *Journal of Sport and Health Science*, 4(1), 47–55. doi: 10.1016/j.jshs.2014.09.003.

Tripp, G., & Wickens, J. R. (2008). Research review: Dopamine transfer deficit: a neurobiological theory of altered reinforcement mechanisms in ADHD. *Journal of Child Psychology and Psychiatry*, 49(7), 691–704. doi: 10.1111/j.1469-7610.2007.01851.x.

Valera, E. M., Faraone, S. V., Murray, K. E., & Seidman, L. J. (2007). Meta-analysis of structural imaging findings in attention-deficit/hyperactivity disorder. *Biological Psychiatry*, 61(12), 1361–1369. doi: 10.1016/j.biopsych.2006.06.011.

van Lieshout, M., Luman, M., Twisk, J. W. R., van Ewijk, H., Groenman, A. P., Thissen, Andrieke J. A. M., . . . Oosterlaan, J. (2016). A 6-year follow-up of a large European cohort of children with attention-deficit/hyperactivity disorder-combined subtype: Outcomes in late adolescence and young adulthood. *European Child and Adolescent Psychiatry*, 1–11. doi: 10.1007/s00787-016-0820-y.

Verret, C., Guay, M.-C., Berthiaume, C., Gardiner, P., & Beliveau, L. (2012). A physical activity program improves behavior and cognitive functions in children with ADHD: An exploratory study. *Journal of Attention Disorders*, 16(1), 71–80. doi: 10.1177/1087054710379735.

Vincent, J. L., Kahn, I., Snyder, A. Z., Raichle, M. E., & Buckner, R. L. (2008). Evidence for a frontoparietal control system revealed by intrinsic functional connectivity. *Journal of Neurophysiology*, 100(6), 3328–3342. doi: 10.1152/jn.90355.2008.

Vitiello, B., Lazzaretto, D., Yershova, K., Abikoff, H., Paykina, N., McCracken, J. T., . . . Riddle, M. A. (2015). Pharmacotherapy of the Preschool ADHD Treatment Study (PATS) children growing up. *Journal of the American Academy of Child and Adolescent Psychiatry*, 54(7), 550–556. doi: 10.1016/j.jaac.2015.04.004.

Wehmeier, P. M., Schacht, A., & Barkley, R. A. (2010). Social and emotional impairment in children and adolescents with ADHD and the impact on quality of life. *Journal of Adolescent Health*, 46(3), 209–217. doi: 10.1016/j.jadohealth.2009.09.009.

Wilens, T. E., Biederman, J., Brown, S., Tanguay, S., Monuteaux, M. C., Blake, C., & Spencer, T. J. (2002). Psychiatric comorbidity and functioning in clinically referred preschool children and school-age youths with ADHD. *Journal of the American Academy of Child and Adolescent Psychiatry*, 41(3), 262–268. doi: 10.1097/00004583-200203000-00005.

Willcutt, E. G., Doyle, A. E., Nigg, J. T., Faraone, S. V., & Pennington, B. F. (2005). Validity of the executive function theory of attention-deficit/hyperactivity disorder: A meta-analytic review. *Biological Psychiatry*, 57(11), 1336–1346. doi: 10.1016/j.biopsych.2005.02.006.

Willoughby, M., Kupersmidt, J., Voegler-Lee, M., & Bryant, D. (2011). Contributions of hot and cool self-regulation to preschool disruptive behavior and academic achievement. *Developmental Neuropsychology*, 36(2), 162–180. doi: 10.1080/87565641.2010.549980.

World Health Organization. (2004). *International statistical classification of diseases and related health problems* (10th revision, 2nd ed.). ICD-10. Geneva: World Health Organization.

Yap, M. B. H., Allen, N. B., & Sheeber, L. (2007). Using an emotion regulation framework to understand the role of temperament and family processes in risk for adolescent depressive disorders. *Clinical Child and Family Psychology Review*, 10(2), 180–196. doi: 10.1007/s10567-006-0014-0.

Yau, P. L., Castro, M. G., Tagani, A., Tsui, W. H., & Convit, A. (2012). Obesity and metabolic syndrome and functional and structural brain impairments in adolescence. *Pediatrics*, 130(4), e856–e864. doi: 10.1542/peds.2012-0324.

Yerkes, R. M., & Dodson, J. D. (1908). The relation of strength of stimulus to rapidity of habit-formation. *Journal of Comparative Neurology and Psychology*, 18(5), 459–482. doi: 10.1002/cne.920180503.

Ziereis, S., & Jansen, P. (2015). Effects of physical activity on executive function and motor performance in children with ADHD. *Research in Developmental Disabilities*, 38, 181–191. doi: 10.1016/j.ridd.2014.12.005.

Zouhal, H., Jacob, C., Delamarche, P., & Gratas-Delamarche, A. (2008). Catecholamines and the effects of exercise, training and gender. *Sports Medicine*, 38(5), 401–423. doi: 10.2165/00007256-200838050-00004.

Chapter 12

The effect of different exercise programmes on cognitive functioning in children and adolescents

Henning Budde, Flora Koutsandréou and Mirko Wegner

Introduction

Current estimates state that children and adolescents growing up in the 21st century will experience a lower life expectancy than previous generations (Olshansky et al., 2005). Lower life expectancy, as well as reduced mental and physical health, may partly be attributed to increasing physical inactivity in industrial countries like the USA (Hillman, Erickson, & Kramer, 2008; Secretary of Health and Human Services and the Secretary of Education, 2007). The harm of this sedentary lifestyle is tremendous (Colditz, 1999; Pratt et al., 2000). Moreover, this inactivity not only decreases health but may also interfere with children's and adolescents' cognitive development (Vaynman & Gomez-Pinilla, 2006). These adverse effects of a physical inactive lifestyle are found, although policy makers may integrate physical activity (PA) and exercise more effectively in different public health sectors (e.g. in schools, programmes in professional companies or health programmes financed by insurance companies).

Previous research has strongly suggested that PA and exercise benefit different areas of mental health (Penedo & Dahn, 2005), including, for example, depression, anxiety, cognitive functioning and psychological well-being in adults (Gauvin & Spence, 1996; Hillman et al., 2008; Wegner, Helmich, Machado, Arias-Carrión, & Budde, 2014) and in children and adolescents (Biddle & Asare, 2011; Donaldson & Ronan, 2006; Lagerberg, 2005; Sibley & Etnier, 2003). The present chapter aims to illustrate how PA and exercise contribute to cognitive functioning in children and adolescents. We will first define the terms PA, exercise and cognitive functioning. Then we will present evidence primarily from high-quality studies (e.g. randomized controlled trials) on the effects of PA and exercise on cognitive functioning, followed by an introduction to the effect of different acute and chronic exercise programmes on cognitive functioning in children and adolescents. In the concluding part of this chapter we will present existing evidence for neurobiological explanations of the benefits of exercise for cognitive functioning that may play a role in children and adolescents (Figure 12.1).

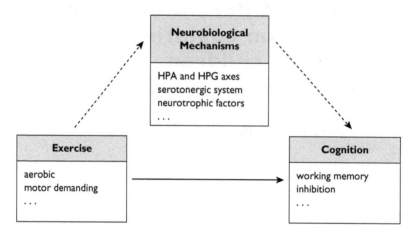

Figure 12.1 Exercise and cognition link and assumed neurobiological mechanisms. HPA, hypothalamic–pituitary–adrenal; HPG, hypothalamic–pituitary–gonadal. (Adapted from Wegner, M., & Budde, H. (in press). The exercise effect on mental health in children and adolescents. In H. Budde & M. Wegner (Eds.), *Exercise and mental health: Neurobiological mechanisms of the exercise effect on depression, anxiety, and well-being.* New York: Taylor and Francis.)

PA refers to body movement that leads to energy expenditure and is initiated by skeletal muscles (Budde et al., 2016; Caspersen, Powell, & Christenson, 1985). *Exercise* has been previously defined as a disturbance of homeostasis through muscle activity resulting in movement and increased energy expenditure (Scheuer & Tipton, 1977). However, the critical difference between the terms refers to the planned and structured nature of exercise (Caspersen et al., 1985). Additionally, a distinction must be made between acute and chronic exercise (Budde et al., 2016). While acute exercise is the physiological response associated with the immediate effects of a single bout of exercise, chronic exercise refers to the repeated performance of acute exercise and is often referred to as training (Scheuer & Tipton, 1977). *Physical fitness* in turn is the result of exercise or a planned, structured and repetitive training process and can typically address health components like cardiorespiratory endurance, strength, muscular and skeletal flexibility or body composition (Blair, Kohl, & Powell, 1987; Howley, 2001).

The term cognition includes processes of perception, attention, thinking/problem solving, memory and language and is typically referred to as how the mind works (Pinker, 1999). Cognitive control processes, also called executive functions, include different cognitive functions such as self-control, selective attention, cognitive inhibition, working memory and cognitive flexibility (Diamond, 2013; Miyake et al., 2000). Executive functions are usually subsumed into the three categories of self-control (also called inhibition), working memory and cognitive flexibility. *Self-control* involves resisting temptations and avoiding impulsive acting. *Working memory* helps to keep information in mind and allows us to work with this information mentally (e.g. to solve a problem). And *cognitive flexibility* refers to the ability to change perspectives on how to solve a problem, and the flexibility to adjust to changing priorities, rules or demands (Diamond, 2013). Executive functions further contribute to the higher-order cognitive processes of planning, problem solving and reasoning and are linked to mental health (Collins & Koechlin, 2012; Diamond, 2013). Individuals suffering from mental disorders (e.g. attention deficit-hyperactivity, conduct disorder, depression) often show decreased executive functioning (Diamond, 2005; Fairchild, van Goozen, Stollery, Aitken, & Savage, 2009; Taylor Tavares et al., 2007).

The exercise effect on cognitive functions in children and adolescents

Three previous meta-analyses illustrated the strength of the link between exercise or PA and cognitive functioning in children and adolescents, showing small to medium effects (0.28–0.52) (Fedewa & Ahn, 2011; Sibley & Etnier, 2003; Verburgh, Königs, Scherder, & Oosterlaan, 2014). Sibley and Etnier (2003) did not find differences between types of exercise on cognition. Fedewa and Ahn (2011), however, found the strongest effect on cognition for aerobic exercise programmes, and PA performed three times per week showed the strongest effects on cognitive performance in children and adolescents. Sibley and Etnier (2003) pointed to an age effect, with 11–13-year-old children benefiting most from exercise interventions followed by very young children aged 4–7 years. However, Verburgh and colleagues (2014) in their meta-analysis found no age effect of exercise on executive functions; thus the effect did not differ between studies examining children, adolescents and young adults. Among the three executive functions they found the strongest effect for self-control/inhibition while the effect on working memory was only marginally significant and that on cognitive flexibility was not significant. Sibley and Etnier (2003) found the strongest effects of exercise on perceptual skills and measures of intelligence. Furthermore, Verburgh et al. (2014) did not find an overall meta-analytic effect for chronic exercise interventions on cognitive function. For acute exercise interventions, however, they found a moderate effect on cognitive functioning. Sibley and Etnier (2003), however, could not find differences regarding the cognition effect between chronic and acute exercise interventions. The following paragraph includes a few examples of recent randomized controlled studies published on the chronic and acute links between exercise and cognition not published earlier than 1990.

Chronic effects

Zervas and colleagues (1991) had $n = 26$ boys (nine pairs of monozygotic twins and eight individuals) aged 11–14 years participate in an exercise programme for 25 weeks. The experiment consisted of two control groups and one experimental group. In the experimental group, one twin of each of the nine pairs performed 90 minutes of interval or continuous running aligned in intensity to their individual anaerobic thresholds three times a week. The other single twins and eight individual boys were part of the control group performing their regular physical education lessons two to three times per week. All participants performed the Cognitrone Test (Schuhfried, 1984) to assess self-control/inhibition before and after the intervention. The authors report that the trained single twins showed an increased number of correct responses in the task, implying improved cognitive performance after the 25-week intervention period when compared to the control groups.

In a study with 92 obese children aged 9–10 years, Davis and colleagues (2007) tested the effects of a low-dose and a high-dose exercise programme compared to a control situation. The programmes lasted 15 weeks. In the low-dose programme children participated in 20 minutes of exercise 5 days per week. In the high-dose programme children performed 40 minutes of exercise on 5 days a week. The Cognitive Assessment System (Naglieri & Das, 1997) was used to assess children's executive functions. The authors found significant improvement in the aspect of planning in the Cognitive Assessment System only in the high-dose group compared to the control group, suggesting that higher doses of exercise are needed to benefit executive functioning in obese children. In a different study by the same research group they confirmed these results, additionally showing that exercise also benefited maths performance in school (Davis et al., 2011).

In a 9-month intervention period, 43 children aged 7–9 years were randomly assigned to either an after-school exercise programme or to a wait-list control group (Kamijo et al., 2011). Children's working memory was measured using a modified Sternberg Task (Sternberg, 1966) before and after the intervention period. Compared to the control group, children in the intervention group significantly improved their working-memory performance over the course of the intervention programme.

Acute effects

Caterino and Polak (1999) reported on a study with 177 participants aged 7–10 years who were assigned to either a classroom activity (control) or a PA including 15 minutes of stretching and aerobic walking. All participants performed the Woodcock–Johnson Test of Concentration (Woodcock & Johnson, 1989) to measure cognitive self-control. The authors reported that only the oldest children (age 9–10 years) benefited significantly from the exercise intervention regarding their performance in the concentration task.

In a study testing the effects of acute exercise intensity on working-memory performance (Letter Digit Span; Gold, Carpenter, Randolph, Goldberg, & Weinberger, 1997), Budde, Voelcker-Rehage et al. (2010) tested 60 adolescents aged 15–16 years and randomly assigned them to two experimental and one control group. In the low-intensity experimental group participants performed 12 minutes of aerobic exercise at 50–65% of their individual maximum heart rate (HR_{max}). In the high-intensity exercise group, participants worked at 70–85% of their individual HR_{max}. The authors found slightly positive effects of moderately intense exercise of 50–65% individual HR_{max} on participants' working-memory performance. This effect was especially pronounced in participants scoring low in the pretest of working memory.

Finally, Niemann and colleagues (2013) investigated $n = 42$ primary school children aged 9–10 years participating in 12 minutes of intensive PA at a heart rate of 180–190 bpm or a control group watching a non-arousing movie. Children performed the d2 test of attention before and after the intervention. The results showed no differences between the experimental groups. All participants gained in their cognitive performance. However, the authors state that participants reporting high levels of PA in their everyday life showed stronger increases from pre- to posttest in their cognitive performance scores, indicating that chronic PA might affect the exercise effect on cognition.

Overall, findings regarding the effects of exercise on different cognitive functions suggest a small positive relationship (Trudeau & Shephard, 2010), with working memory and inhibitory functions (self-control) benefiting most in this age group. More recent findings suggest that cognitively enriched or motor-demanding exercises may additionally benefit cognitive aspects like inhibition and working memory in children and adolescents (Crova et al., 2014).

The effect of different exercise programmes on cognitive functioning in children and adolescents

In the following studies we show some evidence that programmes involving perceptual motor aspects may also positively affect cognitive performance. This point was addressed in several recent studies arguing for the importance of cognitively involving (Crova et al., 2014; Pesce, 2012) or coordinative exercise (Budde, Voelcker-Rehage, Pietrassyk-Kendziorra, Ribeiro, & Tidow, 2008; Koutsandréou, Wegner, Niemann, & Budde, 2016) for improving cognitive performance.

The acute study by Budde et al. (2008) randomly assigned 115 participants aged 13–16 years to an experimental or a control group. In the experimental condition, participants performed 10 minutes of coordinative/ motor-demanding tasks. The control group participated in a regular physical education lesson with no motor focus but with the same intensity for the cardiovascular system (HR of 120 bpm). All participants performed the d2 test of attention (Brickenkamp, 2002) before and after the experimental condition. The authors found a positive effect on cognitive performance in the attention task in favour of the coordinative exercise group.

Recently, a study with 71 children aged 9–10 years was conducted to examine the chronic effects of exercise on working memory (Koutsandréou, Wegner, et al., 2016). Children were randomly assigned to: (1) a cardiovascular exercise group; (2) a motor exercise group; or (3) a control group. The programme lasted 10 weeks. Every week, children participated in this after-school programme for three sessions of 45 minutes each. In the cardiovascular exercise group the children performed aerobic exercise at an intensity of 60–70% of their individual HR_{max}; in the motor exercise group they worked at 55–65% of HR_{max} performing motor-demanding tasks like juggling or balancing. The control group took part in assisted homework sessions at this time. Children's working memory was measured using the Letter Digit Span task (Gold et al., 1997). Results revealed that children's working memory in both exercise groups increased from pre- to posttest while it was not different in the control group. However, only participants in the motor exercise group showed increased working-memory scores compared to the control group after the intervention period, indicating that motor demands may additionally benefit cognitive development.

In a study with 70 lean and obese 9–10-year-old children Crova and colleagues (2014) compared the effects of cognitively demanding and regular physical education programmes. They measured children's inhibition and working-memory skills before and after intervention. The intervention period lasted 6 months. In this study only the overweight but not the lean children benefited from the cognitively enriched physical education programme regarding their inhibition but not their working-memory scores. The regular physical education classes did not foster executive functions in lean or obese children.

The conclusion of the studies on different exercise programmes presented above is that motor-demanding exercise, provided acutely or chronically, is positive for cognitive functioning in children and adolescents and might be even more stimulating than exercise without a focus on coordination.

Physiological mechanisms underlying the positive effects of exercise in children and adolescents

Exercise may positively affect cognition through different neurobiological mechanisms including effects on the functioning of the hypothalamic–pituitary–adrenal (HPA) axis, through effects on testosterone production (hypothalamic–pituitary–gonadal (HPG) axis) and through development in brain regions like the limbic system, the hippocampus and the amygdala.

Is the effect of acute exercise on cognition mediated by steroid hormones?

So far, only a small number of studies exist investigating the link between exercise-related steroid hormone changes and improved cognitive performance due to acute bouts of exercise in children and adolescents. Thus, in this section, we also present research studies investigating psychosocial stressors to activate the HPA and HPG axes and to impact cognition. The first study investigating the impact of acute exercise on cognitive performance and on steroid hormones with 15–16-year-old adolescents failed to show a relationship between cortisol levels and cognitive performance in a working-memory task (Budde, Voelcker-Rehage, et al., 2010). Salivary cortisol was increased after a high-intensity exercise bout (70–85% Vo_{2max}), whereas the performance in a working-memory task mainly benefited from exercising with moderate intensity (65–70% Vo_{2max}). Thus, the enhanced working-memory performance could not be attributed to the increased cortisol concentration.

On the basis of studies by Budde, Voelcker-Rehage, et al. (2010) and Niemann et al. (2013), a recent study tested the effects of 20 minutes of cognitive engaging and playful exercise on executive functions and on cortisol levels in 6–8-year-old children (Jäger, Schmidt, Conzelmann, & Roebers, 2014). Children in the experimental group improved their performance significantly on the inhibition task compared to the control group. Cortisol elevation in the experimental group did not reach significance from pre- to posttest, confirming the results of Budde, Voelcker-Rehage, et al. (2010); nonetheless, in the experimental group cortisol increased significantly between posttest and after 40 minutes and the authors were able to correlate this cortisol change with the performance in the inhibition task. Unfortunately this study has a lack of standardized testing concerning exercise intensity.

Studies with different kinds of stressors, especially psychosocial stress, partly failed (but under certain conditions were able) to demonstrate a relationship between cortisol increases after stress and working memory. In one study cortisol elevation was induced by psychological as well as highly intensive physical stress (Hoffman & al'Absi, 2004). However, the following neuropsychological tests did not result in working-memory improvements. On the other hand, a study by Elzinga and Roelofs (2005), using a psychological stress protocol, could show a link between stress-induced cortisol increases and working-memory performance. They divided participants into cortisol responders and non-responders after a psychological stress phase and found working-memory impairments during the psychosocial stress phase only for the cortisol responders. Additionally, one study found that psychosocial stress impaired working-memory performance at high but not at low working-memory loads (Oei, Everaerd, Elzinga, van Well, & Bermond, 2006).

The previously mentioned results need further exploration. This is also true for the link between exercise-induced cognitive changes and testosterone. In adults many findings point to testosterone as one possible mediator for the effect of exercise on cognition. A study by Moffat and Hampson (1996) demonstrated that intermediate levels of testosterone were linked to better spatial functioning. In another study men with lower testosterone levels showed an increased performance in cognitive tests (Wolf & Kirschbaum, 2002).

Furthermore, a high dose of injected testosterone in elderly men was associated with a decreased performance in a verbal fluency task (Wolf et al., 2000). For adolescents it has also been shown that exercise-induced changes in testosterone concentration are correlated with changes in cognitive performance. A study with adolescents aged 15–16 years found high-intensity exercise-induced increased testosterone levels were negatively related to changes in working-memory performance (Budde, Voelcker-Rehage, et al., 2010). The effects have been attributed to testosterone binding to androgen receptors in the cytoplasm. These androgen receptors are often found in brain areas responsible for memory and learning, such as the hippocampus and the prefrontal cortex (Janowsky, 2006).

Respectively, testosterone levels have been found to be positively related to changes in fine motor skills (Wegner, Koedijker, & Budde, 2014). This is an interesting finding because cognition and motor skills seem to be fundamentally interrelated behaviourally and with regard to the underlying brain structures (Pangelinan et al., 2011).

A possible explanation for exercise and stress-induced testosterone changes being to some extent responsible for enhanced cognitive performance is testosterone-induced synaptogenesis. Testosterone was found to have a neuroprotective function and preserves neurons and synapses (Kurth et al., 2014). Additionally research with animals revealed that testosterone treatment resulted in increased synaptogenesis, which was associated with improved synaptic function (Ziehn et al., 2012). These structural changes of synapses and their associated dendritic spines can appear as fast as minutes to hours after exercise training (Johansen-Berg, Sampaio Baptista, & Thomas, 2012). Synaptic functioning is a well-established electrophysiological biomarker for cognitive function in rodents.

Taken together, this illustrated physiological process can be seen as a further explanation for testosterone as mediating the link between acute exercise and cognitive performance (Figure 12.2). For preadolescent children aged 9–10 years this effect of testosterone on attention could not be confirmed (Niemann et al., 2013). Exercising intensively at a heart rate of

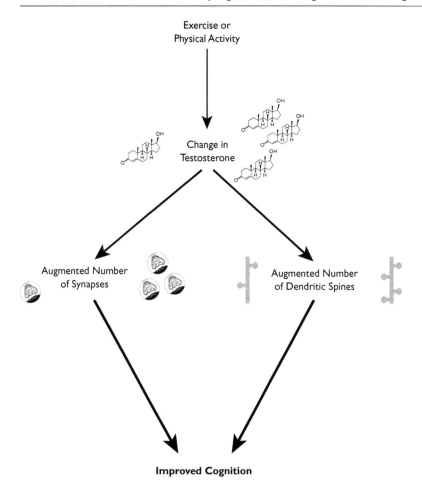

Figure 12.2 Testosterone as a possible mediator for the link between physical activity (or exercise) and cognitive functioning. (Adapted from Koutsandréou, F., Wegner, M., Niemann, C., & Budde, H. (2016). Effects of motor versus cardiovascular exercise training on children's working memory. *Medicine and Science in Sports and Exercise, 48*(6), 1144–1152. doi: 10.1249/MSS.0000000000000869.)

180–190 bpm resulted in larger improvement in selective attention performance (d2 test) compared to a control group, but no increase in testosterone concentration was found. Instead, the habitually less active children showed a significant decrease in testosterone, which was interpreted as a possible disruption of the HPG axis in these children. As outlined above, HPG axis activity and reactivity are still developing in this age group. Children who are less physically active, however, show higher reactivity to stress.

Besides the effect on testosterone, exercise also supports glucocorticoid secretion (Budde, Pietrassyk-Kendziorra, Bohm, & Voelcker-Rehage, 2010; Budde, Voelcker-Rehage, et al., 2010) and changes tissue sensitivity to glucocorticoids (Duclos, Gouarne, & Bonnemaison, 2003). Cortisol responses after acute exercise in physically active individuals are dampened and consumed more quickly than in the physically inactive (Mathur, Toriola, & Dada, 1986; Rudolph & McAuley, 1998). Exercise also increases plasma concentrations in atrial natriuretic peptide (Mandroukas et al., 1995), which has been shown to inhibit the HPA axis (Kellner, Wiedemann, & Holsboer, 1992) and reduce, for example, anxiety (Ströhle, Kellner, Holsboer, & Wiedemann, 2001).

Is the effect of exercise on cognition mediated by changes in brain structure and activity?

Acute studies

On the basis of human brain imaging and animal studies showing that neuronal structures like the cerebellum and the frontal lobe are responsible for coordination as well as cognition (Serrien, Ivry, & Swinnen, 2006), it was hypothesized by Budde et al. (2008) that coordinative exercise would be more effective than the control condition in improving the speed and accuracy of the following concentration and attention task. Picard and Strick (1996) specified that motor complexity co-varies with the pattern of brain activation, and thus the degree of information processing. It has been suggested that automatic motor behaviours, like they were requested during the 10 minutes of exercise without an emphasis on motor coordination, are controlled by the basal ganglia (Dietrich, 2003). The higher the motor demand, the more prefrontal cortex activity is required during the execution of motor tasks (Serrien et al., 2006). Thus, the type of exercise stressed in the coordinative exercise group is believed to require a higher variety of frontal-dependent cognitive processes as compared to completing basic moves at moderate intensity (Serrien, Ivry, & Swinnen, 2007). In addition to activation of neural parts of the brain like the frontal lobes (Hernandez et al., 2002), coordinative exercise is supposed to lead to an excitation of the cerebellum (Diedrichsen, Criscimagna-Hemminger, & Shadmehr, 2007), which is also responsible for mediating cognitive functions (Steinlin, 2007). The results of Budde et al. (2008) suggest that coordinative exercise leads to a facilitation of neuronal networks, resulting in a general pre-activation of consequent cortical activities responsible for cognitive functions like attention. In contrast, a normal sport lesson (without a focus on coordinative exercise) might require the participants to perform more automated movements and in turn prefrontal structures might not be directly required to the same extent as in coordinative tasks.

Chronic studies

The human brain is subject to significant development of different regions from the age of 4 to 21 years (Gogtay et al., 2004; Weir, Zakama, & Rao, 2012). Regarding the effects of exercise on cognition, it was found that children and adolescents with higher fitness levels showed better performances in memory tasks compared to less fit children; this could be linked to an increased volume of the hippocampus (Chaddock, Pontifex, Hillman, & Kramer, 2011). Davis and colleagues (2011) additionally claim that exercise increases activity in the prefrontal cortex and may therefore benefit cognitive performance. Using functional magnetic resonance imaging, chronic exercise programmes were further shown to affect children's brain activation positively in the surrounding areas like the anterior cingulate and superior frontal gyrus that also support executive functioning (Krafft et al., 2014). Regarding the different exercise regimes and their effect on cognition, research with older adults provides possible explanations for these different mechanisms, e.g. different brain activation patterns after training of cardiovascular or motor exercise (Voelcker-Rehage & Niemann, 2013). Furthermore, with regard to brain volume of subcortical structures, motor exercise showed superior effects on volume of the hippocampus and the basal ganglia compared with cardiovascular exercise (Niemann, Godde, & Voelcker-Rehage, 2014). These brain changes may be partly responsible for changed cognitive processes. On the behavioural level, these results provide some support for the argument that motor and cognitive development (particularly executive functions) are fundamentally interrelated (Diamond, 2000; Koziol, Budding, & Chidekel, 2012). Motor training requires perceptual and higher-level cognitive processes that are essential for action and ensuring anticipatory and adaptive aspects of postural control or coordination (Voelcker-Rehage, Godde, & Staudinger, 2011).

As yet, little is known about the exercise–cognitive functioning relationship regarding physiological mechanisms in the young age group. Most of the research suggesting positive effects stems from animal research or studies with adults. Although bidirectional links between exercise and neurobiological activity, exercise and cognitive functioning, as well as neurobiological activity and cognitive functioning have been repeatedly reported, it is seldom that studies identify mediating neurobiological mechanisms for the exercise–cognitive functioning link. Future studies are strongly needed that more closely investigate these mechanisms in children and adolescents.

Conclusion

Our results underline the need for additional acute as well as chronic exercise regimens in schools rather than reductions considering the dual advantages of academic achievement and physical health. Cardiovascular as well as motor exercise regimens should be equally addressed in schools because of the different underlying brain mechanisms, which might benefit more from a variety of activities. This could be included very easily in a school setting because neither sports clothes nor sports facilities are necessary for these types of exercise. By establishing a causal link between exercise and cognition in children, educators and policy makers should carefully consider additional PA programmes in schools.

References

Biddle, S. J. H., & Asare, M. (2011). Physical activity and mental health in children and adolescents: A review of reviews. *British Journal of Sports Medicine, 45,* 886–895. doi: 10.1136/886 bjsports-2011-090185.

Blair, S. N., Kohl, H. W., & Powell, K. E. (1987). Physical activity, physical fitness, exercise, and the public's health. In M. J. Safrit & H. M. Eckert (Eds.), *The cutting edge in physical education and exercise science research.* Champaign, IL: Human Kinetics.

Brickenkamp, R. (2002). *d2-Aufmerksamkeits-Belastungs-Test: Manual [The d2 test of attention: Manual].* Göttingen: Hogrefe.

Budde, H., Pietrassyk-Kendziorra, S., Bohm, S., & Voelcker-Rehage, C. (2010). Hormonal responses to physical and cognitive stress in a school setting. *Neuroscience Letters, 474*(3), 131–134.

Budde, H., Schwarz, R., Velasques, B., Ribeiro, P., Holzweg, M., Machado, S., . . . Wegner, M. (2016). The need for differentiating between exercise, physical activity, and training. *Autoimmunity Reviews, 15,* 110–111. doi: 10.1016/j. autrev.2015.09.004.

Budde, H., Voelcker-Rehage, C., Pietrassyk-Kendziorra, S., Machado, S., Ribeiro, P., & Arafat, A. M. (2010). Steroid hormones in the saliva of adolescents after different exercise intensities and their influence on working memory in a school setting. *Psychoneuroendocrinology, 35*(3), 382–391.

Budde, H., Voelcker-Rehage, C., Pietrassyk-Kendziorra, S., Ribeiro, P., & Tidow, G. (2008). Acute coordinative exercise improves attentional performance in adolescents. *Neuroscience Letters, 441*(2), 219–223.

Caspersen, C. J., Powell, K. E., & Christenson, G. M. (1985). Physical activity, exercise, and physical fitness: Definitions and distinctions for health-related research. *Public Health Reports, 100*(2), 131.

Caterino, M. C., & Polak, E. D. (1999). Effects of two types of activity on the performance of second-, third-, and fourth-grade students on a test of concentration. *Perceptual and Motor Skills, 89*(1), 245–248.

Chaddock, L., Pontifex, M. B., Hillman, C. H., & Kramer, A. F. (2011). A review of the relation of aerobic fitness and physical activity to brain structure and function in children. *Journal of the International Neuropsychological Society, 17,* 1–11. doi: 10.1017/S1355617711000567.

Colditz, G. A. (1999). Economic costs of obesity and inactivity. *Medicine and Science in Sports and Exercise, 31,* 663–667.

Collins, A., & Koechlin, E. (2012). Reasoning, learning, and creativity: Frontal lobe function and human decision-making. *PLoS Biology, 10,* e10011293.

Crova, C., Struzzolino, I., Marchetti, R., Masci, I., Vannozzi, G., Forte, R., & Pesce, C. (2014). Cognitively challenging physical activity benefits executive function in overweight children. *Journal of Sports Sciences, 32*(3), 201–211. doi: 10.1080/02640414.2013.828849.

Davis, C. L., Tomporowski, P. D., Boyle, C. A., Waller, J. L., Miller, P. H., Naglieri, J. A., & Gregoski, M. (2007). Effects of aerobic exercise on overweight children's cognitive functioning: A randomized controlled trial. *Research Quarterly for Exercise and Sport, 78*(5), 510–519. doi: 10.1080/027 01367.2007.10599450.

Davis, C. L., Tomporowski, P. D., McDowell, J. E., Austin, B. P., Miller, P. H., Yanasak, N. E., . . . Naglieri, J. A. (2011). Exercise improves executive function and achievement and alters brain activation in overweight children: A randomized, controlled trial. *Health Psychology, 30*(1), 91–98. doi: 10.1037/a0021766.

Diamond, A. (2000). Close interrelation of motor development and cognitive development and of the cerebellum and prefrontal cortex. *Child Development, 71*(1), 44–56. doi: 10.1111/1467-8624.00117.

Diamond, A. (2005). Attention-deficit disorder (attention-deficit/hyperactivity disorder without hyperactivity): A neurobiologically and behaviorally distinct disorder from attention-deficit/hyperactivity disorder (with hyperactivity). *Developmental Psychopathology, 17*, 807–825.

Diamond, A. (2013). Executive functions. *Annual Review of Psychology, 64*, 135–168. doi: 10.1146/annurev-psych-113011-143750.

Diedrichsen, J., Criscimagna-Hemminger, S. E., & Shadmehr, R. (2007). Dissociating timing and coordination as functions of the cerebellum. *Journal of Neurosciencce, 27*(23), 6291–6301.

Dietrich, A. (2003). Functional neuroanatomy of altered states of consciousness: The transient hypofrontality hypothesis. *Consciousness and Cognition, 12*, 231–256. doi: 10.1016/S1053-8100(02)00046-6.

Donaldson, S. J., & Ronan, K. R. (2006). The effects of sports participation on young adolescents' emotional well-being. *Adolescence, 41*(162), 369–389.

Duclos, M., Gouarne, C., & Bonnemaison, D. (2003). Acute and chronic effects of exercise on tissue sensitivity to glucocorticoids. *Journal of Applied Physiology, 94*(3), 869–875.

Elzinga, B. M., & Roelofs, K. (2005). Cortisol-induced impairments of working memory require acute sympathetic activation. *Behavioral Neuroscience, 119*(1), 98.

Fairchild, G., van Goozen, S. H., Stollery, S. J., Aitken, M. R., & Savage, J. (2009). Decision making and executive function in male adolescents with early-onset or adolescence-onset conduct disorder and control subjects. *Biological Psychiatry, 66*, 162–168.

Fedewa, A. L., & Ahn, S. (2011). The effects of physical activity and physical fitness on children's achievement and cognitive outcomes: A meta-analysis. *Research Quarterly for Exercise and Sport, 82*(3), 521–535. doi: 10.1080/02701367.2011. 10599785.

Gauvin, L., & Spence, J. C. (1996). Physical activity and psychological well-being: Knowledge base, current issues, and caveats. *Nutrition Reviews, 54*(4), S53–S67.

Gogtay, N., Giedd, J. N., Lusk, L., Hayashi, K. M., Greenstein, D., Vaituzis, A. C., . . . Thompson, P. M. (2004). Dynamic mapping of human cortical development during childhood through early adulthood. *Proceedings of the National Academy of Sciences of the USA, 101*(21), 8174–8179.

Gold, J. M., Carpenter, C., Randolph, C., Goldberg, T. E., & Weinberger, D. R. (1997). Auditory working memory and Wisconsin Card Sorting test performance in schizophrenia. *Archives of General Psychiatry, 54*(2), 159–165.

Hernandez, M. T., Sauerwein, H. C., Jambaque, I., De Guise, E., Lussier, F., Lortie, A., . . . Lassonde, M. (2002). Deficits in executive functions and motor coordination in children with frontal lobe epilepsy. *Neuropsychologia, 40*(4), 384–400.

Hillman, C. H., Erickson, K. I., & Kramer, A. F. (2008). Be smart, exercise your heart: Exercise effects on brain and cognition. *Nature Reviews Neuroscience, 9*(1), 58–65.

Hoffman, R., & al'Absi, M. (2004). The effect of acute stress on subsequent neuropsychological test performance. *Archives of Clinical Neuropsychology, 19*(4), 497–506.

Howley, E. T. (2001). Type of activity: Resistance, aerobic and leisure versus occupational physical activity. *Medicine and Science in Sports and Exercise, 33*(6), S364–S369.

Jäger, K., Schmidt, M., Conzelmann, A., & Roebers, C. M. (2014). Cognitive and physiological effects of an acute physical activity intervention in elementary school children. *Frontiers in Psychology: Developmental Psychology, 5*, 1473. doi: 10.3389/fpsyg.2014.01473.

Janowsky, J. S. (2006). Thinking with your gonads: Testosterone and cognition. *Trends in Cognitive Sciences, 10*(2), 77–82.

Johansen-Berg, H., Sampaio Baptista, C., & Thomas, A. G. (2012). Human structural plasticity at record speed. *Neuron, 73*(22), 1058–1060.

Kamijo, K., Pontifex, M. B., O'Leary, K. C., Scudder, M. R., Wu, C. T., Castelli, D. M., & Hillman, C. H. (2011). The effects of an afterschool physical activity program on working memory in preadolescent children. *Developmental Science, 14*(5), 1046–1058.

Kellner, M., Wiedemann, K., & Holsboer, F. (1992). Atrial natriuretic factor inhibits the CRH-stimulated secretion of ACTH and cortisol in man. *Life Sciences, 50*(24), 1835–1842.

Koutsandréou, F., Wegner, M., Niemann, C., & Budde, H. (2016). Effects of motor versus cardiovascular exercise training on children's working memory. *Medicine and Science in Sports and Exercise, 48*(6), 1144–1152. doi: 10.1249/MSS.0000000000000869.

Koziol, L. F., Budding, D. E., & Chidekel, D. (2012). From movement to thought: Executive function, embodied cognition, and the cerebellum. *Cerebellum, 11*(2), 505–525. doi: 10.1007/s12311-011-0321-y.

Krafft, C. E., Schwarz, N. F., Chi, L., Weinberger, A. L., Schaeffer, D. J., Pierce, J. E., . . . McDowell, J. E. (2014). An 8-month randomized controlled exercise trial alters brain activation during cognitive tasks in overweight children. *Obesity, 22*(1), 232–242.

Kurth, F., Luders, E., Sicotte, N. L., Gaser, C., Giesser, B. S., Swerdloff, R. S., . . . Mackenzie-Graham, A. (2014). Neuroprotective effects of testosterone treatment in men with multiple sclerosis. *NeuroImage: Clinical, 4*, 454–460.

Lagerberg, D. (2005). Physical activity and mental health in schoolchildren: A complicated relationship. *Acta Paediatrica, 94*, 1699–1701.

Mandroukas, K., Zakas, A., Aggelopoulou, N., Christoulas, K., Abatzides, G., & Karamouzis, M. (1995). Atrial natriuretic factor responses to submaximal and maximal exercise. *British Journal of Sports Medicine, 29*(4), 248–251.

Mathur, D. N., Toriola, A. L., & Dada, O. A. (1986). Serum cortisol and testosterone levels in conditioned male distance runners and nonathletes after maximal exercise. *Journal of Sports Medicine and Physical Fitness, 26*(3), 245–250.

Miyake, A., Friedman, N. P., Emerson, M. J., Witzki, A. H., Howerter, A., & Wager, T. D. (2000). The unity and diversity of executive functions and their contributions to complex "frontal lobe" tasks: A latent variable analysis. *Cognitive Psychology, 41*(1), 49–100. doi: 10.1006/cogp.1999.0734.

Moffat, S. D., & Hampson, E. (1996). A curvilinear relationship between testosterone and spatial cognition in humans: Possible influence of hand preference. *Psychoneuroendocrinology, 21*(3), 323–337.

Naglieri, J. A., & Das, J. P. (1997). *Cognitive assessment system: Interpretive handbook*. Itasca: Riverside Publishing.

Niemann, C., Godde, B., & Voelcker-Rehage, C. (2014). Not only cardiovascular, but also coordinative exercise increases hippocampal volume in older adults. *Frontiers in Aging Neuroscience, 6*(170), 1–12.

Niemann, C., Wegner, M., Voelcker-Rehage, C., Arafat, A. M., & Budde, H. (2013). Influence of physical activity and acute exercise on cognitive performance and saliva testosterone in preadolescent school children. *Mental Health and Physical Activity, 6*(3), 197–204. doi: 10.1016/j.mhpa.2013.08.002.

Oei, N. Y., Everaerd, W. T., Elzinga, B. M., van Well, S., & Bermond, B. (2006). Psychosocial stress impairs working memory at high loads: An association with cortisol levels and memory retrieval. *Stress, 9*(3), 133–141.

Olshansky, S. J., Passaro, D. J., Hershow, R. C., Layden, J., Carnes, B. A., Brody, J., . . . Ludwig, D. S. (2005). A potential decline in life expectancy of the United States in the 21st century. *New England Journal of Medicine, 352*, 1138–1145.

Pangelinan, M. M., Zhang, G., VanMeter, J. W., Clark, J. E., Hatfield, B. D., & Haufler, A. J. (2011). Beyond age and gender: Relationships between cortical and subcortical brain volume and cognitive-motor abilities in school-age children. *NeuroImage, 54*, 3093–3100.

Penedo, F. J., & Dahn, J. R. (2005). Exercise and well-being: A review of mental and physical health benefits associated with physical activity. *Current Opinion in Psychiatry, 18*(2), 189–193.

Pesce, C. (2012). Shifting the focus from quantitative to qualitative exercise characteristics in exercise and cognition research. *Journal of Sport and Exercise Psychology, 34*, 766–786.

Picard, N., & Strick, P. L. (1996). Motor areas of the medial wall: A review of their location and functional activation. *Cerebral Cortex, 6*(3), 342–353.

Pinker, S. (1999). How the mind works. *Annals of the New York Academy of Sciences, 882*(1), 119–127.

Pratt, M., Macera, M. A., & Wang, G. (2000). Higher direct medical costs associated with physical inactivity. *The Physician and Sportsmedicine, 28*, 63–79.

Rudolph, D. L., & McAuley, E. (1998). Cortisol and affective responses to exercise. *Journal of Sports Sciences, 16*(2), 121–128.

Secretary of Health and Human Services and the Secretary of Education. (2007). *Promoting better health for young people through physical activity and sports.*

Centers for Disease Control and Prevention. Available online at: http://www.cdc.gov/healthyyouth/physicalactivity/promoting_health.

Scheuer, J., & Tipton, C. M. (1977). Cardiovascular adaptations to physical training. *Annual Review of Physiology, 39*, 221–251.

Schuhfried, G. (1984). *Vienna test system: Version 10.85/B – A-2340.* Modling: Schuhfried.

Serrien, D. J., Ivry, R. B., & Swinnen, S. P. (2006). Dynamics of hemispheric specialization and integration in the context of motor control. *Nature Review Neuroscience, 7*(2), 160–166.

Serrien, D. J., Ivry, R. B., & Swinnen, S. P. (2007). The missing link between action and cognition. *Progress in Neurobiology, 82*(2), 95–107.

Sibley, B. A., & Etnier, J. L. (2003). The relationship between physical activity and cognition in children: A meta analysis. *Pediatric Exercise Science, 15*, 243–256.

Steinlin, M. (2007). The cerebellum in cognitive processes: Supporting studies in children. *Cerebellum, 6*(3), 237–241.

Sternberg, S. (1966). High-speed scanning in human memory. *Science, 153*, 652–654.

Ströhle, A., Kellner, M., Holsboer, F., & Wiedemann, K. (2001). Anxiolytic activity of atrial natriuretic peptide in patients with panic disorder. *American Journal of Psychiatry, 158*(9), 1514–1516.

Taylor Tavares, J. V., Clark, L., Cannon, D. M., Erickson, K., Drevets, W. C., & Sahakian, B. J. (2007). Distinct profiles of neurocognitive function in unmedicated unipolar depression and bipolar II depression. *Biological Psychiatry, 62*, 917–924.

Trudeau, F., & Shephard, R. J. (2010). Relationships of physical activity to brain health and the academic performance of schoolchildren. *American Journal of Lifestyle Medicine, 4*, 138–150.

Vaynman, S., & Gomez-Pinilla, F. (2006). Revenge of the "sit": How lifesyle impacts neuronal and cognitive health through molecular systems that interface energy metabolism with neuronal plasticity. *Journal of Neuroscience Research, 84*, 699–715.

Verburgh, L., Königs, M., Scherder, E. J. A., & Oosterlaan, J. (2014). Physical exercise and executive functions in preadolescent children, adolescents and young adults: A meta-analysis. *British Journal of Sports Medicine, 48*(12), 973–979. doi: 10.1136/bjsports-2012-091441.

Voelcker-Rehage, C., Godde, B., & Staudinger, U. M. (2011). Cardiovascular and coordination training differentially improve cognitive performance and neural processing in older adults. *Frontiers in Human Neuroscience, 5*, 26.

Voelcker-Rehage, C., & Niemann, C. (2013). Structural and functional brain changes related to different types of physical activity across the life span. *Neuroscience and Biobehavioral Reviews, 37*(9), 2268–2295.

Wegner, M., Helmich, I., Machado, S., Arias-Carrión, O., & Budde, H. (2014). Effects of exercise on anxiety and depression disorders: Review of meta-analyses and neurobiological mechanisms. *CNS and Neurological Disorders – Drug Targets, 13*(6), 1002–1014. doi: 10.2174/1871527313666140612102841.

Wegner, M., Koedijker, J. M., & Budde, H. (2014). The effect of acute exercise and psychosocial stress on fine motor skills and testosterone concentration in the saliva of high school students. *PloS One, 9*(3), e92953.

Weir, J. M., Zakama, A., & Rao, U. (2012). Developmental risk I: Depression and the developing brain. *Child and Adolescent Psychiatric Clinics of North America, 21*(2), 237–259.

Wolf, O. T., & Kirschbaum, C. (2002). Endogenous estradiol and testosterone levels are associated with cognitive performance in older women and men. *Hormones and Behavior, 41*(3), 259–266.

Wolf, O. T., Preut, R., Hellhammer, D. H., Kudielka, B. M., Schurmeyer, T. H., & Kirschbaum, C. (2000). Testosterone and cognition in elderly men: A single testosterone injection blocks the practice effect in verbal fluency, but has no effect on spatial or verbal memory. *Biological Psychiatry, 47*(7), 650–654.

Woodcock, R. N., & Johnson, M. B. (1989). *Revised tests of cognitive ability, test 10. Standard and supplemental batteries.* Allen: DLM Teaching Resources.

Zervas, Y., Danis, A., & Klissouras, V. (1991). Influence of physical exertion on mental performance with reference to training. *Perceptual and Motor Skills, 72,* 1215–1221.

Ziehn, M. O., Avedisian, A. A., Dervin, S. M., Umeda, E. A., O'Dell, T. J., & Voskuhl, R. R. (2012). Therapeutic testosterone administration preserves excitatory synaptic transmission in the hippocampus during autoimmune demyelinating disease. *Journal of Neuroscience, 32,* 12312–12324.

Chapter 13

The integrative neuroscience of physical activity, fitness and academic proficiency

R. Davis Moore, Jacob J. Kay and Eric S. Drollette

Introduction

The last two decades witnessed an unprecedented increase in morbidities associated with sedentary lifestyles (Institute of Medicine of the National Academies, 2013). Concomitantly, children are increasingly sedentary, and opportunities for physical activity during the school day are being diminished (Donnelly et al., 2016; Institute of Medicine of the National Academies, 2013). Given these unfortunate trends, it is essential to delineate the health benefits resulting from cardiorespiratory fitness and physical activity (PA) during development. One area gaining attention is the relation of fitness and PA to neurocognitive health and development. Research reveals that increased cardiorespiratory fitness and PA are associated with improved cognitive health across the lifespan (Colcombe et al., 2004a, b; Hillman et al., 2005, 2006; Kramer et al., 2006; Pontifex et al., 2009; Smith et al., 2010; Erickson et al., 2011; see Hillman et al., 2008, for review). With regard to children, fitness and PA are positively associated with the structural and functional integrity of the brain areas and networks supporting cognitive development (Buck et al., 2008; Chaddock et al., 2011; Moore et al., 2013; Pontifex et al., 2011; Voss et al., 2011), including the acquisition and maintenance of higher-cognitive functions (Buck et al., 2008; Castelli et al., 2007; Moore et al., 2013; Pontifex et al., 2011; Sibley & Etnier, 2003; Tomporowski, 2003).

Accordingly, increasing research examines the relation between fitness and PA to academic achievement and the acquisition of scholastic skills. Indeed, for years school teachers have noted that children who are physically active tend do better in the classroom (Donnelly et al., 2016). This longstanding notion has gained considerable momentum in the scientific community over the past few decades, with accumulating evidence demonstrating the important contribution of fitness and PA to scholastic performance in children (Castelli et al., 2014). Large-scale cross-sectional and intervention studies point to a positive relation between fitness and PA and linguistic and arithmetic metrics of academic achievement (California

Department of Education, 2001, 2005; Castelli et al., 2007; Chomitz et al., 2009; Cottrell et al., 2007; Hillman et al., 2014; Moore et al., 2014; Scudder et al., 2014; Wittberg et al., 2012). Further, PA interventions appear to improve or maintain in-class academic performance (Donnelly et al., 2009; Sallis et al., 1999) and reduce off-task behaviours (Mahar et al., 2006). Thus, increased fitness and PA during development appear to influence positively skills and behaviours necessary for successfully navigating the academic environment.

Although these studies provide promising results, behavioural measures alone fail to isolate the specific underlying neural and cognitive processes responsible for successful academic performance. Little research has sought to provide this integrative neuroscience perspective regarding how specific neural and cognitive changes (induced by fitness/PA) translate into particular mathematical, linguistic and problem-solving abilities. As such, this chapter will provide an integrative neuroscience perspective on how fitness and PA directly translate into changes in scholastic skills. It will begin by outlining some of the specific neurobiological changes associated with fitness and PA which result in structural and functional alterations in key cortical and subcortical areas subserving higher-cognition and academic skills. Then, the key functional changes in neurotransmission and how they relate to changes in brain potentials during cognitive and arithmetic task performance will be discussed. An integrative summary will then be provided, followed by a summary of current knowledge gaps and suggestions for future research.

Neurobiology and neuroanatomy

One proposed mechanism underlying exercise-induced changes in cognition and academic skills is the upregulation of cell proliferation molecules, known as *growth factors* (Cotman et al., 2007; Gomez-Pinilla & Hillman, 2013). Animal models and human studies demonstrate that fitness and regular PA are associated with the upregulation of essential growth factors including (among others) brain-derived neurotrophic factor (BDNF), insulin-related growth factor-1 (IGF-1) and vascular endothelial growth factor (VEGF). Across the lifespan, these growth factors support a variety of structural and functional changes throughout the brain by stimulating neurogenesis and angiogenesis, as well as playing critical roles in facilitating long-term potentiation and synaptic plasticity (van Praag et al., 2005; Viboolvorakul & Patumraj, 2014). Neurogenesis is the physiological phenomenon of new cell proliferation and integration, and angiogenesis is the process of vascular outgrowth which occurs to supply these newly formed and integrated cells (Gomez-Pinilla & Feng, 2012). Although these phenomena occur throughout the brain, neurogenesis disproportionately influences the hippocampus, which supports learning and memory (Gomez-Pinilla & Feng, 2012).

Acute and chronic PA have a strong regulatory effect on these growth factors, increasing their central and peripheral bioavailability (Gomez-Pinilla & Feng, 2012), and together these factors support the proliferation of new neurons (BDNF), the integration of new cells into existing circuits (IGF-1) and the maintenance of their function once established (VEGF; Fabel et al., 2003; Kim et al., 2010, Lou et al., 2008; Trejo et al., 2001). So integral are these three factors that inhibition of any one of these molecules obstructs neurogenesis. For example, BDNF knockout mice fail to exhibit exercise-induced neurogenesis (Rossi et al., 2006), and administration of IGF-1 antiserum abolishes hippocampal neurogenesis following exercise (Trejo et al., 2001). Further, administration of VEGF antagonist also blocks hippocampal neurogenesis (Fabel et al., 2003). Attenuating the action of these growth factors has also been shown to interfere with communication between neurons and cognitive performance (O'Callaghan et al., 2009; Vaynman et al., 2004). For example, Vaynman and colleagues (2004) found that antagonizing BDNF disrupted spatial learning and memory on the Morris Water Maze (MWM), and Ding and colleagues (2006a) found that blocking IGF-1 negates memory retention on the MWM task. Additionally, Kerr and colleagues (2010) found that blocking VEGF action also disrupts performance on the MWM. Therefore, these factors not only orchestrate important morphological changes within the brain, but directly affect the acquisition and maintenance of new information. Accordingly, in humans, exercise-induced changes in these growth factors (i.e. BDNF) demonstrate similar modulatory patterns with improvements in neurocognitive function observed in older adults (Erickson et al., 2012; Leckie et al., 2014).

Beyond cellular genesis, these growth factors are integral to adaptive modulation at the synapse. For example, BDNF and specific brain monoamines synergize to regulate several important cell functions, including neurite outgrowth and synaptogenesis (Martinowich & Lu, 2008). Further, both synaptophysin and synapsin I increase as a result of exercise (Ding et al., 2002, 2003; Gomez-Pinilla et al., 2002), and several molecular chaperones (e.g. heat shock protein 8 (HSP8), HSP60) and cytoskeletal proteins (e.g. β-tubulin, α-internexin, glial fibrillary acid protein) have been found to increase in exercise-trained animals (Ding et al., 2006b). The downstream effect of these BDNF-mediated events is exercise-induced increases in dendritic arborization and spine density, as well as synaptogenesis (Gomez-Pinilla & Feng, 2012). Thus, these growth factors not only promote the creation, integration and vascularization of new neurons, but also act to alter existing neurons structurally.

Together, the modulatory effects of PA on these growth factor-related processes result in gross neuroanatomical changes throughout the brain. Accordingly, morphological differences are observed in more fit and active children, relative to their sedentary peers (Donnelly et al., 2016; Gomez-Pinilla & Hillman, 2013). With regard to white matter, fitness and regular PA influence white-matter volume and diffusivity across the lifespan (Burzynska et al., 2014; Svatkova et al., 2015; Voss et al., 2012). For example, Chaddock-Heyman and colleagues (2014) measured the relation between fitness (in developing children) and fractional anisotropy (FA), which is an index of white-matter integrity (i.e. fibre density; Voss et al., 2012). These authors observed that fitter children exhibit greater FA in sections of the corpus callosum, corona radiata and superior longitudinal fasciculus, compared to less fit children. In another study, Herting and colleagues (2014) observed fitness-related differences in FA in both the corticospinal tract and the anterior corpus callosum, and FA values systematically varied with fitness level.

With respect to grey matter, neuroimaging studies provide substantial evidence that fitness and PA interventions are associated with increased volume in the prefrontal cortex and the anterior cingulate cortex, which support attention, executive functions, error detection and correction and problem solving (Chaddock et al., 2010a, b, 2011; Chaddock-Heyman et al., 2016; Flöel et al., 2010; Gordon et al., 2008). Volumetric differences are also observed in the cerebellum (involved in the coordinated execution of movement, language and attention; Buckner, 2013) in physically active children compared to sedentary controls (Chaddock-Heyman et al., 2014; Flöel et al., 2010). Further, convergent research indicates that fitness and PA increase hippocampal volume, and fitness-related differences are associated with enhanced working memory (Chaddock et al., 2010a; Herting & Nagel, 2012). In addition, fitness and PA interventions are related to volumetric changes in the basal ganglia, with volumetric changes associated with greater inhibitory/impulse control (Chaddock et al., 2010b, 2012).

Perhaps the strongest evidence, however, comes from Chaddock-Heyman and colleagues (2016). These authors observed a dose–response, whereby regular participation in moderate-to-vigorous PA was associated with increased grey-matter thickness in various cortical and subcortical areas, including the prefrontal cortex. Further, these cortical changes were associated with superior mathematic and linguistic achievement scores. Thus, PA and fitness appear to facilitate the structural connections and integrity of key brain areas supporting higher-cognition and academic skills.

Lastly, exercise-induced growth and plasticity of the cerebrovascular system – as measured by changes in cerebral blood flow – are also observed during development. For example, higher fitness is associated with increased blood flow in the hippocampus during relational memory performance (Chaddock et al., 2011), and higher fitness is associated with greater efficiency in cerebral blood flow during development. Specifically, the brains of fitter children exhibit more efficient blood flow, with increases to brain areas such as the prefontal and posterior parietal cortex during conditions of increased cognitive demands, and decreases to these areas during conditions of lower cognitive demand (Chaddock et al., 2011). Beyond fitness, haemodynamic evaluations before and after a 9-month PA intervention revealed a dose–response increase in blood flow to the frontal cortex during a flanker task, which requires multiple aspects of attention and executive function (Chaddock-Heyman et al., 2013). Thus, fitness and PA facilitate blood flow as well as the efficient modulation of blood flow to brain areas subserving higher-cognitive process.

Together, the available research makes a strong argument that fitness and PA serve to upregulate key growth factors resulting in the creation, integration and maintenance of new neurons. These factors also serve to change the structure of existing neurons and their connections. These processes result in gross volumetric changes in grey and white matter which are directly related to enhancements in aspects of higher-cognition and academic skills. Lastly, the increased vascularization of these areas also facilitates blood flow, as well as the efficient modulation of blood flow according to environmental demands.

Neurobiology and neurophysiology

In addition to gross anatomical changes, exercise exerts a potent influence on the functional properties of neurons (i.e. electrical activity, neurotransmission). Indeed, one of the strongest effects of exercise is to alter the intrinsic variability of neurons by lowering and sustaining excitatory thresholds (Gomez-Pinilla & Feng, 2012). In doing so, exercise facilitates long-term potentiation (LTP) and synaptic plasticity (Wang & van Praag, 2012). LTP is the physiological process underlying most forms of learning and memory (Wang & van Praag, 2012). LTP is heavily mediated by the phasic firing of glutamate and the BDNF-mediated expression of specific ionotropic and metabotropic glutamate receptors (Farmer et al., 2004). Both acute and regular PA increase the bioavailability of glutamate in key areas such as the anterior cingulate cortex and hippocampus (Maddock et al., 2016; Wang & van Praag, 2012), as well as the BDNF-mediated expression of ionotropic and metabotropic glutamate receptors, such as N-methyl-D-aspartate and $mGluR_5$ (Gomez-Pinilla & Feng, 2012; Wang & van Praag, 2012). Thus, PA promotes the acquisition of new skills by facilitating LTP.

Beyond LTP, exercise also exerts a strong effect on the release of monoamines (serotonin (5-HT), dopamine (DA), noradrenaline (norepinephrine; NE), etc.; Dishman et al., 2006). For example, exercise increases the activation of several 5-HT subreceptors, including the $5\text{-}HT_{2A}Rs$ subreceptor which is involved in object memory, fear memory and spatial cognition (Zhang & Stackman, 2015). Stimulation of this receptor elevates cyclic adenosine monophosphate levels, which is a second messenger essential to learning and memory (Lin & Kuo, 2013). Exercise also enhances DA synthesis, and the binding of the DA receptors (Foley & Fleshner, 2008; Sutoo & Akiyama,

2003). DA is believed to act in concert with 5-HT to alter the electrical activity and communication of neurons in the striatum (Eddy et al., 2014), and disruption of either impairs learning and memory (Gonzalez-Burgos & Feriavelasco, 2008). DA is involved in motivation and reward (Adcock et al., 2006; Wittmann et al., 2005), as well as learning and executive control (Brown & Braver, 2005). Thus, exercise-induced changes in DA availability and binding may exert a strong influence on a variety of behaviours.

Lastly, exercise has been shown to increase levels of NE in the brain (Wang et al., 2013). Changes in the locus coeruleus NE system are believed to underlie many of the cognitive benefits of fitness and PA observed in humans (Dishman et al., 2006; Gomez-Pinilla & Hillman, 2013). Specifically, exercise is believed to optimize the tonic and phasic firing of the locus coeruleus NE system, which projects to areas involved in higher-cognitive processes such as the prefrontal cortex, orbitofrontal cortex and the posterior parietal cortex (Nieuwenhuis et al., 2005). Accordingly, NE is heavily involved in higher-level attention, and executive functions (e.g. working memory, inhibition, mental flexibility), and suppression of NE activity impairs executive functions and the allocation of attention during goal-directed behaviour (McGaughy et al., 2008; Milstein et al., 2007). Thus, fitness and PA likely influence many higher-cognitive processes by optimizing activity of the locus coeruleus NE systems.

Psychophysiology of academic skills

Together, the available research indicates that fitness and PA optimize the electrical properties of neurons and facilitate the firing of monoamine systems. These functional adaptations result in changes in brain potentials which can been measured via electroencephalography, and the event-related potential (ERP) technique. ERPs are voltage fluctuations measured at the scalp (i.e. summation of postsynaptic potentials) which are time-locked to a specific stimulus or response. Unlike overt behaviour, ERPs provide a continuous millisecond-by-millisecond measure of neural functions, affording a real-time measure of information processing (Luck, 2005). That is, ERPs allow researchers to decompose the information-processing stream into its constituent components, enabling the identification of where and how two groups or conditions differ. Changes in ERP components' amplitude and latency have been used to provide a more integrative understanding of fitness/PA and academic skills (Hillman et al., 2012a, b; Moore et al., 2014; Scudder et al., 2014).

For example, Hillman and colleagues (2012a, b) sought to clarify the importance of PA-related changes in the P3b ERP component to academic achievement in preadolescent children. The P3b ERP component is generated by the locus coeruleus NE system (Nieuwenhuis et al., 2005), and reflects the allocation of attentional resources during the updating of working memory

(Polich, 2007). After controlling for IQ scores and grade level, the change in P3b amplitude was significantly related to both mathematic and linguistic achievement scores. In a separate investigation, the authors measured this ERP component before and after a 9-month PA intervention, and observed that P3b ERP amplitude was significantly increased following the intervention (Hillman et al., 2014). Thus, it appears that regular PA increases the ability to allocate attention during tasks requiring working memory, which carries direct implications for positively influencing mathematic and linguistic proficiency.

To delineate further the influence of fitness on mathematic competency, Moore and colleagues (2014) evaluated the behavioural and neural indices of arithmetic cognition in preadolescent children. On the behavioural level, the authors observed that fitter children were superior at detecting correct and rejecting incorrect problem solutions during an arithmetic verification task. Fitter children also utilized more advanced problem-solving strategies relative to their less fit counterparts, relying on more automated decomposition and retrieval strategies, rather than finger counting and lower-level decomposition. On the neural level, fitter children exhibited greater N170 amplitude, which reflects the encoding and transfer of meaningful visual features into semantic networks (Ince et al., 2016; Maurer, Zevin, & McCandliss, 2008). Children also exhibited larger N400 amplitude, when presented with incorrect solutions, and amplitudes were related to task performance. The N400 is an index assessing meaningful information from semantic memory (Kutas & Federmeier, 2011). Thus, in addition to employing more efficient mathematical problem-solving strategies, fitter children exhibit enhanced encoding and retrieval of numeric information from semantic memory, allowing them to differentiate efficiently between correct and incorrect problem solutions.

With respect to linguistic proficiency, Scudder and colleagues (2014) employed an experimental sentence-processing task while ERPs were recorded. Similarly to Moore and colleagues, fitter children exhibited greater N400 amplitudes during semantically incongruous sentences. Fitter children also exhibited greater P600 (an index of language structure processing; Kutas & Federmeier, 2011) during syntactic violations compared to less fit children. Accordingly, fitter children were also better able to detect erroneous sentence structure on the behavioural level. Therefore, fitness appears to be associated with a richer network of words and their meanings, and a greater ability to detect and/or repair syntactic errors.

Beyond scholastic paradigms, fitness and PA are associated with differences in dopaminergic brain potentials during tasks requiring attention and executive functions (Hillman et al., 2014; Kamijo et al., 2011). For example, fitter children exhibit increased N2 ERP amplitude, which is a neural index of response inhibition during an impulse control task (Kamijo et al., 2012).

Furthermore, Pontifex and colleagues (2011) observed greater error-related negativity (ERN) amplitudes in fitter vs. less fit children following the commission of an erroneous response. Generated by dopaminergic volleying emanating from the anterior cingulate cortex, the ERN is an index of a person's ability to monitor his/her actions, and reflects the activation of top-down compensatory control following an erroneous response (Gehring & Knight, 2000; Nieuwenhuis et al., 2001). Accordingly, the ERN is strongly related to real-time error detection and correction (Nieuwenhuis et al., 2001). Thus, in addition to academic specific processes, PA/fitness facilitates impulse control and the ability to detect and correct errors, further supporting that fitness and PA facilitate neurocognitive processes essential for academic success.

An integrative perspective

Together, the available research makes a strong argument that fitness and PA serve to upregulate key growth factors resulting in the creation, integration and maintenance of new neurons. These factors also serve to change the structure of existing neurons and their connections. These processes result in gross volumetric changes in grey and white matter which are directly related to enhancements in aspects of higher-cognition and academic skills. Lastly, the increased vascularization of these areas also facilitates blood flow, as well as the efficient modulation of blood flow according to environmental demands. In addition, fitness and PA appear to promote the acquisition and retention of new skills by facilitating LTP, and optimizing glutamate and monoamine neurotransmission. This in turn results in enhanced neuroelectric activity during performance of cognitive and academic tasks: specifically, ERPs which index response inhibition (N2), attention/working memory (P3b), and action monitoring (ERN), as well as visual expertise for numbers/words (N170), access to mathematic and linguistic networks (N400) and recognition of erroneous sentence structures (P600). Thus, the ultimate effect of exercise-induced neurobiological alterations is the expedited development of higher-cognitive processes underlying academic success.

Indeed, beyond the neurocognitive benefits observed during academic paradigms, more generalized benefits of PA and fitness on higher cognitive functions, such as attention and working memory, carry direct implications for academic success. Not only do the neural signatures of these functions (P3b) correlate with achievement scores (Hillman et al., 2012a, b), but deficiencies in these functions are believed partially to underlie learning disabilities in various academic subjects (Gathercole et al., 2006; Geary et al., 2004; Peng & Fuchs, 2014; Wang & Gathercole, 2013;). For example, children with working-memory impairments exhibit high levels of inattentiveness and distractibility, fail to monitor the quality of their classroom performance effectively and exhibit difficulty in problem-solving abilities (Alloway et al., 2009; Geary et al., 2004; Peng & Fuchs, 2014). Thus, differences in these functions may also explain, in part, why more active and fitter children outperform their sedentary peers in terms of academic achievement. When viewed in concert with the other academic-specific enhancements observed in number encoding, access to mathematic and linguistic networks, recognition of erroneous sentence structures and more advanced problem-solving strategies, PA and fitness appear to have a multifactorial benefit on the skills necessary for academic success.

Limitations and future directions

Although the findings described herein illustrate an appealing picture of the influence of fitness/PA on the neurocognitive processes underlying academic skills, there are several limitations to consider. For example, although consistent benefits are observed on the neural and psychophysiological levels, the benefits of PA/fitness on standardized measures of academic achievement are inconsistent. That is, some studies find associations between fitness or PA and maths and reading, while others find associations for spelling or science, but not maths and reading. Indeed, the large variability of research methods and designs utilized prevents a more coherent understanding of the influence of fitness and PA on achievement. Further, we are still beginning to understand how the mode, intensities and frequency of exercise may differentially influence the acquisition and maintenance of academic skills and account for variability between studies. Also, there are few longitudinal studies, and the question of whether fitness or PA is what changes neurocognition and academic skills is hotly debated (Donnelly et al., 2016). In addition, key factors such as genetic profiles, socioeconomic status, body mass index, IQ, sex and age all exert individual influences on neurocognitive development and academic achievement, but we are just beginning to understand how the factors interact with fitness and PA to moderate neurocognition and academic competency (Donnelly et al., 2016). Lastly, social and motivational factors also influence academic achievement, but are seldom addressed by those studying fitness and PA. Thus, although researchers are off to a promising start, there is still much to be deciphered before we have a truly integrative understanding of the influence of fitness and PA on academic achievement.

Future research should continue to address these issues diligently, as recent research demonstrates that several of these factors (i.e. exercise intensity, IQ, body mass index, sex, etc.) do indeed interact with fitness or PA to modulate neurocognitive and academic development. Further, given the widespread variability in research methodology, more concerted efforts for multisite trials using the same procedures should be undertaken. Lastly, as in most areas of health science, we are in need of more longitudinal interventions and randomized controlled trials. Together, taking these steps will foster our understanding of who derives what benefits from fitness/ PA, and how best to tailor an intervention to maximize neurocognitive and scholastic development.

References

Adcock, R. A., Thangavel, A., Whitfield-Gabrieli, S., Knutson, B., & Gabrieli, J. D. (2006). Reward-motivated learning: Mesolimbic activation precedes memory formation. *Neuron, 50*(3), 507–517. doi: 10.1016/j.neuron.2006.03.036.

Alloway T. P., Gathercole S. E., Kirkwood H., & Elliott J. (2009). The cognitive and behavioral characteristics of children with low working memory. *Child Development, 80*, 606–621. 10.1111/j.1467–8624.2009.01282.x.

Brown, J. W., & Braver, T. S. (2005). Learned predictions of error likelihood in the anterior cingulate cortex. *Science, 307*, 1118–1121. doi: 10.1126/science.1105783.

Buck, S. M., Hillman, C. H., & Castelli, D. M. (2008). The relation of aerobic fitness to Stroop task performance in preadolescent children. *Medicine and Science in Sports and Exercise, 40*, 166–172. doi: 10.1249/mss.0b013e318159b035.

Buckner, R. (2013). The cerebellum and cognitive function: 25 years of insight from anatomy and neuroimaging. *Neuron, 80*(3), 807–815. doi: 10.1016/j.neuron. 2013.10.044.

Burzynska, A. Z., Chaddock-Heyman, L., Voss, M. W., Wong, C. N., Gothe, N. P., Olson, E. A., . . . Kramer, A. F. (2014). Physical activity and cardiorespiratory fitness are beneficial for white matter in low-fit older adults. *PLoS One, 9*, e107413. doi: 10.1371/journal.pone.0107413.

California Department of Education. (2001). *California physical fitness test: Report to the Governor and legislature*. Sacramento, CA: California Department of Education Standards and Assessment Division.

California Department of Education. (2005). *California physical fitness test: Report to the Governor and legislature*. Sacramento, CA: California Department of Education Standards and Assessment Division.

Castelli, D. M., Carson, R. L., & Hodeges Kulinna P. (2014). Special issues: Comprehensive school physical activity programmes. *Journal of Teacher Education, 33*, 435–439.

Castelli, D. M., Hillman, C. H., Buck, S. M., & Erwin, H. E. (2007). Physical fitness and academic achievement in third- and fifth-grade students. *Journal of Sport Exercise Psychology, 29*, 239–252.

Chaddock, L., Erickson, K. I., Prakash, R. S., Kim, J. S., Voss, M. W., Vanpatter, M., . . . Kramer, A. F. (2010a). A neuroimaging investigation of the association between aerobic fitness, hippocampal volume, and memory performance in preadolescent children. *Brain Research, 1358*, 172–183. doi: 10.1016/j. brainres.2010.08.049.

Chaddock, L., Erickson, K. I., Prakash, R. S., VanPatter, M., Voss, M. W., Pontifex, M. B., . . . Kramer, A. F. (2010b). Basal ganglia volume is associated with aerobic fitness in preadolescent children. *Developmental Neuroscience, 32*(3), 249–256. doi: 10.1159/000316648.

Chaddock, L., Erickson, K. I., Prakash, R. S., Voss, M. W., VanPatter, M., Pontifex, M. B., . . . Kramer, A. F. (2012). A functional MRI investigation of the association between childhood aerobic fitness and neurocognitive control. *Biological Psychology, 89*(1), 260–268. doi: 10.1016/j.biopsycho.2011.10.017.

Chaddock, L., Hillman, C. H., Buck, S. M., & Cohen, N. J. (2011). Aerobic fitness and executive control of relational memory in preadolescent children. *Medicine and Science in Sports and Exercise, 43*(2), 344–349. doi: 10.1249/MSS.0b013e3181e9af48.

Chaddock-Heyman, L., Erickson, K. I., Chappell, M. A., Johnson, C. L., Kienzler, C., Knecht, A., . . . Kramer, A. F. (2016). Aerobic fitness is associated with greater hippocampal cerebral blood flow in children. *Developmental Cognitive Neuroscience, 20*, 52–58. doi: http://dx.doi.org/10.1016/j.dcn.2016.07.001.

Chaddock-Heyman, L., Erickson, K. I., Holtrop, J. L., Voss, M. W., Pontifex, M. B., Raine, L. B., . . . Kramer, A. F. (2014). Aerobic fitness is associated with greater white matter integrity in children. *Frontiers in Human Neuroscience, 8*, 584. doi: http://doi.org/10.3389/fnhum.2014.00584.

Chaddock-Heyman, L., Erickson, K. I., Voss, M. W., Knecht, A. M., Pontifex, M. B., Castelli, D. M., . . . Kramer, A. F. (2013). The effects of physical activity on functional MRI activation associated with cognitive control in children: A randomized controlled intervention. *Frontiers in Human Neuroscience, 7*, 2–13.

Chomitz, V. R., Slining, M. M., McGowan, R. J., Mitchell, S. E., Dawson, G. F., & Hacker, K. A. (2009). Is there a relationship between physical fitness and academic achievement? Positive results from public school children in the northeastern United States. *Journal of School Health, 79*, 30–37. doi: 10.1111/j.1746-1561.2008.00371.x.

Colcombe, S. J., Kramer, A. F., Erickson, K. I., Scalf, P., McAuley, E., Cohen, N. J., . . . Elavsky, S. (2004a). Cardiovascular fitness, cortical plasticity, and aging. *Proceedings of the National Academy of Sciences U.S.A, 101*, 3316–3321. doi: 10.1073/pnas.0400266101.

Colcombe, S. J., Kramer, A. F., McAuley, E., Erickson, K. I., & Scalf, P. (2004b). Neurocognitive aging and cardiovascular fitness. *Journal of Molecular Neuroscience, 24*, 9–14. doi: 10.1385/JMN:24:1:009.

Cotman, C. W., Berchtold, N. C., & Christie, L. (2007). Exercise builds brain health: Key roles of growth factor cascades and inflammation. *Trends in Neurosciences, 30*, 464–472. doi: 10.1016/j.tins.2007.06.011.

Cottrell, L. A., Northrup, K., & Wittberg, R. (2007). The extended relationship between child cardiovascular risks and academic performance measures. *Obesity, 15*, 3170–3177. doi: 10.1038/oby.2007.377.

Ding, Q., Vaynman, S., Akhavan, M., Ying, Z., & Gomez-Pinilla, F. (2006a). Insulin-like growth factor I interfaces with brain-derived neurotrophic factor-mediate synaptic plasticity to modulate aspects of exercise-induced cognitive function. *Neuroscience, 140*, 823–833. doi: 10.1016/j.neuroscience.2006.02.084.

Ding, Y., Li, J., Clark, J., Diaz, F. G., & Rafols, J. A. (2003). Synaptic plasticity in the thalamic nuclei enhanced by motor skill training in rat with transient middle cerebral artery occlusion. *Neurological Research, 25*, 189–194. doi: 10.1179/016164103101201184.

Ding, Y., Li, J., Lai, Q., Azam, S., Rafols, J. A., & Diaz, F. G. (2002). Functional improvement after motor training is correlated with synaptic plasticity in rat thalamus. *Neurological Research, 24*, 829–836. doi: 10.1179/016164102101200816.

Ding, Y. H., Li, J., Zhao, Y., Rafols, J. A., Clarck, J. C., & Ding, Y. (2006b). Cerebral angiogenesis and expression of angiogenic factors in aging rats after exercise. *Current Neurovascular Research, 3*, 15–23.

Dishman, R. K., Berthoud, H. R., Booth, F. W., Cotman, C. W., Edgerton, V. R., Fleshner, M. R., . . . Zigmond, M. J. (2006). Neurobiology of exercise. *Obesity, 14*, 345–356. doi: 10.1038/oby.2006.46.

Donnelly, J. E., Greene, J. L., Gibson, C. A., Smith, B. K., Washburn, R. A., & Sullivan, D. K. (2009). Physical activity across the curriculum (PAAC): A randomized controlled trial to promote physical activity and diminish overweight and obesity in elementary children. *Preventive Medicine, 49*, 336–341. doi: 10.1016/j. ypmed.2009.07.02.

Donnelly, J. E., Hillman, C. H., Castelli, D., Etnier, J. L., Lee, S., Tomporowski, P., . . . Szabo-Reed, A. N. (2016). Physical activity, fitness, cognitive function, and academic achievement in children: A systematic review. *Medicine and Science in Sports and Exercise, 48*, 1223–1224. doi: 10.1249/ MSS.0000000000000966.

Eddy, M. C., Stansfield, K. J., & Green, J. T. (2014). Voluntary exercise improves performance of a discrimination task through effects on the striatal dopamine system. *Learning and Memory, 21*, 334–337. doi: 10.1101/lm.034462.114.

Erickson, K. I., Miller, D. L., & Roecklein, K. A. (2012). The aging hippocampus: Interactions between exercise, depression, and BDNF. *Neuroscientist, 18*, 82–97.

Erickson, K. I., Voss, M. W., Prakash, R. S., Basak, C., Szabo, A., Chaddock, L., . . . Kramer, A. F. (2011). Exercise training increases size of hippocampus and improves memory. *Proceedings of the National Academy of Sciences U.S.A., 108*, 3017–3022. doi: 10.1073/pnas.1015950108.

Fabel, K., Fabel, K., Tam, B., Kaufer, D., Baiker, A., Simmons, N., . . . Palmer, T. D. (2003). VEGF is necessary for exercise-induced adult hippocampal neurogenesis. *European Journal of Neuroscience, 18*, 2803–2812. doi: 10.1111/j.1460-9568.2003.03041.x.

Farmer, J., Zhao, X., van Praag, H., Wodtke, K., Gage, F. H., & Christie, B. R. (2004). Effects of voluntary exercise on synaptic plasticity and gene expression in the dentate gyrus of adult male Sprague–Dawley rats in vivo. *Neuroscience, 124*, 71–79. doi: 10.1016/j.neuroscience.2003.09.029.

Flöel, A., Ruscheweyh, R., Krüger, K., Willemer, C., Winter, B., Völker, K., . . . Knecht, S. (2010). Physical activity and memory functions: Are neurotrophins and cerebral gray matter volume the missing link? *Neuroimage, 49*, 2756–2763.

Foley, T. E., & Fleshner, M. (2008). Neuroplasticity of dopamine circuits after exercise: Implications for central fatigue. *NeuroMolecular Medicine, 10*, 67–80. doi: 10.1007/s12017-008-8032-3.

Gathercole, S. E., Alloway, T. P., Willis, C. S., & Adams, A. M. (2006). Working memory in children with reading disabilities. *Journal of Experimental Child Psychology, 93*, 265–281.

Geary, D. C., Hoard, M. K., Byrd-Craven, J., & DeSoto, M. C. (2004). Strategy choices in simple and complex addition: Contributions of working memory and counting knowledge for children with mathematical disability. *Journal of Experimental Child Psychology, 88*, 121–151. doi: 10.1016/j.jecp.2004.03.002.

Gehring, W. J., & Knight, R. T. (2000). Prefrontal–cingulate interactions in action monitoring. *Nature Neuroscience, 3*, 516–520.

Gomez-Pinilla, F., & Feng, C. (2012). Molecular mechanisms for the ability of exercise supporting cognitive abilities and counteracting neurological disorders. In *Functional neuroimaging in sport and exercise science* (pp. 25–43). New York: Springer.

Gomez-Pinilla, F., & Hillman, C. (2013). The influence of exercise on cognitive abilities. *Comprehensive Physiology, 3*, 403–428. doi: 10.1002/cphy.c110063.

Gomez-Pinilla, F., Ying, Z., Roy, R. R., Molteni, R., & Edgerton, R. (2002). Voluntary exercise induces a BDNF-mediated mechanism that promotes neuroplasticity. *Journal of Neurophysiology, 88*, 2187–2195.

Gonzalezburgos, I., & Feriavelasco, A. (2008). Serotonin/dopamine interaction in memory formation. *Progress in Brain Research Serotonin–Dopamine Interaction: Experimental Evidence and Therapeutic Relevance, 172*, 603–623. doi: 10.1016/S0079-6123(08)00928-X.

Gordon, B. A., Rykhlevskaia, E. I., Brumback, C. R., Lee, Y., Elavsky, S., Konopack, J. F., . . . Fabiani, M. (2008). Neuroanatomical correlates of aging, cardiopulmonary fitness level, and education. *Psychophysiology, 45*, 825–838. 10.1111/j.1469-8986.2008.00676.x.

Herting, M. M., Colby, J. B., Sowell, E. R., & Nagel, B. J. (2014). White matter connectivity and aerobic fitness in male adolescents. *Developmental Cognitive Neuroscience, 7*, 65–75.

Herting, M. M., & Nagel, B. J. (2012). Aerobic fitness relates to learning on a virtual Morris water task and hippocampal volume in adolescents. *Behavioural Brain Research, 233*, 517–525. doi: http://dx.doi.org/10.1016/j.bbr.2012.05.012.

Hillman, C. H., Castelli, D. M., & Buck, S. M. (2005). Aerobic fitness and neuro-cognitive function in healthy preadolescent children. *Medicine and Science in Sports and Exercise, 37*, 1967–1974. doi: 10.1249/01.mss.0000176680.79702.ce.

Hillman, C. H., Erickson, K. I., & Kramer, A. F. (2008). Be smart, exercise your heart: effects on brain and cognition. *Nature Reviews Neuroscience, 9*, 58–65.

Hillman, C. H., Motl, R. W., Pontifex, M. B., Posthuma, D., Stubbe, J. H., Boomsma, D. I., . . . De Geus, E. J. C. (2006). Physical activity and cognitive function in a cross-section of younger and older community-dwelling individuals. *Health Psychology, 25*, 678–687. doi: 10.1037/0278-6133.25.6.678.

Hillman, C. H., Kamijo, K., & Pontifex, M. B. (2012a). The relation of ERP indices of exercise to brain health and cognition. In *Functional neuroimaging in sport and exercise science* (pp. 419–446). New York: Springer.

Hillman, C. H., Pontifex, M. B., Castelli, D. M., Khan, N. A., Raine, L. B., Scudder, M. R., . . . Kamijo, K. (2014). Physical activity intervention improves cognitive and brain health in children. *Pediatrics, 134*, e1063–e1071.

Hillman, C. H., Pontifex, M. B., Motl, R. W., O'Leary, K. C., Johnson, C. R., Scudder, M. R., . . . Castelli, D. M. (2012b). From ERP's to academics. *Developmental Cognitive Neuroscience, 2S*, S90–S98.

Ince, R. A., Jaworska, K., Gross, J., Panzeri, S., Van Rijsbergen, N. J., Rousselet, G. A., & Schyns, P. G. (2016). The deceptively simple N170 reflects network information processing mechanisms involving visual feature coding and transfer across hemispheres. *Cerebral Cortex, 26*(11), 4123–4135.

Institute of Medicine of the National Academies. (2013). *Educating the student body: Taking physical activity and physical education to school.* Washington, DC: The National Academies Press.

Kamijo, K., Pontifex, M. B., Khan, N. A., Raine, L. B., Scudder, M. R., Drollette, E. S., . . . Hillman, C. H. (2012). The association of childhood obesity to neuroelectric indices of inhibition. *Psychophysiology, 49*, 1361–1371. doi: 10.1111/j.1469-8986.2012.01459.x. Epub 2012 Aug 22.

Kamijo, K., Pontifex, M. B., O'Leary, K. C., Scudder, M. R., Wu, C.-T., Castelli, D. M., & Hillman, C. H. (2011). The effects of an afterschool physical activity program on working memory in preadolescent children. *Developmental Science, 14*, 1046–1058.

Kerr, A. L., Steuer, E. L., Pochtarev, V., & Swain, R. A. (2010). Angiogenesis but not neurogenesis is critical for normal learning and memory acquisition. *Neuroscience, 171*, 214–226. doi: 10.1016/j.neuroscience.2010.08.008.

Kim, S. E., Ko, I., Kim, B. K., Shin, M., Cho, S., Kim, C. G., . . . Jee, Y. (2010). Treadmill exercise prevents aging-induced failure of memory through an increase in neurogenesis and suppression of apoptosis in rat hippocampus. *Experimental Gerontology, 45*, 357–365. doi: 10.1016/j.exger.2010.02.005.

Kramer, A. F., Erickson, K. I., & Colcombe, S. J. (2006). Exercise, cognition, and the aging brain. *Journal of Applied Physiology, 101*, 1237–1242. doi: 10.1152/japplphysiol. 00500.2006.

Kutas, M., & Federmeier, K. D. (2011). Thirty years and counting: Finding meaning in the N400 component of the event-related brain potential (ERP). *Annual Review of Psychology, 62*, 621–647.

Leckie, R. L., Oberlin, L. E., Voss, M. W., Prakash, R. S., Szabo-Reed, A., Chaddock-Heyman, L., . . . Erickson, K. I. (2014). BDNF mediates improvements in executive function following a 1-year exercise intervention. *Frontiers in Human Neuroscience, 8*, 985.

Lin, T., & Kuo, Y. (2013). Exercise benefits brain function: The monoamine connection. *Brain Sciences, 3*, 39–53. doi: 10.3390/brainsci3010039.

Lou, S., Liu, J., Chang, H., & Chen, P. (2008). Hippocampal neurogenesis and gene expression depend on exercise intensity in juvenile rats. *Brain Research, 1210*, 48–55. doi: 10.1016/j.brainres.2008.02.080.

Luck, S. J. (2005). *An introduction to the event-related potential technique* (p. 388). Cambridge, MA: The MIT Press.

Maddock, R. J., Casazza, G. A., Fernandez, D. H., & Maddock, M. I. (2016). Acute modulation of cortical glutamate and GABA content by physical activity. *Journal of Neuroscience, 36*(8), 2449–2457. doi: 10.1523/JNEUROSCI. 3455-15.2016.

Mahar, M. T., Murphy, S. K., Rowe, D. A., Golden, J., Shields, A. T., & Raedeke, T. D. (2006). Effects of a classroom-based program on physical activity and on-task behavior. *Medicine and Science in Sports and Exercise, 38*, 2086–2094. doi: 10.1249/01.mss.0000235359.16685.a3.

Martinowich, K., & Lu, B. (2008). Interaction between BDNF and serotonin: Role in mood disorders. *Neuropsychopharmacology, 33*, 73–83. doi: 10.1038/sj.npp.1301571.

Maurer U., Zevin J. D., & McCandliss, B. D. (2008). Left-lateralized N170 effects of visual expertise in reading: Evidence from Japanese syllabic and logographic scripts. *Journal of Cognitive Neuroscience, 20,* 1878–1891. doi: 10.1162/jocn.2008.20125.

McGaughy, J., Ross, R. S., & Eichenbaum, H. (2008). Noradrenergic, but not cholinergic, deafferentation of prefrontal cortex impairs attentional set-shifting. *Neuroscience, 153,* 63–71. doi: 10.1016/j.neuroscience.2008.01.064.

Milstein, J. A., Lehmann, O., Theobald, D. E., Dalley, J. W., & Robbins, T. W. (2007). Selective depletion of cortical noradrenaline by anti-dopamine beta-hydroxylase-saporin impairs attentional function and enhances the effects of guanfacine in the rat. *Psychopharmacology, 190*(1), 51–63. doi: 10.1007/s00213-006-0594-x.

Moore, R. D., Drollette, E. S., Scudder, M. R., Bharij, A., & Hillman, C. H. (2014). The influence of cardiorespiratory fitness on strategic, behavioral, and electrophysiological indices of arithmetic cognition in preadolescent children. *Frontiers in Human Neuroscience, 8,* 258. doi: 10.3389/fnhum.2014.00258.

Moore, R. D., Wu, C. T., Pontifex, M. B., O'Leary, K. C., Scudder, M. R., Raine, L. B., & Hillman, C. H. (2013). Aerobic fitness and intra-individual variability of neurocognition in preadolescent children. *Brain and Cognition, 82,* 43–57. doi: 10.1016/j.bandc.2013.02.006.

Nieuwenhuis, S., Aston-Jones, G., & Cohen, J. (2005). Decision making, the P3, and the locus coeruleus-norepinephrine system. *Psychological Bulletin, 131,* 510–532.

Nieuwenhuis, S., Ridderinkhof, K. R., Blom, J., Band, G. P. H., & Kok, A. (2001). Error-related brain potentials are differentially related to awareness of response errors: Evidence from an antisaccade task. *Psychophysiology, 38,* 752–760.

O'Callaghan, R. M., Griffin, E. W., & Kelly, A. M. (2009). Long-term treadmill exposure protects against age-related neurodegenerative change in rat hippocampus. *Hippocampus, 19,* 1019–1029. doi: 10.1002/hipo.20591.

Peng, P., & Fuchs, D. (2014). A meta-analysis of working memory deficits in children with learning difficulties: Is there a difference between verbal domain and numerical domain? *Journal of Learning Disabilities, 49*(1), 3–20. doi: 10.1177/0022219414521667.

Polich, J. (2007). Updating P300: An integrative theory of P3a and P3b. *Clinical Neurophysiology, 118*(10), 2128–2148.

Pontifex, M. B., Hillman, C. H., & Polich, J. (2009). Age, physical fitness, and attention: P3a and P3b. *Psychophysiology, 46,* 379–387. doi: 10.1111/j.1469-8986.2008.00782.x.

Pontifex, M. B., Raine, L. B., Johnson, C. R., Chaddock, L., Voss, M. W., Cohen, N. J., & Hillman, C. H. (2011). Cardiorespiratory fitness and the flexible modulation of cognitive control in preadolescent children. *Journal of Cognitive Neuroscience, 23,* 1332–1345. doi: 10.1162/jocn.2010.21528.

Rossi, C., Angelucci, A., Costantin, L., Braschi, C., Mazzantini, M., Babbini, F., Fabbri, M. E., . . . Caleo, M. (2006). Brain-derived neurotrophic factor (BDNF) is required for the enhancement of hippocampal neurogenesis following environmental enrichment. *European Journal of Neuroscience, 24,* 1850–1856. doi: 10.1111/j.1460-9568.2006.05059.x.

Sallis, J. F., Prochaska, J. J., Taylor, W. C., Hill, J. O., & Geraci, J. C. (1999). Correlates of physical activity in a national sample of girls and boys in grades 4 through 12. *Health Psychology, 18,* 410–415.

Scudder, M. R., Federmeier, K. D., Raine, L. R., Direito, A., Boyd, J., & Hillman, C. H. (2014). The association between aerobic fitness and language processing in children: Implications for academic achievement. *Brain and Cognition, 87C,* 140–152. doi: 10.1016/j.bandc.2014.03.016.

Sibley, B. A., & Etnier, J. L. (2003). The relationship between physical activity and cognition in children: A meta-analysis. *Pediatric Exercise Science, 15,* 243–256.

Smith, P. J., Blumenthal, J. A., Hoffman, B. M., Cooper, H., Strauman, T. A., & Welshbohmer, K. (2010). Aerobic exercise and neurocognitive performance: A meta-analytic review of randomized controlled trials. *Psychosomatic Medicine, 72,* 239–252. doi: 10.1097/PSY.0b013e3181d14633.

Sutoo, D., & Akiyama, K. (2003). Regulation of brain function by exercise. *Neurobiology of Disease, 13,* 1–14. doi: 10.1016/S0969-9961(03)00030-5.

Svatkova, A., Mandl, R. C., Scheewe, T. W., Cahn, W., Kahn, R. S., & Pol, H. E. (2015). Physical exercise keeps the brain connected: Biking increases white matter integrity in patients with schizophrenia and healthy controls. *Schizophrenia Bulletin, 41,* 869–878. doi: 10.1093/schbul/sbv033.

Tomporowski, P. D. (2003). Effects of acute bouts of exercise on cognition. *Acta Psychologica. 112,* 297–324. doi: 10.1016/S0001-6918(02)00134-8.

Trejo, J. L., Carro, E., & Torres-Aleman, I. (2001). Circulating insulin-like growth factor I mediates exercise-induced increases in the number of new neurons in the adult hippocampus. *The Journal of Neuroscience, 21*(5), 1628–1634.

van Praag, H., Shubert, T., Zhao, C., & Gage, F. H. (2005). Exercise enhances learning and hippocampal neurogenesis in aged mice. *Journal of Neuroscience, 25,* 8680–8685. doi: 10.1523/JNEUROSCI.1731-05.2005.

Vaynman, S., Ying, Z., & Gomez-Pinilla, F. (2004). Hippocampal BDNF mediates the efficacy of exercise on synaptic plasticity and cognition. *European Journal of Neuroscience, 20*(10), 2580–2590. doi: 10.1111/j.1460-9568.2004. 03720.x.

Viboolvorakul, S., & Patumraj, S. (2014). Exercise training could improve age-related changes in cerebral blood flow and capillary vascularity through the upregulation of VEGF and eNOS. *BioMed Research International, 2014,* 1–12. doi: 10.1155/2014/230791.

Voss, M. S., Chaddock, L., Kim, J. S., VanPatter, M., Pontifex, M. B., Raine, L. B., & Kramer, A. F. (2011). Aerobic fitness is associated with greater efficiency of the network underlying cognitive control in preadolescent children. *Neuroscience, 199,* 166–176. doi: 10.1016/j.neuroscience.2011.10.009.

Voss, M. W., Heo, S., Prakash, R. S., Erickson, K. I., Alves, H., Chaddock, L., . . . Kramer, A. F. (2012). The influence of aerobic fitness on cerebral white matter integrity and cognitive function in older adults: Results of a one-year exercise intervention. *Human Brain Mapping, 34,* 2972–2985. doi: 10.1002/hbm.22119.

Wang, J., Chen, X., Zhang, N., & Ma, Q. (2013). Effects of exercise on stress-induced changes of norepinephrine and serotonin in rat hippocampus. *The Chinese Journal of Physiology, 56,* 245–252. doi: 10.4077/CJP.2013.BAB097.

Wang, S., & Gathercole, S. E. (2013). Working memory deficits in children with reading difficulties: Memory span and dual task coordination. *Journal of Experimental Child Psychology, 115,* 188–197.

Wang, Z., & van Praag, H. (2012). Exercise and the brain: Neurogenesis, synaptic plasticity, spine density, and angiogenesis. In *Functional neuroimaging in exercise and sport sciences* (pp. 3–24). New York: Springer.

Wittberg, R. A., Northrup, K. L., & Cottrell, L. A. (2012). Children's aerobic fitness and academic achievement: A longitudinal examination of students during their fifth and seventh grade years. *American Journal of Public Health, 102,* 2303–2307. doi: 10.2105/AJPH.2011.300515.

Wittmann, B. C., Schott, B. H., Guderian, S., Frey, J. U., Heinze, H., & Düzel, E. (2005). Reward-related fMRI activation of dopaminergic midbrain is associated with enhanced hippocampus-dependent long-term memory formation. *Neuron, 45,* 459–467. doi: 10.1016/j.neuron.2005.01.010.

Zhang, G., & Stackman, R. W. (2015). The role of serotonin 5-HT2A receptors in memory and cognition. *Frontiers in Pharmacology, 6,* eCollection 2015. doi: 10.3389/fphar.2015.00225.

Chapter 14

Coupling our plough of thoughtful moving to the star of children's right to play

From neuroscience to multisectoral promotion

Caterina Pesce, Avery D. Faigenbaum,
Marios Goudas and Phillip Tomporowski

Merely moving for expending calories or moving for improving? Neuroscience perspective

The multifaceted benefits of physical activity (PA) for children's physical, mental and socioemotional healthy development and the pivotal role of physical education and school sport are well acknowledged (Bailey et al., 2009; Pate et al., 2006; Poitras et al., 2016; Society of Health and Physical Education, 2016). However, over the past century, there has been a rise and fall of attention to the different facets of PA outcomes due to reasons that range from cultural and epidemiological trends to methodological advancements in research areas critical to PA advocacy.

The worldwide obesity epidemic has led to a disproportional focus on encouraging PA to ensure health-appropriate levels of caloric expenditure. Given the early onset of overweight and obesity during development (Centers for Disease Control and Prevention, 2015; Ogden et al., 2016), PA advocacy targeted to children and adolescents has been predominantly driven by an antiobesity discourse (European Commission, 2007a; World Health Organization, 2014). Central to PA advocacy is the call for synergistic efforts by sports organizations and public health groups (European Commission, 2007b; World Health Organization, 2010). However, it is questionable if the prevalently performance-oriented approach to sport specialization is appropriate for pursuing goals of long-term PA participation and health development (Malina, 2010; Myer, Jayanthi, et al., 2015). Indeed, actions such as the introduction of the Youth Olympic Games in 2010 seem not coherent with the declared motivation to contribute, in this way, to solving the universal problem of increasing sedentariness and obesity in youths. This rather highlights the low capacity of the sport system to implement educational policies different from early sport specialization that is linked with a growing incidence of overuse injuries in specialized young athletes (DiFiori et al., 2014).

Thus, mainly linking PA promotion for children and youths either to the battle against obesity, emphasizing PA quantity at the expense of its quality, or to the competitive goals of the sport system, building on talent development, involves the risk of neglecting the role of PA for holistic development. Warning against this risk, Bailey and colleagues (Bailey, Hillman, Arent, & Petitpas, 2013) proposed the Human Capital Model, in which the goals of PA – specifically sport-related forms of PA – go beyond the common discourse about getting children moving merely linked to energy expenditure. PA promotion is conceived as an investment capable of delivering wider-reaching outcomes in multiple domains.

This model is the expression of an ongoing shift in priority that rebalances the importance attributed to the different outcomes of PA to advocate for it. Exercise sciences have long been characterized by a predominantly medical perspective ('exercise is medicine', American College of Sports Medicine, 2016, and 'PA vital sign', Sallis et al., 2016) and by the examination of dose–response relations between PA and health outcomes (Lee, 2008) in childhood and adolescence – not dissimilar to young and old adulthood. The current shift in trade-off set point between PA quantity and quality (Garber et al., 2011) leads from the primary search of the 'right dose' of PA just for balancing calories in and out and ensuring health-related fitness to the attempt to 'qualify' PA quantity for an improvement in multiple life domains, especially the cognitive domain (Pesce, 2012; Tomporowski, McCullick, Pendelton, & Pesce, 2015). The provocative title of an article by Myer, Faigenbaum, et al. (2015, p. 1), Sixty minutes of what?, exemplifies this cultural trend, mainly prompted by methodological advances in neuroscientific research, which have acted as a catalyst of converging efforts from different research lines on the neural correlates and outcomes of PA and underlying mechanisms.

In the last decade, there has been an exponential growth of exercise and cognition research with a neuroscientific approach by exercise and sport scientists (McMorris, 2016). The application of neurosciences to sport and exercise research started with sport (Zani & Rossi, 1991), prompted by the interest in sport expertise and performance optimization that is central to the expert performance approach (Williams & Ericsson, 2005). Like sport itself, sport-related neuroscience was therefore 'adult-born', since it started with the study of adult athletes. The extension of the use of neuroscientific research tools to the study of physical exercise effects on the brain beyond the narrow view on expert sport performers was the natural consequence of the propagation of the health and wellness movement and the growth of exercise psychology. Exercise and cognition research was adult-born too, or even old-adult-born, as the priority was understanding how and why physical exercise could counteract the age-related decline in cognitive functioning, thus contributing to mental health and wellness (Bherer, Erikson, & Liu-Ambrose, 2013; Colcombe & Kramer, 2003;

Gajewski & Falkenstein, 2016). Instead, the interest in the beneficial effects of PA on healthy brain development in childhood and adolescence emerged later (Khan & Hillman, 2014; Pesce & Ben-Soussan, 2016; Tomporowski, Lambourne, & Okumura, 2011).

Cross-sectional evidence consistently shows the functional and structural brain benefits of being physically fit in childhood (Chaddock, Pontifex, Hillman, & Kramer, 2011; Donnelly et al., 2016; Hillman, Kamijo, & Scudder, 2011; Khan & Hillman, 2014) and, even though less investigated, in adolescence (Herting, Colby, Sowell, & Nagel, 2014; Herting & Nagel, 2012, 2013; Lee et al., 2014). Interventional research mostly shows that, following PA programmes, there are functional changes in the brain that, with few exceptions (Krafft et al., 2014), are paralleled by enhancements in cognitive function (Chaddock-Heyman et al., 2013; Chang, Tsai, Chen, & Hung, 2013; Davis et al., 2011; Hillman et al., 2014; Kamijo et al., 2011).

There also is specific evidence on the neural changes and cognitive benefits elicited by PA in overweight children (Crova et al., 2014; Davis et al., 2007, 2011; Krafft et al., 2014). This evidence, embedded in the bigger picture of the interrelations between PA, obesity and cognition (Chang, Chu, Chen, Hung, & Etnier, 2017), helps broaden the narrow antiobesity discourse in PA advocacy, pushing it to the higher level of a holistic perspective on mind–body outcomes. In sum, although literature with children and adolescents is still in need of more well-powered randomized controlled trials (Prakash, Voss, Erickson, & Kramer, 2015), cross-sectional and interventional research together offers objective arguments to advocate for more PA for children, suggesting that by promoting quality PA, we can 'fill two needs with one deed': physical and brain health (Donnelly et al., 2016).

Quality physical activity as a unique form of enrichment impinging on brain development

The majority of exercise and cognition research with a neuroscience approach has focused on exercise quantity, exercise-related fitness and dose–response relations. Thus, similarly to research on the physical benefits of PA, it is still dominated by the attempt to understand 'how much' exercise is appropriate to reap the greatest cognitive benefits and what changes are induced in the brain by the metabolic demands of PA (Gomez-Pinilla & Hillman, 2013). In this way, however, it is not possible to draw conclusions on whether cardiovascular fitness gains and/or other metabolic, neurophysiological and neurotrophic mechanisms influencing the integrity of the neural 'hardware' are the only mechanisms through which PA may affect cognitive functioning during development.

Thus, the current state of the art does not allow us to go beyond the quantitative approach to PA for children and adolescents. Only recently, there has been a first call to move toward a 'quality–response' relationship

(Pesce, 2012), based on the notion that physical exercise tasks may differ not only in intensity, duration and frequency, but also in coordinative and cognitive complexity, which affects the efficiency of the neural 'software'. This call has been followed by attempts – in behavioural, but still not in neuroscientific studies – to identify what qualitative characteristics of exercise, complementary to its quantity, may impact brain sculpturing and cognitive functioning during development (Vazou, Pesce, Lakes, & Smiley-Owen, 2016).

This perspective change in exercise and cognition research – specifically as regards children and adolescents – is welcome by developmental neuroscientists in search of effective interventions aiding cognitive development. Looking at comprehensive reviews of one of the leading spokespeople in this scientific area, Adele Diamond, it becomes clear that a growing priority consideration is given to PA as one of the most powerful means of promoting the development of the 'orchestra leader' of our mind, executive function (Diamond & Lee, 2011; Diamond & Ling, 2016). Executive function is an umbrella term for those high-level cognitive functions that are responsible for cognitive flexibility and adaptability of goal-oriented behaviour (Diamond, 2013). An intriguing aspect is that Diamond and Ling (2016) clearly de-emphasize the role played by the metabolic demands of PA, highlighting that to reap benefits for the developing brain and particularly for the areas subtending executive function, PA must be cognitively challenging, emotionally loaded and socially engaging.

There are relevant implications, from an applied perspective of educational research and practice, of the fact that exercise and cognition scientists and developmental neuroscientists are progressively complementing the focus on exercise dosage with a new focus on its qualitative characteristics (Pesce, 2012; Pesce & Ben-Soussan, 2016). This offers relevant arguments to advocate not only for more PA in educational settings, but also for a shift 'from simply moving to moving with thought' (Diamond, 2015, p. 1). The convergence of exercise and cognition scientists and developmental neuroscientists on thoughtful moving further intersects with the interest areas of motor developmentalists and motor learning researchers (Pesce, Croce, et al., 2016).

Different lines of research foster awareness, in the scientific community, of the role played by motor development and learning for brain sculpturing. Prospective studies indicate that motor development is predictive of positive trajectories of cognitive development and, particularly, of executive function (van der Fels et al., 2015), which in turn is crucial for development across multiple behavioural and socioemotional domains (Diamond, 2013; Moriguchi, Chevalier, & Zelazo, 2016). This is particularly relevant for PA advocacy if we consider the selective and disproportionately larger benefits that PA exerts on executive function (Etnier & Chang, 2009). Indeed, the primary brain substrate of executive function, the prefrontal cortex, seems one of the loci of selective PA effects on the developing brain (Khan & Hillman, 2014), probably thanks to its protracted development that extends the window of opportunity – that is of brain responsiveness to environmental enrichment as PA is – until late adolescence (Andersen, 2003; Casey, Getz, & Galvan, 2008).

The evidence that the development and acquisition of motor competence contribute to promoting the development of an efficient brain might seem not relevant to PA advocacy within public health policies typically concerned with the physical diseases provoked by physical inactivity. Instead, following seminal works (Barnett, Van Beurden, Morgan, Brooks, & Beard, 2008; Stodden et al., 2008) on the predictive role of motor competence in childhood for the development of an active and healthy lifestyle later in life, this research line has generated evidence that has definitively pushed motor competence into the public health arena (Robinson et al., 2015). Motor skill competence and muscular strength development offer a 'synergistic adaptation' (Faigenbaum, Lloyd, & Myer, 2013), with a driving force attributed to prerequisite levels of strength, which is needed to perform complex motor skills properly and remain injury-free (Faigenbaum, Lloyd, MacDonald, & Myer, 2016). This renders even more alarming the secular trends that show children currently being less skilled and weaker than the previous generation (Cohen et al., 2011; Runhaar et al., 2010), or their fundamental motor skill competence remaining poor despite incremental trends (Hardy, Barnett, Espinel, & Okely, 2013).

Also when linked to the fight against obesity, PA advocacy can take advantage of evidence from PA interventions tailored to motor skill development and learning, since overweight children are at risk of both poor motor development and poor cognition (D'Hondt et al., 2013; Reinert, Po'e, & Barkin, 2013). These arguments strongly justify the call, from paediatric exercise scientists, to develop integrative exercise approaches that include and attribute a central role to motor skill development and learning, while not neglecting that the driving cog of integrative training is a threshold level of strength (Faigenbaum et al., 2016; Myer, Faigenbaum et al., 2015; Figure 14.1).

One more piece of the puzzle is an emerging line of motor learning research focused on the acquisition of complex motor skills in ecological PA and sport settings as a means of cognitive training (Moreau & Conway, 2014; Pesce, Croce, et al., 2016). It has been claimed and demonstrated that purposefully designed motor/sports training offers ecologically optimal conditions for cognitive enhancement (Green & Bavelier, 2008; Moreau, 2015; Moreau, Morrison, & Conway, 2015), due to the coordinative and cognitive demands of complex motor tasks (Best, 2010; Pesce, 2012). The challenge for educators and practitioners is to understand how to exploit all these facets of quality PA and motor skill learning as a unique form of enrichment that impinges on the developing brain.

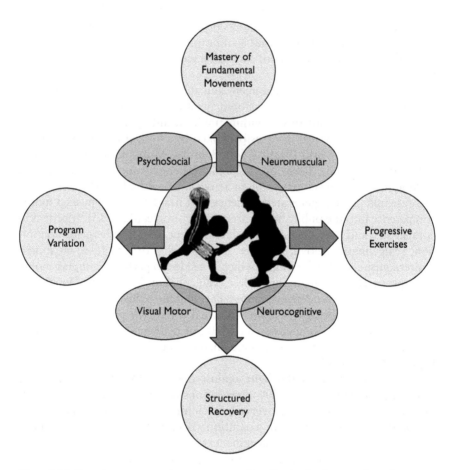

Figure 14.1 Complex programming components for effective implementation of integrative neuromuscular training by qualified educators. Reprinted with permission from Myer, G. D., Kushner, A. M., Faigenbaum, A. D., Kiefer, A., Kashikar-Zuck, S., & Clark, J. F. (2013). Training the developing brain, part I: Cognitive developmental considerations for training youth. *Current Sports Medicine Reports, 12*, 304–310. doi: 10.1097/01.CSMR.0000434106.12813.69.

Translating neuroscientific evidence into designed physical activity games: key concepts

European guidelines for health-enhancing PA include recommendations on educational PA, highlighting that it should be grounded on innovative learning theories and 'incorporate the best-known practices derived from research into teaching experiences and education programmes that maximise opportunities for learning and success for all' (European Union, 2008, p. 24).

Following this recommendation, we propose that the next step for transitioning theory into practice is to capitalize on neuroscience as a tool in the service of education, by translating neuroscientific evidence into cognitively challenging PA games for children. We propose to structure PA games that, tuning repetition and change to match children's developmental level and stage of learning, generate a challenge point that is needed for successful learning and cognitive improvement. Key concepts for this translation emerge at the intersection point between motor and cognitive development and learning areas.

Novelty and diversity of motor coordination patterns, as well as cognitive effort and success of the learning experience seem essential to impinge on brain plasticity and cognitive development (Moreau and Conway, 2014; Pesce, Croce, et al., 2016). Interventional studies with children demonstrate that both motor coordination training (Chang et al., 2013; Koutsandreou, Wegner, Niemann, & Budde, 2016) and cognitively complex PA (Schmidt, Jäger, Egger, Roebers, & Conzelmann, 2015; van der Niet et al., 2016) specifically benefit executive function in children. Moreover, Pesce, Masci et al. (2016) demonstrated that the extent to which children improve their motor coordination through diversified and cognitively engaging PA experiences is a mechanism that explains why they also gain executive function. It is proposed that coordinative exercise, if it is novel and diversified, not highly repetitive and automatized, involves cognitively challenging motor skill learning. The crucial role of task complexity and cognitive effort in skill learning for inducing changes in brain and cognition is supported by evidence from both human and animal models.

Neural changes that subserve skilful motor performance occur when a learning task is challenging and leads to successful outcomes (Carey, Bhatt, & Nagpal, 2005). Moreover, skill learning increases the number of newly generated neurons that survive in the hippocampus (Shors, 2014), the substrate of memory performance that is capable of neurogenesis along the whole life and is sensitive to PA as early as childhood (Chaddock et al., 2011). Cognitive effort is also a necessary ingredient for aiding the development of executive function. Children who perform a task repeatedly without experiencing challenge because there are no increments in task complexity do not gain executive function (Diamond & Lee, 2011). Motor learning typically progresses toward automaticity that no longer requires cognitive effort. A way of avoiding a reduction of cognitive effort and therefore the derecruitment of executive function is to introduce alterations into the ongoing learning task to keep the child 'on the learning curve' (Tomporowski, McCullick, & Horvat, 2010), or require the child to apply the skill learned in a constant environment to varying situations (Tomporowski, McCullick, & Pesce, 2015).

A further step to exploit the full potential of PA for aiding executive function development is to understand what 'dose' and 'type' of coordinative and cognitive demands of PA tasks are appropriate to gain maximum benefits.

As regards the dose, we refer to the notion of optimal challenge point that has been coined in motor learning research (Guadagnoli & Lee, 2004) and applied to the field of exercise and cognition research (Pesce, Crova, et al., 2013) to finetune cognitive engagement through movement to age and individual skill level. Pesce et al. found that cognitively enriched PA games elicit higher gains in executive function in typically rather than atypically developing children, with the latter improving best with PA games which match their needs.

As regards the type of qualitative demands of PA tasks, we move from the general view on how to generate cognitive effort in PA to a more differentiated view on how to design PA games that specifically engage individual executive functions ('gross-motor cognitive training', Pesce, 2012). To this aim, it has been proposed to feature PA games in specific ways that match the principles of neuropsychological executive function tasks and exploit, for cognitive training purposes, the principles of variability of practice that have been developed in motor learning research (Pesce, Croce, et al., 2016; Tomporowski, McCullick, & Pesce, 2015). Variability of practice refers to a set of ways to vary practice sequences in motor/sports training (Schmidt & Wrisberg, 2008), or to manipulate the environmental and task constraints (Vereijken & Boongardt, 1999), as opposed to repetitive trials in stable learning environments. When the trials within a practice sequence are varied or random, or when the environmental conditions or task demands are changing, the learner must inhibit behavioural routines, update information held in working memory according to changing rules and use cognitive flexibility to switch between practice schedules or adapt to emerging needs of the learning environment. Inhibition, working memory and cognitive flexibility are core executive functions that are highly predictive of successful achievements (Diamond, 2013).

Beyond this core, higher-level executive functions come into play in goal-oriented achievement behaviours, such as planning and problem solving (Diamond, 2013), which overlap or are intertwined with metacognitive functions (Tomporowski, McCullick, Pendleton, et al., 2015) and life skills (Pesce, 2012). Metacognition reflects the understanding and conscious and thoughtful use of strategies to solve problems and self-regulate behaviour. Problem solving and self-regulation also belong to those life skills that the World Health Organization (1999) recognizes as cornerstones of personal and social competence protecting against risk behaviours in youths. Life skills are trainable and strategies have been tailored to develop them through specifically tailored sports and PA programmes (Danish & Forneris, 2008; Goudas, 2010; Gould & Carson, 2008).

Despite clear intersections, the two areas of life skills and executive functions have a different theoretical background – social cognitive and neurocognitive, respectively – and the intervention programmes to promote their development have therefore grown on separate tracks. However, intriguing commonalities show that they are getting closer, with the most evident

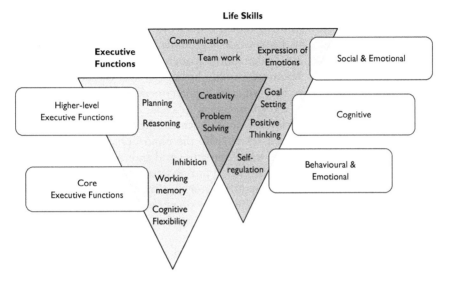

Figure 14.2 Contiguities and intersections between executive functions and life skills, proposed as a common framework to operationalize the notion of 'moving for improving'.

convergence on self-regulation (Pesce, 2012), a life skill that relies on behavioural inhibition and self-control resources. From a life skills perspective, European experts are moving towards self-regulation training and self-regulated learning in PA (Goudas, Kolovelonis, & Dermitzaki, 2012). From a neuroscience perspective, Diamond (2015) highlights the value of thoughtfulness in PA programmes centred on self-regulation training, such as martial arts and yoga (Lakes & Hoyt, 2004). From an exercise and cognition perspective, Audiffren and André (2015) propose a theoretical framework centred on self-control and self-regulation as a less metabolic and more psychological mechanism to explain the exercise–cognition relation. Thus, novel attempts to train life skills and executive functions jointly (Pesce, Marchetti, et al., 2016) and to synthesize within a common framework existing evidence on PA interventions that aid executive function, metacognition, life skills and academic performance (Álvarez-Bueno et al., 2016) represent further building blocks to operationalize the notion of 'moving for improving' in a holistic manner (Figure 14.2).

Designed physical activity within the brain–body– environment system: ecological approach

To move on from neuroscience to good practices, we adopt an ecological approach that may help design PA interventions for children that not only target, as previously discussed, the two needs of brain and body development in one deed, but also emphasize the entire brain–body–environment system. To this aim, we refer to the theoretical framework of radical embodied cognitive neurosciences. This framework is grounded in a neurophilosophy of education (Thompson, 2007) that 'shifts from a Cartesian notion of cognition as consisting of a homunculus-like, little person in the head, isolated phenomenon that occurs in brains, to a phenomenon that spans multiple scales across brain, body, and environment' (Favela, 2014, p. 2). In developmental exercise and cognition research, Pesce and Ben-Soussan (2016) have proposed that we distance ourselves from the philosophical proposition of Descartes (Cartesius), 'I think, therefore I am', and embrace the objection by his coeval Gassendi, 'I walk, therefore I am', because, as stated almost four centuries later in the light of scientific evidence, 'travel broadens the mind' (Campos et al., 2000, p. 1). In this way, we do not share the prioritization of cognition over movement and ground our cognitively challenging PA games for children on embodied cognition.

Embodied cognition posits that the brain evolved for the control of action rather than for cognition per se. Thus, cognition is viewed as subserving action and having its origins in sensorimotor interaction (Engel, Maye, Kurthen, & König, 2013). In the last century, Jean Piaget proposed a sensorimotor stage during cognitive development, thus attributing a key role to children's hands-on engagement (Piaget, 1952). This embodied cognition perspective has received renewed attention in recent years, together with a reconsideration of the role of the cerebellum. In previous sections, we have highlighted how cortical regions typically considered responsible for cognitive operations may be recruited when performing new and complex motor skills (Serrien, Ivry, & Swinnen, 2007). Conversely, regions such as the cerebellum, mainly deemed responsible for sensorimotor processes in movement execution and regulation, are also involved in cognitive processes (Buckner, 2013; Koziol, Budding, & Chidekel, 2012).

Models of the 'cognitive cerebellum' support the usefulness of PA experiences for children centred on problem solving and creativity. In fact, in creative processes the cerebellum is thought to model cognitive routines to be fed back to the cortex to enhance its efficiency, in the same way that it models routines for the control of repetitive, well-coordinated bodily movements to be fed back to the cortex responsible for action control and adaptation (Vandervert, Schimpf, & Liu, 2007). A problem-solving approach to motor learning in PA is ecological in nature, because it emphasizes the role played by the environment within the inextricable linkages among individual, task and environmental constraints (Renshaw, Chow, Davids, & Hammond, 2010). Newell (1986) has defined constraints as the boundaries that shape the emergence and stabilization of movement patterns, as developmental status and skill level (individual constraints), time pressure or accuracy requirements (task constraints), and contextual conditions specific to given PA or sports training experiences (environmental constraints).

However, stabilization of movement patterns is not the endpoint of motor learning, particularly, as we have discussed in the previous section, if we want to train executive function and therefore avoid the derecruitment that occurs in the course of movement automatization. To explain the role played by the environment, we introduce the concept of affordances as opportunities for action at a given moment under a given set of conditions. If, in a PA game, we purposefully organize the set of conditions of the game environment, we can help children progress from reacting to the perceived constraints to adapting movements in advance of opportunities by exerting prospective control on action (Fajen, Riley, & Turvey, 2008). The adaptability of action to the environment relies on both the availability of an appropriately large repertoire of motor behaviours that the cerebellum contributes to coordinate and the development of cognitive control that allows routine behaviours to be overcome in favour of actions directed by goal representations in the frontal – specifically prefrontal – cortex (Munakata, Snyder, & Chatham, 2012).

The focus on how to design PA experiences that recruit executive function should not lead to excessive trade automaticity and skilled routine behaviours for maximizing proactive control of action. Flexibility that derives from the use of proactive control has costs that must be taken into account, as it may limit learning of regularities and use of routine behaviours (Munakata, Snyder, & Chatham, 2013). Indeed, in motor learning, movement adaptability is accompanied by lower stability to external perturbations (Seidler, 2004). Thus, Pesce, Croce, et al. (2016) have proposed that PA experiences should be designed that capitalize on the circular relationship between stability and flexibility in motor behaviour. This proposal is grounded on dual-tiered models of the complementary role of automaticity and proactive control of goal-oriented behaviour (Koziol et al., 2012) depicted in the always relevant metaphor of the obedient horse and the quick-witted rider, first published by N. A. Bernstein in his monography on dexterity in the 1940s and resurrected 50 years later (1996, p. 157).

In sum, to adopt an ecological approach that encompasses the brain–body–environment system, we have intersected, in a multidisciplinary and interdisciplinary manner, evidence belonging to the two areas of cognitive and motor development and learning (Pesce, Croce, et al., 2016). Cognitive psychology is needed to understand when and how executive and metacognitive functions come online and neuroscience to explore the neural substrate of such changes; motor development and learning sciences are needed to understand transitions in motor skills development and learning and sports pedagogy to identify teaching methods most appropriate to transition such an evidence base into good practice (Figure 14.3). The role of qualified professionals, able to translate such an evidence base into effective teaching

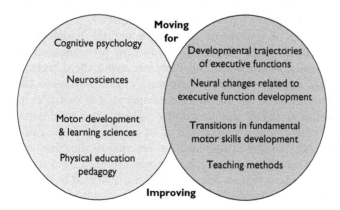

Figure 14.3 Common framework showing how the two areas of cognitive and motor development and learning provide evidence to ground the notion of 'moving for improving' on interdisciplinarity.

and programme design, is crucial if we consider current trends that, with few exceptions, still focus on academics and not physical education and the uneven presence and large absence of national strategies and large-scale initiatives to promote PA in education (European Commission, 2013; Society of Health and Physical Education, 2016).

Active play and designed games for the provision of child's right to play and to health

From the above multidisciplinary perspective, we examine developmental models of school-based PA and sport that can aid cognitive development and their relation to children's free play, anchoring them to a common denominator: the provision of the child's right to play and to health. The amount of developmental exercise and cognition studies that have been performed in the school context is growing (Centers for Disease Control and Prevention, 2010) and their type is increasingly differentiated, focusing on the metabolic-aerobic, coordinative, or cognitive demands, or a combination of them (Vazou et al., 2016). The context of such studies ranges from physical education to classroom-based PA, recess and extracurricular PA. Classroom-based PA includes activity breaks that are short bouts of pure PA interspersed in the sitting learning time and integrated PA that is related to the study content and intended to promote learning by moving. There is evidence that both activity breaks (Fedewa, Ahn, Erwin, & Davis, 2015) and integrated PA (Vazou & Smiley-Owen, 2014) may positively impact cognition and academic achievement in children (Donnelly & Lambourne, 2011), as well as active recess (Hill et al., 2010).

Also youth sport participation has the potential to promote cognitive development (Verburgh, Scherder, van Lange, & Oosterlaan, 2014). Nevertheless, early sport specialization cannot allow the full potential of the circular relationship between stability and flexibility to be exploited, because it prioritizes the stabilization and automatization of highly specific movement patterns, especially in closed-skill sports. There are developmental models of sport participation which propose alternative solutions to early sport specialization. Without hindering the way to the top for elite athletes (Baker, 2003), multisports models of early diversification allow the pursuit of goals of long-term adherence of non-competitive practisers to PA and sport in the frame of a healthy lifestyle. Such models, including wide sports sampling in childhood (Kirk, 2005; Myer, Jayanthi et al., 2016), have also been applied in primary and junior high school contexts (Gallotta, Marchetti, Baldari, Guidetti, & Pesce, 2009; Pesce, Faigenbaum, Crova, Marchetti, & Bellucci, 2013). Initial evidence exists that a school-based multisports approach improves cognitive function of senior high school students (Pesce, Marchetti, et al., 2016) when coupled with content and implementation strategies of life skills training (Goudas, 2010; Hodge, Danish, & Martin, 2012).

Early diversification can also aid cognitive development when applied to training in open-skill sports such as ball games, which inherently exercise the circular relationship between technical stability and tactical flexibility. In fact, a sport enrichment programme in ball games training involving diversified motor coordination and tactical components from different team ball sports promotes the development of creative thinking (Memmert, 2006). Moreover, time spent in diversified, unstructured play activities in childhood and youth is predictive of athletes' creativity later in life (Memmert, Baker, & Bertsch, 2010). The relation of free active play to the development of creativity – a metacognitive competence that relies on executive function (Dietrich, 2004) – is in line with evidence that time spent in non-structured activities may promote executive function during childhood (Barker et al., 2014) and playful and enjoyable features are essential for any activity to impact positively executive function development (Diamond & Lee, 2011).

While playfulness is inherent in free active play of young children, it mostly gets lost along the way to adolescent and adult sport participation, especially when children undergo early sport specialization. Early diversification models are instead characterized by high amounts of enjoyable deliberate play (Myer, Jayanthi, et al., 2016). Deliberate play is defined as activity done for its own sake, characterized by flexibility and enjoyment and targeted to bridge the spontaneous play by young children and the deliberate practice of structured sports by older children and adolescents (Côté, Baker, & Abernethy, 2007; Côté, Lidor, & Hackfort, 2009). Probably in response to an excessive dichotomization of deliberate play for fun and deliberate practice for performance, Côté and Hancock (2016) have proposed a common framework to reconcile them and Giblin, Collins, MacNamara, and Kiely (2014) an intermediate form of play and practice of fundamental movement skills – deliberate preparation – that bridges the two extremes.

Pesce, Masci, et al. (2016) have tailored a mixture of deliberate play and preparation to pursue goals of cognitive development in physical education. Well-designed PA games joining the variable and enjoyable problem-solving conditions of deliberate play and the diversified fundamental motor skills demands of deliberate preparation elicited improvements in motor coordination that mediated those in executive function. An aspect of Pesce et al.'s findings relevant for informing policy development is that a large amount of outdoor free play by children acted as an amplifier of the effects of the enriched physical education. This is evidence in favour of the claim to consider school-based and environment-based policies jointly, capitalizing on active play for healthy development that goes beyond mere 'fitness and fatness' arguments (Alexander, Frohlich, & Fusco, 2014; Burdette & Whitaker, 2005; Faigenbaum & Myer, 2012).

Evidence into policy or policy into evidence? A multisectoral issue

The last step of our 'storytelling' addresses how evidence-based guidelines of quality PA for children and adolescents may be delivered, adopted and implemented and what barriers may render multisectoral implementation unsuccessful. In recent years, many of the neuroscientific studies that have provided evidence of the beneficial impact of PA on the brain during development started off with general statements on public health concerns and costs of the early onset of physical inactivity and concluded highlighting the relevance of evidence of exercise effects on children's brain for public health and education policies. Indeed, the accumulating evidence obtained with neuroscientific measures of brain biochemistry, structure and function has a high level of objectivity. Thus, the American College of Sports Medicine has published its first up-to-date Position Stand on the association of PA and fitness with cognitive function and academic achievement in children (Donnelly et al., 2016). However, as Donnelly et al. (2016) state, more research is still necessary to translate neuroscientific findings obtained in laboratory research into policies and good practices, particularly in the school environment, where all children may be given equal opportunities to 'improve by moving'.

To derive practice recommendations useful for policy makers, it is not sufficient to perform more research on the cognitive outcomes of PA in the school context and meta-analyses of largely or solely efficacy studies. Even well-powered interventional research is biased toward reporting on internal validity issues rather than generalizability. The current trend of publishing in advance the study protocol of large-scale school-based PA interventions offers the opportunity to report detailed information on representativeness and implementation, especially at the level of settings and intervention agents. However, the focus of such PA promotion protocols is still on inactivity and overweight reduction (Martínez-Vizcaino et al., 2015; Zahner et al., 2006), or also includes academic achievement outcomes but merely pursued through enhanced PA quantity (Resaland et al., 2015), while a focus on PA quality and whole-child development is still the exception (Piek et al., 2010). Still underrepresented in interventional exercise and cognition research is process evaluation that is the post hoc evaluation of whether a programme works and is sustainable over time when delivered and implemented under real-world conditions (Pesce, Leone, Motta, Marchetti, & Tomporowski, 2016).

Thus, it is necessary to shift research efforts from efficacy to effectiveness. This means shifting from testing the capacity of quality PA interventions to impact children's brain and body (efficacy) to evaluating the possibility of disseminating efficacious PA interventions effectively, by adopting and implementing them in different contexts (effectiveness). This need is not specific to interventional exercise and cognition research, but generalizes to the whole area of health promotion research (Glasgow, Lichtenstein, & Marcus, 2003; Rychetnik et al., 2012). Until now, 'translational' research addressing the effectiveness of PA intervention programmes for children and adolescents by means of internationally recognized quantitative evaluation metrics (RE-AIM – Reach, Effectiveness, Adoption, Implementation, Maintenance; Estabrooks & Glasgow, 2006) is exclusively targeted to enhance PA levels for obtaining physical health outcomes (McGoey, Root, Bruner, & Law, 2015, 2016). If, instead, the targeted outcomes also encompass brain health and other developmental outcomes that are elicited by the qualitative characteristics of designed PA and there is a complex and multifaceted process of implementation of delivery strategies, it is essential to complement quantitative metrics with the evaluation of qualitative implementation aspects (Pesce, Leone, et al., 2016). Particularly, we need to monitor knowledge transfer and supervision of content and delivery fidelity by networked programme planners, local service providers and other synergistic actors from public and private sectors.

Currently, there is not only a gap between a larger availability of evidence-based PA guidelines based on the relation of PA quantity to physical health indicators and a smaller availability of guidelines on the relation of PA quality to both physical and brain health. There is also a paucity of evidence on the characteristics of or threats to successful adoption, implementation and delivery of PA guidelines in specific settings. To fill this gap, there are attemps to identify some mechanisms through which PA guidelines are adopted in different policy sectors – health, education, sport, urban planning and transport – and barriers that can hinder their implementation by policy makers and professionals. Firstly, there is an overordered problem of low synergy in PA and sport policies among health, education and sport sectors in EU plans and documents (Daugbjerg et al., 2009). As specifically regards children's free active play, urban planners have a pivotal role in rendering the environment more walkable and conducive to active play (Dill & Howe, 2011). However, a barrier is represented by a self-referential concept of knowledge and narrowly defined methodological 'gold standard' in medical sciences (Weaver et al., 2002). This may lead to neglecting non-medical evidence on the built environment relevant for public health, also due to a very small overlap between medical and built environment or social science databases (Ogilvie, Egan, Hamilton, & Petticrew, 2005). As regards the school environment, barriers to implementing PA include budget constraints, lack of specialist physical education teachers at preschool and primary school levels and perceived time constraints by school personnel (Fedewa, Candelaria, Erwin, & Clark, 2013). The steeply increasing evidence that PA is beneficial to cognitive development and academic achievement – in any case, not detrimental (Donnelly & Lambourne, 2011) – may positively inform policy development, helping PA in schools leave behind its 'Cinderella' status.

Conclusions

In the title of this chapter, it was not our intention to echo rhetorically the Swahili proverb that 'We should hitch our plough to a star'. At the end, we can unwrap its concreteness (Figure 14.4). We not only need to put more evidence into policy, providing policy makers with a stronger evidence base. We also need to put more policy into evidence. If research is not driven by a north star, but narrowly informed (and granted) by unisectoral needs – like that of the health system to limit the costs of pandemic inactivity – researchers can only draw straight, and maybe effective, but conventional and non-creative furrows. To put more policy into evidence search, we propose hitching the plough of PA promotion to the child's right to play and be physically active (United Nations, 2013).

This is grounded in the increasing awareness of the public health and social value of play and purposely designed PA by authoritative institutions (European Union, 2008; Milteer et al., 2012). Putting more policy into evidence means broadening the research focus, being aware that the two fields of human rights and public health ethics can jointly contribute to strengthen global health actions (Nixon & Forman, 2008) and, referring to our developmental interest, to ensure the provision of the child's right to play and be physically active as a health determinant. Indeed, by playing – freely or deliberately – and being physically active within well-designed PA experiences, children may develop foundational strength and motor skills early in life, intertwined with each other and with physical and mental health. In this light, our plough could not be merely operationalized

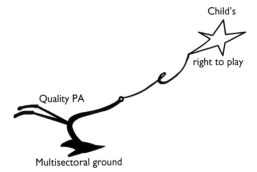

Figure 14.4 'We should hitch our plough to a star' (Swahili proverb). The child's right to play can enlighten our efforts to promote quality physical activity (PA), transitioning neuroscientific evidence stepwise into multisectoral policies and practices.

as a health-enhancing amount of PA, but as 'thoughtful moving' grounded in developmental neuroscience and implemented, within multisectoral contexts, as enjoyable free and deliberate play and sports sampling, for children to achieve their full potential.

'The very nature of executive functions that makes them vulnerable is also a source of untapped opportunities' (Garon, Bryson, & Smith, 2008, p. 52): let's further explore these opportunities within the developmental window, joining our plough of thoughtful moving to the star of children's right to play.

References

Alexander, S. A., Frohlich, K. L., & Fusco, C. (2014). Playing for health? Revisiting health promotion to examine the emerging public health position on children's play. *Health Promotion International, 29*, 155–164. doi: 10.1093/heapro/das042.

Álvarez-Bueno, C., Pesce, C., Cavero-Redondo, I., Sánchez-López, M., Pardo-Guijarro, M. J., & Martínez-Vizcaíno, V. (2016). Association of physical activity with cognition, metacognition and academic performance in children and adolescents: A protocol for systematic review and meta-analysis. *BMJ Open, 6*, e011065. doi: 10.1136/bmjopen-2016-011065.

American College of Sports Medicine. (2016). *Exercise is medicine: A global health initiative.* http://www.exerciseismedicine.org/.

Andersen, S. L. (2003). Trajectories of brain development: Point of vulnerability or window of opportunity? *Neuroscience and Biobehavioral Reviews, 27*, 3–18. doi: 10.1016/S0149-7634(03)00005-8.

Audiffren, M., & André, N. (2015). The strength model of self-control revisited: Linking acute and chronic effects of exercise on executive functions. *Journal of Sport and Health Science, 4*, 30–46. doi: 10.1016/j.jshs.2014.09.002.

Bailey, R. P., Armour, K., Kirk, D., Jess, M., Pickup, I., & Sandford, R. (2009). The educational benefits claimed for physical education and school sport: An academic review. *Research Papers in Education, 24*, 1–27.

Bailey, R. P., Hillman, C., Arent, S., & Petitpas, A. (2013). Physical activity: An underestimated investment in human capital? *Journal of Physical Activity and Health, 10*, 289–308.

Baker, J. (2003). Early specialization in youth sport: A requirement for adult expertise? *High Ability Studies, 14*, 85–94. doi: 10.1080/13032000093526.

Barker, J. E., Semenov, A. D., Michaelson, L., Provan, L. S., Snyder, H. R., & Munakata, Y. (2014). Less-structured time in children's daily lives predicts self-directed executive functioning. *Frontiers in Psychology, 5*, 593. doi: 10.3389/fpsyg.2014.00593.

Barnett, L. M., Van Beurden, E., Morgan, P. J., Brooks, L. O., & Beard, J. R. (2008). Does childhood motor skill proficiency predict adolescent fitness? *Medicine and Science in Sports and Exercise, 40*, 2137–2144. doi: 10.1249/MSS.0b013e31818160d3.

Bernstein, N. A. (1996). On dexterity and its development. In M. L. Latash & M. T. Turvey (Eds.), *Dexterity and its development* (pp. 3–244). Mahwah, NJ: Lawrence Erlbaum.

Best, J. R. (2010). Effects of physical activity on children's executive function: Contributions of experimental research on aerobic exercise. *Developmental Review, 30*, 331–351. doi: 10.1016/j.dr.2010.08.001.

Bherer, L., Erickson, K., & Liu-Ambrose, T. (2013). A review of the effects of physical activity and exercise on cognitive and brain functions in older adults. *Journal of Aging Research, 2013*, 657508. doi: 10.1155/2013/657508.

Buckner, R. L. (2013). The cerebellum and cognitive function: 25 years of insight from anatomy and neuroimaging. *Neuron, 80*, 807–815. doi: 10.1016/j.neuron.2013.10.044.

Burdette, H. L., & Whitaker, R. C. (2005). Resurrecting free play in young children looking beyond fitness and fatness to attention, affiliation, and affect. *Archives of Pediatric and Adolescent Medicine, 159*, 46–50. doi: 10.1001/archpedi.159.1.46.

Campos, J. J., Anderson, D. I., Barbu-Roth, M. A., Hubbard, E. M., Hertenstein, M. J., & Witherington, D. (2000). Travel broadens the mind. *Infancy, 1*, 149–219. doi: 10.1207/S15327078IN0102_1.

Carey, J. R., Bhatt, E., & Nagpal, A. (2005). Neuroplasticity promoted by task complexity. *Exercise and Sport Sciences Reviews, 33*, 24–31.

Casey, B. J., Getz, S., & Galvan, A. (2008). The adolescent brain. *Developmental Review, 28*, 62–77. doi: 10.1016/j.dr.2007.08.003.

Centers for Disease Control and Prevention. (2010). *The association between school-based physical activity, including physical education, and academic performance.* Atlanta, GA: U.S. Department of Health and Human Service. http://www.cdc.gov/healthyschools/health_and_academics/pdf/pa-pe_paper.pdf.

Centers for Disease Control and Prevention. (2015). *Childhood obesity facts.* https://www.cdc.gov/healthyschools/obesity/facts.htm.

Chaddock, L., Pontifex, M. B., Hillman, C. H., & Kramer, A. F. (2011). A review of the relation of aerobic fitness and physical activity to brain structure and function in children. *Journal of International of the Neuropsychological Society, 17*, 1–11. doi: 10.1017/S1355617711000567.

Chaddock-Heyman, L., Erickson, K. I., Voss, M. W., Knecht, A. M., Pontifex, M. B., Castelli, D., . . . Kramer, A. F. (2013). The effects of physical activity on functional MRI activation associated with cognitive control in children: A randomized controlled intervention. *Frontiers in Human Neuroscience, 7*, 72, 1–13. doi: 10.3389/fnhum.2013.000727.

Chang, Y. K., Chu, C. H., Chen, F. T., Hung, T. M., & Etnier, J. L. (2017). Combined effects of physical activity and obesity on cognitive function: Independent, overlapping, moderator, and mediator models. *Sports Medicine, 47*(3), 449–468.

Chang, Y. K., Tsai, Y. J., Chen, T. T., & Hung, T. M. (2013). The impacts of coordinative exercise on executive function in kindergarten children: An ERP study. *Experimental Brain Research, 225*, 187–196. doi: 10.1007/s00221-012-3360-9.

Cohen, D. D., Voss, C., Taylor, M. J., Delextrat, A., Ogunleye, A. A., & Sandercock, G. R. (2011). Ten-year secular changes in muscular fitness in English children. *Acta Paediatrica, 100*, 175–177. doi: 10.1111/j.1651-2227.2011.02318.x.

Colcombe, S. J., & Kramer, A. F. (2003). Fitness effects on the cognitive function of older adults: A meta-analytic study. *Psychological Science, 14*, 125–130. doi: 10.1111/1467-9280.t01-1-01430.

Côté, J., Baker, J., & Abernethy, B. (2007). Play and practice in the development of sport expertise. In G. Tenenbaum & R. C. Eklund (Eds.), *Handbook of sport psychology* (pp. 184–202). Hoboken, NJ: John Wiley.

Côté, J., & Hancock, D. J. (2016). Evidence-based policies for youth sport programmes. *International Journal of Sport Policy and Politics. 8*, 51–65. doi: 10.1080/19406940.2014.919338.

Côté, J., Lidor, R., & Hackfort. D. (2009). ISSP position stand: To sample or to specialize? Seven postulates about youth sport activities that lead to continued participation and elite performance. *International Journal of Sport and Exercise Psychology, 7*, 7–17.

Crova, C., Struzzolino, I., Marchetti, R., Masci, I., Vannozzi, G., Forte, R., & Pesce, C. (2014). Benefits of cognitively challenging physical activity in overweight children. *Journal of Sports Sciences, 32*, 201–211. doi: 10.1080/02640414.2013.828849.

Danish, S. J., & Forneris, T. (2008). Promoting positive development and competency across the lifespan. In S. D. Brown & R. W. Lent (Eds.), *Handbook of counseling psychology* (4th ed., pp. 500–517). Hoboken, NJ: Wiley.

Daugbjerg, S. B., Kahlmeier, S., Racioppi, F., Martin-Diener, E., Martin, B., Oja, P, & Bull, F. (2009) Promotion of physical activity in the European region: Content analysis of 27 national policy documents. *Journal of Physical Activity and Health, 6*, 805–817.

Davis, C. L., Tomporowski, P. D., Boyle, C. A., Waller, J. L., Miller, P. H., Naglieri, J. A., & Gregoski, M. (2007). Effects of aerobic exercise on overweight children's cognitive functioning: A randomized controlled trial. *Research Quarterly for Exercise and Sport, 78*, 510–519.

Davis, C. L., Tomporowski, P. D., McDowell, J. E., Austin, B. P., Miller, P. H., Yanasak, N. E., . . . Naglieri, J. A. (2011). Exercise improves executive function and achievement and alters brain activation in overweight children: A randomized, controlled trial. *Health Psychology, 30*, 91–98. doi: 10.1037/a0021766.

D'Hondt, E., Deforche, B., Gentier, I., De Bourdeaudhuij, I., Vaeyens, R., Philippaerts, R., & Lenoir, M. (2013). A longitudinal analysis of gross motor coordination in overweight and obese children versus normal-weight peers. *International Journal of Obesity, 37*, 61–67. doi: 10.1038/ijo.2012.55.

Diamond, A. (2013). Executive functions. *Annual Review of Psychology, 64*, 135–168. doi: 10.1146/annurev-psych-113011-143750.

Diamond, A. (2015). Effects of physical exercise on executive functions: Going beyond simply moving to moving with thought. *Annuals of Sports Medicine and Research, 2*, 1011.

Diamond, A., & Lee, K. (2011). Interventions shown to aid executive function development in children 4 to 12 years old. *Science, 333*, 954–969. doi: 10.1126/science.1204529.

Diamond, A., & Ling, D. S. (2016). Conclusions about interventions, programs, and approaches for improving executive functions that appear justified and those that, despite much hype, do not. *Developmental Cognitive Neuroscience, 18*, 34–48. doi: 10.1016/j.dcn.2015.11.005.

Dietrich, A. (2004). The cognitive neuroscience of creativity. *Psychonomic Bulletin and Review, 11*, 1011–1026. doi: 10.3758/BF03196731.

DiFiori, J. P., Benjamin, H. J., Brenner, J., Gregory, A., Jayanthi, N., Landry, G. L., & Luke, A. (2014). Overuse injuries and burnout in youth sports: A position statement from the American Medical Society for Sports Medicine. *Clinical Journal of Sport Medicine, 24*, 3–20.

Dill, J., & Howe, D. (2011). The role of health and physical activity in the adoption of innovative land use policy: Findings. *Journal of Physical Activity and Health, 8*(Suppl 1), S116–S124.

Donnelly, J. E., Hillman, C. H., Castelli, D., Etnier, J. L., Lee, S., Tomporowski, P., . . . Szabo-Reed, A. N. (2016). Physical activity, fitness, cognitive function, and academic achievement in children: A systematic review. *Medicine and Science in Sports and Exercise, 48*, 1197–1222. doi: 10.1249/MSS.0000000000000901.

Donnelly, J. E., & Lambourne, K. (2011). Classroom-based physical activity, cognition, and academic achievement. *Preventive Medicine 52*, S36–S42. doi: 10.1016/j.ypmed.2011.01.021.

Engel, A. K., Maye, A., Kurthen, M., & König, P. (2013). Where's the action? The pragmatic turn in cognitive science. *Trends in Cognitive Science, 17*, 202–209. doi: 10.1016/j.tics.2013.03.006.

Estabrooks, P. A., & Glasgow, R. E. (2006). Translating effective clinic-based physical activity interventions into practice. *American Journal of Preventive Medicine, 31*(Suppl 4), S45–S56.

Etnier, J. L., & Chang, Y. K. (2009). The effect of physical activity on executive function: A brief commentary on definitions, measurement issues, and the current state of the literature. *Journal of Sport and Exercise Psychology, 31*, 469–483.

European Commission. (2007a). *White Paper on a strategy for Europe on nutrition, overweight and obesity related health issues.* COM(2007)279 final. 30 May 2007. http://ec.europa.eu/health/ph_determinants/life_style/nutrition/documents/nutrition_wp_en.pdf.

European Commission. (2007b). *White Paper on sport.* COM (2007)391 final. 11 July 2007.http://eur-lex.europa.eu/legal-content/EN/TXT/?uri=CELEX:52007DC0391.

European Commission. (2013). *Physical education and sport at school in Europe. Eurydice report.* Luxembourg: Publications Office of the European Union. doi: 10.2797/49648. http://eacea.ec.europa.eu/education/eurydice.

European Union. (2008). *EU physical activity guidelines. Recommended policy actions in support of health-enhancing physical activity.* Brussels: European Union. http://ec.europa.eu/sport/library/policy_documents/eu-physical-activity-guidelines-2008_en.pdf.

Faigenbaum, A. D., Lloyd, R. S., MacDonald, J., & Myer, G. D. (2016). Citius, altius, fortius: Beneficial effects of resistance training for young athletes. *British Journal of Sports Medicine, 50*(1), 3–7. doi: 10.1136/bjsports-2015-094621.

Faigenbaum, A. D., Lloyd, R. S., & Myer, G. D. (2013). Youth resistance training: Past practices, new perspectives, and future directions. *Pediatric Exercise Science, 25,* 591–604.

Faigenbaum, A. D., & Myer, G. D. (2012). Exercise deficit disorder in youth: Play now or pay later. *Current Sports Medicine Reports, 11,* 196–200. doi: 10.1249/JSR.0b013e31825da961.

Fajen, B. R., Riley, M. A., & Turvey, M. T. (2008). Information, affordances, and the control of action in sport. *International Journal of Sport Psychology, 40,* 79–107.

Favela, L. H. (2014). Radical embodied cognitive neuroscience: Addressing "grand-challenges" of the mind sciences. *Frontiers in Human Neuroscience, 8*(796), 1–10. doi: 10.3389/fnhum.2014.00796.

Fedewa, A. L., Ahn, S., Erwin, H., & Davis, M. C. (2015). A randomized controlled design investigating the effects of classroom-based physical activity on children's fluid intelligence and achievement. *School Psychology International, 36,* 135–153.

Fedewa, A. L., Candelaria, A., Erwin, H. E., & Clark, T. P. (2013). Incorporating physical activity into schools using a 3-tiered approach. *Journal of School Health, 83,* 290–297. doi: 10.1111/josh.12029.

Gajewski, P. D., & Falkenstein, M. (2016). Physical activity and neurocognitive functioning in aging – a condensed updated review. *European Review of Aging and Physical Activity, 13,* 1. doi: 10.1186/s11556-016-0161-3.

Gallotta, M. C., Marchetti, R., Baldari, C., Guidetti, L., & Pesce, C. (2009). Linking coordinative and fitness training in physical education settings. *Scandinavian Journal of Medicine and Science in Sports, 19,* 412–418.

Garber, C. E., Blissmer, B., Deschenes, M. R., Franklin, B. A., Lamonte, M. J., & Lee, I.-M., American College of Sports Medicine. (2011). Quantity and quality of exercise for developing and maintaining cardiorespiratory, musculoskeletal, and neuromotor fitness in apparently healthy adults: guidance for prescribing exercise. Position stand. *Medicine and Science in Sports and Exercise, 43,* 1334–1359.

Garon, N., Bryson, S., & Smith, I. M. (2008). Executive function in preschoolers: A review using an integrative framework. *Psychological Bulletin, 134,* 31–60. doi: 10.1037/0033-2909.134.1.31.

Giblin, S., Collins, D., MacNamara, Á., & Kiely, J. (2014). "Deliberate preparation" as an evidence-based focus for primary physical education. *Quest, 66,* 385–395. doi: 10.1080/00336297.2014.944716.

Glasgow, R. E., Lichtenstein, E., & Marcus, A. C. (2003). Why don't we see more translation of health promotion research to practice? Rethinking the efficacy-to-effectiveness transition. *American Journal of Public Health, 93,* 1261–1267.

Gomez-Pinilla, F., & Hillman, C. H. (2013). The influence of exercise on cognitive abilities. *Comparative Physiology, 1,* 403–428. doi: 10.1002/cphy.c110063.

Goudas, M. (2010). Prologue: A review of life skills teaching in sport and physical education. *Hellenic Journal of Psychology, 7*, 241–258.

Goudas, M., Kolovelonis, A., & Dermitzaki, I. (2012). Implementation of self-regulation interventions in physical education and sports contexts. In H. Bembenutty, T. J. Cleary, & A. Kitsantas (Eds.), *Applications of self-regulated learning across diverse disciplines* (pp. 383–415). Charlotte, NC: Information Age Publishing.

Gould, D., & Carson, S. (2008). Life skills development through sport: Current status and future directions. *International Review of Sport and Exercise Psychology, 1*, 58–78. doi: 10.1080/17509840701834573.

Green, C. S., & Bavelier, D. (2008). Exercising your brain: A review of human brain plasticity and training-induced learning. *Psychology of Aging, 23*, 692–701. doi: 10.1037/a0014345.

Guadagnoli, M. A., & Lee, T. D. (2004). Challenge point: A framework for conceptualizing the effects of various practice conditions in motor learning. *Journal of Motor Behavior, 36*, 212–224.

Hardy, L. L., Barnett, L., Espinel, P., & Okely, A. D. (2013). Thirteen-year trends in child and adolescent fundamental movement skills: 1997–2010. *Medicine and Science in Sports and Exercise, 45*, 1965–1970. doi: 10.1249/MSS.0b013e318295a9fc.

Herting, M. M., & Nagel, B. J. (2012). Aerobic fitness relates to learning on a virtual Morris Water Task and hippocampal volume in adolescents. *Behavioral Brain Research, 233*, 517–525. doi: 10.1016/j.bbr.2012.05.012.

Herting, M. M., & Nagel, B. J. (2013). Differences in brain activity during a verbal associative memory encoding task in high- and low-fit adolescents. *Journal of Cognitive Neuroscience, 25*, 595–612. doi: 10.1162/jocn a 00344.

Herting, M. M., Colby, J. B., Sowell, E. R., & Nagel, B. J. (2014). White matter connectivity and aerobic fitness in male adolescents. *Developmental Cognitive Neuroscience, 7*, 65–75. doi:10.1016/j.dcn.2013.11.003.

Hill, L., Williams, J. H. G., Aucott, L., Milne, J., Thomson, J., Greig, J., . . . Mon-Williams, M. (2010). Exercising attention within the classroom. *Developmental Medicine and Child Neurology, 52*, 929–934. doi: 10.1111/j.1469-8749.2010.03661.x.

Hillman, C. H., Kamijo, K., & Scudder, M. R. (2011). A review of chronic and acute physical activity participation on neuroelectric measures of brain health and cognition during childhood. *Preventive Medicine, 52*, 21–28. doi: 10.1016/j.ypmed.2011.01.024.

Hillman, C. H., Pontifex, M. B., Castelli, D. M., Khan, N. A., Raine, N. B., Scudder, M. R., . . . Kamijo, K. (2014). Effects of the FITKids randomized controlled trial on executive control and brain function. *Pediatrics, 134*, e1063. doi: 10.1542/peds.2013-3219.

Hodge, K., Danish, S., & Martin, J. (2012). Developing a conceptual framework for life skills interventions. *The Counseling Psychologist, 20*, 1–28. doi: 10.1177/0011000012462073.

Kamijo, K., Pontifex, M. B., O'Leary, K. C., Scudder, M. R., Wu, C-T., Castelli, D. M., & Hillman, C. H. (2011). The effects of an afterschool physical activity program on working memory in preadolescent children. *Developmental Science, 14*, 1046–1058. doi: 10.1111/j.1467-7687.2011.01054.x.

Khan, N. A., & Hillman, C. H. (2014). The relation of childhood physical activity and aerobic fitness to brain function and cognition: A review. *Pediatric Exercise Science, 26*, 138–146. doi: 10.1123/pes.2013-0125.

Kirk, D. (2005). Physical education, youth sport and lifelong participation: The importance of early learning experiences. *European Physical Education Review, 11*, 239–255. doi: 10.1177/1356336X05056649.

Koutsandreou, F., Wegner, M., Niemann, C., & Budde, H. (2016). Effects of motor vs. cardiovascular exercise training on children's working memory. *Medicine and Science in Sports and Exercise, 48*, 1144–1152. doi: 10.1249/MSS.0000000000000869.

Koziol, L. F., Budding, D. E., & Chidekel, D. (2012). From movement to thought: Executive function, embodied cognition, and the cerebellum. *Cerebellum, 11*, 505–525. doi: 10.1007/s12311-011-0321-y.

Krafft, C. E., Schwarz, N. F., Chi, L., Weinberger, A. L., Schaeffer, D. J., Pierce, J. E., . . . McDowell, J. E. (2014). An 8-month randomized controlled exercise trial alters brain activation during cognitive tasks in overweight children. *Obesity, 22*, 232–242. doi: 10.1002/oby.20518.

Lakes, K. D., & Hoyt, W. T. (2004). Promoting self-regulation through school-based martial arts training. *Applied Developmental Psychology, 25*, 283–302. doi: 10.1016/j.appdev.2004.04.002.

Lee, I.-M. (2008). Current issues in examining dose–response relations between physical activity and health outcome. In I.-M. Lee (Ed.), *Epidemiologic methods in physical activity studies* (pp. 56–76). New York: Oxford.

Lee, T. M. C., Wong, M. L., Lau, B. W-M., Lee, J. C-D., Yau, S. Y., & So, K. F. (2014). Aerobic exercise interacts with neurotrophic factors to predict cognitive functioning in adolescents. *Psychoneuroendocrinology, 39*, 214–224. doi: 10.1016/j.psyneuen.2013.09.019.

Malina, R. M. (2010). Early sport specialization: Roots, effectiveness, risks. *Current Sports Medicine Reports, 9*, 364–371. doi: 10.1249/JSR.0b013e3181fe3166.

Martínez-Vizcaino, V., Mota, J., Solera-Martínez, M., Notario-Pacheco, B., Arias-Palencia, N., García-Prieto, J. C., . . . Sánchez-López, M. on behalf of the MOVI-KIDS group (2015). Rationale and methods of a randomised cross-over cluster trial to assess the effectiveness of MOVI-KIDS on preventing obesity in pre-schoolers. *BMC Public Health, 15*, 176. doi: 10.1186/s12889-015-1512-0.

McGoey, T., Root, Z., Bruner, M. W., & Law, B. (2016). Evaluation of physical activity interventions in children via the reach, efficacy/effectiveness, adoption, implementation, and maintenance (RE-AIM) framework: A systematic review of randomized and non-randomized trials. *Preventive Medicine, 82*, 8–19. doi: 10.1016/j.ypmed.2015.11.004.

McGoey, T., Root, Z., Bruner, M. W., & Law, B. (2015). Evaluation of physical activity interventions in youth via the reach, efficacy/effectiveness, adoption, implementation, and maintenance (RE-AIM) framework: A systematic review of randomised and non-randomized trials. *Preventive Medicine, 76*, 58–67. doi: 10.1016/j.ypmed.2015.04.006.

McMorris, T. (2016). *Exercise–cognition interaction: Neuroscience perspectives.* London: Elsevier.

Memmert, D. (2006). Developing creative thinking in a gifted sport enrichment program and the crucial role of attention processes. *High Ability Studies, 17*, 101–115. doi: 10.1080/13598130600947176.

Memmert, D., Baker, J., & Bertsch, C. (2010). Play and practice in the development of sport-specific creativity in team ball sports. *High Ability Studies, 21*, 3–18. doi: 10.1080/13598139.2010.488083.

Milteer, R. M., Ginsburg, K. R., Council on Communications and Media Committee on Psychosocial Aspects of Child and Family Health, & Mulligan, D. A. (2012). The importance of play in promoting healthy child development and maintaining strong parent child bond: Focus on children in poverty. *Pediatrics, 129*, e204. doi: 10.1542/peds.2011-2953.

Moreau, D. (2015). Unreflective actions? Complex motor skill acquisition to enhance spatial cognition. *Phenomenology Cognitive Science, 14*, 349–359. doi: 10.1007/s11097-014-9376-9.

Moreau, D., & Conway, A. R. A. (2014). The case for an ecological approach to cognitive training. *Trends in Cognitive Training, 18*, 334–336. doi: 10.1016/j.tics.2014.03.009.

Moreau, D., Morrison, A. B., & Conway, A. R. A. (2015). An ecological approach to cognitive enhancement: Complex motor training. *Acta Psychologica, 157*, 44–55. doi: 10.1016/j.actpsy.2015.02.007.

Moriguchi, Y., Chevalier, N., & Zelazo, P. D. (2016). Editorial: Development of executive function during childhood. *Frontiers in Psychology, 7*, 6. doi: 10.3389/fpsyg.2016.00006.

Munakata, Y., Snyder, H. R., & Chatham, C. H. (2012). Developing cognitive control: Three key transitions. *Current Directions in Psychological Sciences, 21*, 71–77. doi: 10.1177/0963721412436807.

Munakata, Y., Snyder, H. R., & Chatham, C. H. (2013). Developing cognitive control: The costs and benefits of active, abstract representations. In P. D. Zelazo & M. D. Sera (Eds.), *Developing cognitive control processes: Mechanisms, implications, and interventions*. West Sussex: Wiley. doi: 10.1002/9781118732373.ch3.

Myer, G. D., Faigenbaum, A. D., Edwards, N. M., Clark, J. F., Best, T. M., & Sallis, R. E. (2015). Sixty minutes of what? A developing brain perspective for activating children with an integrative exercise approach. *British Journal of Sports Medicine, 49*, 1510–1516. doi: 10.1136/bjsports-2014-093661.

Myer, G. D., Jayanthi, N., DiFiori, J. P., Faigenbaum, A. D., Kiefer, A. W., Logerstedt, D., & Micheli, L. J. (2015). Sport specialization, part I: Does early sports specialization increase negative outcomes and reduce the opportunity for success in young athletes? *Sports Health, 7*, 437–442. doi: 10.1177/1941738115598747.

Myer, G. D., Jayanthi, N., DiFiori, J. P., Faigenbaum, A. D., Kiefer, A. W., Logerstedt, D., & Micheli, L. J. (2016). Sports specialization, part II: Alternative solutions to early sport specialization in youth athletes. *Sports Health, 8*, 65–73. doi: 10.1177/1941738115614811.

Newell, K. (1986). Constraints on the development of coordination. In M. G. Wade & H. T. Whiting (Eds.), *Motor development in children: Aspects of coordination and control* (pp. 341–360). Dordrecht, Netherlands: Nijhoff.

Nixon, S., & Forman, L. (2008). Exploring synergies between human rights and public health ethics: A whole greater than the sum of its parts. *BMC International Health and Human Rights, 8*, 2. doi: 10.1186/1472-698X-8-2.

Ogden, C. L., Carroll, M. D., Lawman, H. G., Fryar, C. D., Kruszon-Moran, D., Kit, B. K., & Flegal, K. M. (2016). Trends in obesity prevalence among children and adolescents in the United States, 1988–1994 through 2013–2014. *JAMA, 315*, 2292–2299. doi: 10.1001/jama.2016.6361.

Ogilvie, D., Egan, M., Hamilton, V., & Petticrew, M. (2005). Theory and methods of systematic reviews of health effects of social interventions: 2. Best available evidence: How low should you go? *Journal of Epidemiology and Community Health, 59*, 886–892.

Pate, R. R., Davis, M. G., Robinson, T. N., Stone, E. J., McKenzie, T. L., & Young, J. C.; American Heart Association Council on Nutrition, Physical Activity, and Metabolism (Physical Activity Committee); Council on Cardiovascular Disease in the Young; Council on Cardiovascular Nursing (2006). Promoting physical activity in children and youth: A leadership role for schools. *Circulation, 114*, 1214–1224. doi: 10.1161/CIRCULATIONAHA.106.177052.

Pesce, C. (2012). Shifting the focus from quantitative to qualitative exercise characteristics in exercise and cognition research. *Journal of Sport and Exercise Psychology, 34*, 766–786.

Pesce, C., & Ben-Soussan, T. D. (2016). 'Cogito ergo sum' or 'ambulo ergo sum'? New perspectives in developmental exercise and cognition research. In T. McMorris (Ed.), *Exercise–cognition interaction: Neuroscience perspectives.* London: Elsevier.

Pesce, C., Croce, R., Ben-Soussan. T. D., Vazou, S., McCullick, B., Tomporowski, P. D., & Horvat, M. (2016). Variability of practice as an interface between motor and cognitive development. *International Journal of Sport and Exercise Psychology.* doi: 10.1080/1612197X.2016.1223421 (published online: 19 Aug 2016).

Pesce, C., Crova, C., Marchetti, M., Struzzolino, I., Masci, I., Vannozzi, G., & Forte, R. (2013). Searching for cognitively optimal challenge point in physical activity for children with typical and atypical motor development. *Mental Health and Physical Activity, 6*, 172–180. doi: 10.1016/j.mhpa.2013.07.001.

Pesce, C., Faigenbaum, A. D., Crova, C., Marchetti, R., & Bellucci, M. (2013). Benefits of multisports physical education in the elementary school context. *Health Education Journal, 72*, 326–336. doi: 10.1177/0017896912444176.

Pesce, C., Leone, L., Motta, A., Marchetti, R., & Tomporowski, P. D. (2016). From efficacy to effectiveness of a "whole child" initiative of physical activity promotion. *Translational Journal of the ACSM, 1*, 18–29.

Pesce, C., Marchetti, R., Forte, R., Crova, C., Scatigna, M., Goudas, M., & Danish, S. J. (2016). Youth life skills training: Exploring outcomes and mediating mechanisms of a group-randomized trial in physical education. *Sport, Exercise, and Performance Psychology.* Advance online publication, 4 February 2016. doi: 10.1037/spy0000060.

Pesce, C., Masci, C., Marchetti, R., Vazou, S., Sääkslahti, A., & Tomporowski, P. D. (2016). Deliberate play jointly benefits motor and cognitive development: Direct and indirect effects of cognitive stimulation by movement. *Frontiers in Psycholog, 7*, 349. doi: 10.3389/fpsyg.2016.00349.

Piaget, J. (1952). *The origins of intelligence in children.* New York: International Universities Press.

Piek, J. P., Straker, L. M., Jensen, L., Dender, A., Barrett, N. C., McLaren, S., . . . Elsley, S. (2010). Rationale, design and methods for a randomised and controlled trial to evaluate "Animal Fun" – a program designed to enhance physical and mental health in young children. *BMC Pediatrics 2010, 10*, 78. doi: 10.1186/1471-2431-10-78.

Poitras, V. J., Gray, C. E., Borghese, M. M., Carson, V., Chaput, J. P., Janssen, I., . . . Tremblay, M. S. (2016). Systematic review of the relationships between objectively measured physical activity and health indicators in school-aged children and youth. *Applied Physiology, Nutrition, and Metabolism, 41*(Suppl 3), S197–S239. doi: 10.1139/apnm-2015-0663.

Prakash, R. S., Voss, M. V., Erickson, K. I., & Kramer, A. F. (2015). Physical activity and cognitive vitality. *Annual Reviews of Psychology, 66*, 769–797. doi: 10.1146/annurev-psych-010814-015249.

Reinert, K. R. S., Po'e, E. K., & Barkin, S. L. (2013). The relationship between executive function and obesity in children and adolescents: A systematic literature review. *Journal of Obesity, 2013*, 820956. doi: 10.1155/2013/820956.

Renshaw, I., Chow, J. Y., Davids, K., & Hammond, J. (2010). A constraints-led perspective to understanding skill acquisition and game play: A basis for integration of motor learning theory and physical education praxis? *Physical Education and Sport Pedagogy, 15*, 117–137. doi: 10.1080/17408980902791586.

Resaland, G. K., Moe, V. F., Aadland, E., Steene-Johannessen, J., Glosvik, Ø., Andersen, J. R., . . . Anderssen, S. A. and on behalf of the ASK study group (2015). Active Smarter Kids (ASK): Rationale and design of a cluster-randomized controlled trial investigating the effects of daily physical activity on children's academic performance and risk factors for non-communicable diseases. *BMC Public Health, 15*, 709. doi: 10.1186/s12889-015-2049-y.

Robinson, L. E., Stodden, D. F., Barnett, L. M., Lopes, V. P., Logan, S. W., Rodrigues, L. P., & D'Hondt, E. (2015). Motor competence and its effect on positive developmental trajectories of health. *Sports Medicine, 45*, 1273–1284. doi: 10.1007/s40279-015-0351-6.

Runhaar, J., Collard, D. C. M., Singh, A. S., Kemper, H. C., van Mechelen, W., & Chin A Paw, M. J. M. (2010). Motor fitness in Dutch youth: Differences over a 26-year period (1980–2006). *Journal of Science and Medicine in Sport, 13*. 323–328.

Rychetnik, L., Bauman, A., Laws, R., King, L., Rissel, C., Nutbeam, D., . . . Caterson, I. (2012). Translating research for evidence-based public health: Key concepts and future directions. *Journal of Epidemiology and Community Health, 66*, 1187–1192. doi: 10.1136/jech-2011-200038.

Sallis, R. E., Matuszak, J. M., Baggish, A. L., Franklin, B. A., Chodzko-Zajko, W., Fletcher, B. J., . . . Williams, J. (2016). Call to action on making physical activity assessment and prescription a medical standard of care. *Current Sports Medicine Reports, 15*, 207–214. doi: 10.1249/JSR.0000000000000249.

Schmidt, M., Jäger, K., Egger, F., Roebers, C. M., & Conzelmann, A. (2015). Cognitively engaging chronic physical activity, but not aerobic exercise, affects executive functions in primary school children: A group-randomized controlled trial. *Journal of Sport and Exercise Psychology, 37*, 575–591. doi: 10.1123/jsep.2015-0069.

Schmidt, R. A., & Wrisberg, C. A. (2008). *Motor learning and performance*. Champaign, IL: Human Kinetics.

Seidler, R. D. (2004). Multiple motor learning experiences enhance motor adaptability. *Journal of Cognitive Neuroscience, 16*, 65–73.

Serrien, D. J., Ivry, R. B., & Swinnen, S. P. (2007). The missing link between action and cognition. *Progress in Neurobiology, 82*, 95–107. doi: 10.1016/j.pneuro bio.2007.02.003.

Shors, T. J. (2014). The adult brain makes new neurons, and effortful learning keeps them alive. *Current Directions in Psychological Science, 23*, 311–318. doi: 10.1177/0963721414540167.

Society of Health and Physical Education. (2016). *2016 Shape of the nation. Status of physical education in the USA.* http://www.shapeamerica.org/advocacy/son/2016/upload/Shape-of-the-Nation-2.

Stodden, D., Goodway, J., Langendorfer, S., Robertson, M., Rudisill, M., & Garcia, C. (2008). A developmental perspective on the role of motor skill competence in physical activity: An emergent relationship. *Quest, 60*, 290–306.

Thompson, E. (2007). *Mind in life: Biology, phenomenology, and the sciences of the mind.* Cambridge, MA: Belknap Press of Harvard University Press.

Tomporowski, P. D., Lambourne, K., & Okumura, M. S. (2011). Physical activity interventions and children's mental function: An introduction and overview. *Preventive Medicine, 52*, 3–9. doi: 10.1016j.ypmed.2011.01.028.

Tomporowski, P. D., McCullick, B. A., & Horvat, M. (2010). *Role of contextual interference and mental engagement on learning.* New York: Nova Science.

Tomporowski, P. D., McCullick, B., Pendelton, D. M., & Pesce, C. (2015). Exercise and children's cognition: The role of exercise characteristics and a place for metacognition. *Journal of Sport and Health Science, 4*, 47–55. doi: 10.1016/j.jshs.2014.09.003.

Tomporowski, P. D., McCullick, B., & Pesce, C. (2015). *Enhancing children's cognition with physical activity games.* Champaign, IL: Human Kinetics.

United Nations. (2013). *Committee on the rights of the child, general comment no. 17. The right of the child to rest, leisure, play, Recreational activities, cultural life and the arts* (Article 31). CRC/C/GC/17. New York: UN Committee on the Rights of the Child.

van der Fels, I. M., Te Wierike, S. C., Hartman, E., Elferink-Gemser, M. T., Smith, J., & Visscher, C. (2015). The relationship between motor skills and cognitive skills in 4–16 year old typically developing children: A systematic review. *Journal of Science and Medicine in Sport, 18*, 697–703. doi: 10.1016/j.jsams.2014.09.007.

van der Niet, A. G., Smith, J., Oosterlaan, J., Scherder, E. J. A., Hartman, E., & Visschera, C. (2016). Effects of a cognitively demanding aerobic intervention during recess on children's physical fitness and executive functioning. *Pediatric Exercise Science, 28*, 64–70. doi: 10.1123/pes.2015-0084.

Vandervert, L. R., Schimpf, P. H., & Liu, H. (2007). How working memory and the cerebellum collaborate to produce creativity and innovation. *Creativity Research Journal, 19*, 1–18. doi: 10.1080/10400410709336877.

Vazou, S., Pesce, C., Lakes, K., & Smiley-Owen, A. (2016). More than one road leads to Rome: A narrative review and meta-analysis of physical activity intervention effects on cognition in youth. *International Journal of Sport and Exercise Psychology.* doi: 10.1080/1612197X.2016.1223423 [Published online: 17 Sep 2016].

Vazou, S., & Smiley-Oyen, A. (2014). Moving and academic learning are not antagonists: Acute effects on executive function and enjoyment. *Journal of Sport and Exercise Psychology, 36*, 474–485. doi: 10.1123/jsep.2014-0035.

Verburgh, L., Scherder, E. J. A., van Lange, P. A., & Oosterlaan, J. (2014). Executive functioning in highly talented soccer play-ers. *PLoS One, 9*(3), e91254. doi: 10.1371/journal.pone.0091254.

Vereijken, B., & Boongardt, R. (1999). Complex motor skill acquisition. In Y. V. Auweele, F. Bakker, S. Biddle, M. Durand, & R. Selier (Eds.), *Psychology for physical educators* (first ed., pp. 233–256). Champaign, IL: Human Kinetics.

Weaver, N., Williams, J. L., Weightman, A. L., Kitcher, H. N., Temple, J. M., Jones P., & Palmer, S. (2002). Taking STOX: developing a cross disciplinary methodology for systematic reviews of research on the built environment and the health of the public. *Journal of Epidemiology and Community Health, 56*, 48–55.

Williams, A. M., & Ericsson, K. A. (2005). Perceptual-cognitive expertise in sport: Some considerations when applying the expert performance approach. *Human Movement Science, 24*, 283–307. doi: 10.1016/j.humov.2005.06.002.

World Health Organization. (1999). *Partners in life skills education. Conclusions from a United Nations inter-agency meeting.* Geneva: World Health Organization, Department of Mental Health. http://www.who.int/mental_health/media/en/30. pdf.

World Health Organization. (2010). *Global recommendations on physical activity for health.* Geneva: World Health Organization. http://www.who.int/dietphysical activity/factsheet_recommendations/en/.

World Health Organization. (2014). *Global strategy on diet, physical activity and health. Commission on Ending Childhood Obesity.* Geneva: World Health Organization. http://www.who.int/dietphysicalactivity/strategy/eb11344/strategy_ english_web.pdf.

Zahner, L., Puder, J. J., Roth, R., Schmid, M., Guldimann, R., Pühse, U., . . . Kriemler, S. (2006). A school-based physical activity program to improve health and fitness in children aged 6–13 years ("Kinder-Sportstudie KISS"): Study design of a randomized controlled trial [ISRCTN15360785]. *BMC Public Health, 6*, 147. doi: 10.1186/1471-2458-6-147.

Zani, A., & Rossi, B. (1991). Cognitive psychophysiology as an interface between cognitive and sport psychology. *International Journal of Sport and Exercise Psychology, 22*, 376–398.

Part III

Education and evaluation

A review of school-based studies on the effect of acute physical activity on cognitive function in children and young people

Andy Daly-Smith, Jim McKenna, Greta Defeyter and Andrew Manley

Introduction

Since the 1990s, a body of literature has emerged investigating the impact of single acute bouts of physical activity on cognitive function. To establish the underlying mechanisms, studies were first conducted on mice before progressing to humans in laboratory-based studies (Hillman et al., 2009). Recently, work has focused on settings with potential for establishing translational merit; testing the impact of acute bouts of physical activity delivered in schools. This research has focused on classroom exercise breaks and aerobic exercise or cognitively engaging physical activity outside of the classroom environment.

This chapter reviews literature regarding the impact of different physical activity modes on cognition within the school environment. First, a definition of cognition will be provided along with an outline of the underlying cognitive processes. Next, current issues in physical activity will be discussed with specific reference to quantifying the participant experience. Each of the three acute intervention types will be discussed in turn: *classroom exercise breaks, aerobic exercise outside of the classroom* and *cognitively engaging physical activity outside of the classroom*. The chapter concludes with a summary, drawing conclusions based on existing evidence, followed by recommendations for practice and future research.

Cognition in the 21st-century school

Cognition refers to 'a series of mental processes that contribute to perception, memory, intellect and action' (Donnelly et al., 2016, p. 1198). Within school, these processes are essential to processing new information, manipulating information in the mind and goal-directed behaviours.

It is assumed that acute exercise improves cognition through metabolic changes which occur both during and after exercise (Tomporowski, McCullick, Pendleton, & Pesce, 2015). While these effects are unlikely to endure, enhanced learning may occur through increased processing speed and/or accuracy. Demonstrating these effects very precisely will be important to galvanize the energy of teachers to promote physical activity throughout the school day. Given the scale of need in many schools today to engage 21st-century children, these issues are given even greater prominence. Prior to reviewing the current literature, it is important to understand which tasks provide a measure of each cognitive process.

Confusingly, many studies assess one aspect of cognition and will wrongly assert that exercise 'does/does not improve cognitive function'. While the majority of cognitive tasks use multiple concurrent processes rather than a single one, more precise reporting is required than within some of the individual studies summarized in the following review; this enhanced precision will aid the understanding of practitioners and researchers alike. A further limitation is that measures such as speed and accuracy only provide indirect evidence about internal cognitive processes. While they clearly demonstrate children's response to an imposed task, they do not explain how internal processes occur to facilitate learning. Despite these limitations, cognitive psychologists have developed strategies to discover the cognitive processes involved in a number of commonly used cognitive tasks.

For teachers and practitioners to understand fully the role of physical activity in cognition, it is important to express what we grasp about cognition and how physical activity might make a difference. We begin by focusing on human memory, the distinction between short-term and long-term memory, working memory and the central executive. Many prominent psychologists have argued that the central executive is the most important component of working memory. Establishing how physical activity plays a role in extending working memory will refine understanding of its relevance to 21st-century learning.

Baddeley and Hitch (1974) argued that short-term memory is essential to performance on a number of complex tasks that are not explicitly memory tasks. A good example is that of mental mathematics. Mentally adding a string of numbers together requires that each addition results in a new total that must be remembered to generate the next number. This process continues to establish the final answer. Based on this thinking, Baddeley and Hitch (1974) replaced the concept of short-term memory with that of working memory. This is essential for any young person to thrive in contemporary learning environments.

As an example of the complexity in this area, their latest memory model has four components: a central executive; a phonological loop; a visuospatial sketchpad; and an episodic buffer (Baddeley, 2012). With four distinctive areas this gives an indication of the many ways in which physical activity might play a role in enhancing cognition in young people. The central executive itself does not store information, but acts as an 'attentional system' and is a vital component in nearly all complex cognitive activities commonly faced by children in the classroom, including multitasking and problem solving. The phonological loop processes and temporarily stores information in a phonological form, which may be a challenge for schools with high linguistic diversity. The visuospatial sketchpad processes and temporarily stores spatial and visual information, which may have relevance for children who lack spatial awareness. Finally, information from the phonological loop and the visuospatial sketchpad is stored in the episodic buffer. Clearly anything that expands the episodic buffer will benefit learning.

Even though the central executive has been claimed by many to be the most important, it does not store information; rather it resembles an attentional system. Baddeley (2012) acknowledged that the central executive is associated with a number of executive processes: focusing attention, dividing attention, switching attention and interfacing with long-term memory are examples. To date there is no overall consensus amongst scientists on the number of executive processes. While there is no agreement, it is important to understand the processes that play a role in completing the tasks that are used to indicate cognitive performance.

Expanding one framework from among many provides an insight into learning in humans. Within the framework of Miyake et al. (2000), the term 'executive function' is used to account for what is common to the three functions they identified: inhibition, shifting and updating. Typically, inhibition is used to resist distraction, a familiar problem for many pupils. An excellent example of use of this function is in the well-known Stroop task in which, rather than name a colour word, people have to name the colour in which it is printed. This is easy when the colour name and the colour of the ink are congruent (e.g. RED printed in red) as no inhibition is required. However, in cases where the dominant response needs to be inhibited (e.g. the word RED printed in yellow), it is far more difficult. The shifting function is used to switch attention between tasks often seen within classroom lessons. Common assessment of shifting includes the more-odd task or modified flanker test (Chen, Yan, Yin, Pan, & Chang, 2014; Jäger, Schmidt, Conzelmann, & Roebers, 2015). Updating, as usually measured by n-back tests, monitors rapid addition or deletion of working-memory contents (Jäger, Schmidt, Conzelmann, & Roebers, 2014, 2015).

While working memory is important, the role of long-term memory in storing information is equally important. This schematic knowledge is extensively used during language comprehension, for example, when a pupil attempts to follow instructions provided by physical education (PE) teachers. Although there are some similarities between episodic and semantic memory, it is generally accepted that they form separate memory systems, giving rise to speculation about specific physical activity effects. Recognition and recall are commonly used to assess episodic memory. Recognition memory is often tested by presenting a list of words or pictures and then later presenting the same stimuli alongside distractor items and simply asking participants if they have seen the item before. Typically, pictures are remembered better than words – the so-called 'picture superiority effect' (Defeyter, Russo, & McPartlin, 2009). There are three forms of recall memory test: serial recall, free recall and cued recall. Better understanding of the nuances of working and long-term memory and how physical activity plays a role in affecting these processes will be important for teachers preparing pupils for assessment and exams.

Another example of a title that has many facets is attention. This is a well-researched area due to its importance in everyday life and prediction of school achievement (Steinmayr, Ziegler, & Träuble, 2010). Although attention is cross-modal, the majority of researchers have examined the effects of physical activity on visual attention. Posner (1980) proposes visual attention acts as a spotlight, while others have suggested a more flexible approach using the analogy of a zoom lens (Eriksen & St James, 1986). A third, and less well-supported, approach uses the analogy of multiple spotlights, where attention can be split between two or more regions of space not adjacent to each other (Awh & Pashler, 2000). Essential to learning, visual attention enables an individual to process information while resisting distractors within a single task or across multiple tasks.

In the cognitive psychology literature, it is important to distinguish between selective – or focused – attention, divided attention, sustained attention and mental shifting. Selective attention, as measured by the d2 test of attention (Schmidt, Egger, & Conzelmann, 2015), is the most assessed cognitive process within studies investigating the impact of acute physical activity on cognition. Within the test, participants are required to highlight correct letters presented among a string of distractors. In divided-attention tasks, participants are also presented two or more stimuli at the same time, responding to all of the stimuli – rather like multitasking in everyday life. The distinction between selective and divided-attention tasks is important as the former provides information on the nature of the selection process and the role of distractors, while the latter provides information about processing capacity and limitations. Sustained attention refers to the ability to maintain attention and respond consistently to a stimulus during a repetitive or continuous activity. Finally, altering attention or mental shifting is the process of shifting attention from one task to another as required.

In addition to being able to attend to stimuli in the external world, it is important for humans to be able to plan efficiently. Planning, a higher-order executive function, refers to the formation and management of goal-directed behaviour (Diamond, 2013). An essential facet of educational achievement, planning supports organizing a study timetable or the management and completion of school projects. Currently, only a limited number of studies have investigated the impact of acute physical activity on planning within the school environment, providing opportunity for further investigation. Common tests to assess planning function include the Trail-Making Test and the dot task (Kubesch et al., 2009; Pirrie & Lodewyk, 2012).

Summary

The core thread of this chapter is that, while it is inappropriate to use a single label for cognitive processes that have multiple dimensions, it is equally inappropriate to use single tests to represent whole systems as complex as cognition. Researchers need to be cautious of attributing performance on cognitive tasks to one specific cognitive process and carefully consider the effect of cognitive load. Furthermore, researchers also need to ensure that cognitive tasks use age-appropriate stimuli and instructions, and that chronological age groups are theoretically underpinned in the cognitive developmental literature, rather than being based purely on opportunistic sampling. Further research is required to examine the effects of moderate-to-vigorous physical activity (MVPA) on a wider range of cognitive processes. While the above section has focused on linking cognition to the school environment and the role teachers may play in supporting this, parents and sports coaches also need to be aware of the role of cognition in the development of children and young people, enabling them to reach their potential.

Acute study physical activity considerations

A recent systematic review (Donnelly et al., 2016) found that single bouts of physical activity positively impact children's cognitive performance. Closer inspection of the contributing studies and subsequent literature makes our interpretation more cautious. Prior to reviewing the contribution of each study, it is essential to present a physical activity framework within which the school-based literature can be analysed and more clearly understood. When designing a single bout of physical activity, many authors refer to the quantitative and qualitative aspects of exercise (Pesce, 2012).

Distinctive from the incidental activity associated with 'physical activity', 'quantitative exercise' is the subset of activity that is planned, structured and repetitive (Shephard & Balady, 1999). Using the American College of Sports Medicine (ACSM) FITT-VP principle (frequency, intensity, time and type – volume and progression), this focuses on the intensity and time (duration of bout). Exercise mode requires minimal skill, focusing on rhythmic movement such as walking, jogging, running or aerobic circuits. As the activity requires minimal skill, participants are able to focus on maintaining the prescribed intensity, often moderate to vigorous in nature (ACSM, 2014). Examples of this approach within the research include steady-state jogging (Chen et al., 2014), dance videos (Altenburg, Chinapaw, & Singh, 2016) and aerobic circuits (Gallotta et al., 2015).

In recent years, researchers have developed interventions to assess the impact of cognitively enhanced physical activity on cognition (Budde, Voelcker-Rehage, Pietrabyk-Kendziorra, Ribeiro, & Tidow, 2008; Jäger et al., 2015; Schmidt et al., 2015). Termed 'qualitative exercise' (Pesce, 2012), this involves physical activities that also impose cognitive demands on individuals. Cognitive load is achieved through a range of modes. Recent studies by Jäger and colleagues (2014, 2015) used cognitively enhanced games focused on activating one or more executive processes. Alternatively, Gallotta et al. (2015) used activities which combined gross motor, manipulative control and perceptual motor adaptation abilities.

Such varied approaches produce two challenges in interpreting study outcomes. First, the cognitive demands of such activities may not be clear (Furley & Wood, 2016). Currently with no body of literature that details how activities link to different cognitive processes, it is difficult to interpret the specific cognitive impact. Second, while the focus of qualitative exercise sessions may be to engage young people in cognitively demanding physical activity, there are still quantitative outcomes such as duration and intensity to address. To confirm the qualitative effects, a comparator quantitative experience, equal in duration and intensity, might be included within studies. To date, few investigations have deployed this design (Budde et al., 2008; Jäger et al., 2015).

Comparing the different studies gives rise to a final challenge. In laboratory studies, researchers using steady-state exercise assess treatment fidelity through heart rate (HR), often presented as group means (Hillman et al., 2009). This approach has been transferred, seemingly unquestioningly, to studies within school environments. Due to the intermittent nature of young people's physical activity experiences, this poses challenges for interpreting the quantitative demands of the session (Bailey et al., 1995). First, HR has a delayed response to changes in the mechanical demands of exercise (Rowlands & Eston, 2007). Second, during game-based sessions, exercise is often intermittent in nature with a high degree of interindividual variation. The result is that two individuals may engage very differently within the same acute bout. Within translational physical activity research with children and young people, accelerometers are increasingly regarded as the gold-standard assessment tool, providing accurate interpretation of activity patterns, intensity and duration (Corder, Ekelund, Steele, Wareham, & Brage, 2008).

Figure 15.1 shows physical activity profiles, collected through accelerometry, of two different children taking part in the same game-based PE session. On average, the two individuals accumulated 11 minutes of MVPA. Closer inspection of the physical activity traces shows a high degree of variability between the two individuals regarding total time engaged in moderate intensity or above. A recent meta-analysis found that a minimum engagement of 11 minutes at moderate intensity resulted in significant improvements in cognitive engagement (Chang, Labban, Gapin, & Etnier, 2012). In Figure 15.1, child A achieved 5 minutes of MVPA, while child B achieved 17 minutes. Monitoring this individual variability and then factoring this into the statistical analyses is fundamental to developing a precise understanding of how acute physical activity bouts impact on cognition.

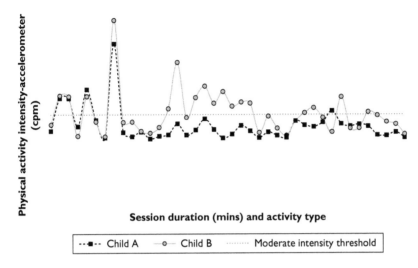

Figure 15.1 Accelerometer-determined physical activity profiles of two participants (high active and low active) within a physically active games session.

Warm-up: participants follow coned path, walking, jogging and running, followed by stretching. **Four corners:** participants were divided into four teams of three or four. Each team had one hoop in the corner of the playing area; a central hoop contained beanbags. Participants ran to the centre hoop, one at a time, collected a beanbag and returned it to their hoop. The game was progressed by allowing participants to raid other teams' hoops to take beanbags. **Active story:** participants sat in a large circle and received a number from one to five. When a number was called in the story, participants stood up, ran around the circle and returned to their place. **Cool down:** participants performed a range of static stretches.

It is also important to consider the type of activity, as indicated along the *x*-axis within Figure 15.1, when analysing and interpreting such statistical data. During the first activity that focused on steady-state walking, jogging and running, the intensity and duration profiles are similar. Within the second activity, a team game, there is high individual variability in both the duration and the intensity of the exercise. In the final activity, an active story, a large degree of variability in activity duration and intensity is again observed. Within the review which follows, identification of the physical activity profiles and corresponding modes of activity will provide an opportunity to evaluate the trustworthiness of study outcomes.

Summary

In summary, the current literature can divide studies into quantitative and qualitative exercise. Quantitative exercise focuses on predetermined intensity and duration and is often moderate to vigorous in nature. Qualitative physical activity has a direct or indirect cognitive requirement; often this arises from the activity being specifically designed to include cognitive challenges, and may include playing sport or learning new skills. The following sections will review current literature on acute bouts of physical activity within the school environment, discussing the potential consequences of the issues raised on the cognitive outcomes.

Review of the literature

To identify relevant articles, a two-step search strategy was used. First, a search of relevant databases (SPORTDiscus and PubMed) was undertaken. Second, a manual search of the reference lists of all included papers was completed. Studies were included if they met the following criteria: (1) the study was conducted within the school environment with children or young people (<17 years of age); (2) an acute bout of physical activity was compared to a control condition; and (3) one or more cognitive assessments were performed. The temporal threshold for including papers in this review was 2006, producing 20 studies over a particularly important decade of new work. This was justified by finding the first important study in 2008 followed by a mushrooming of work to the present day. These 20 studies were then divided into three subcategories: (1) classroom-based exercise breaks (CEB); (2) aerobic exercise outside of the classroom; and (3) cognitively enhanced physical activity outside of the classroom (CEPA-OC). A number of studies appeared in more than one subcategory due to multiple treatment interventions.

In the following subsections, for the physical activity and cognitive tests, we refer readers to the original source for the description and validity of the respective methods.

Classroom-based exercise breaks

Summarizing Table 15.1

Four peer-reviewed papers were identified that examined the impact of an acute classroom exercise break on cognition (Table 15.1, studies 1–4). Across the four papers, sample size varied from 88 (Ma, Le Mare, & Gurd, 2015) to 1,224 (Hill et al., 2010), with a mean of 368 participants (girls = 52%) per study. All studies focused on children aged 8–13 years old. Two studies were conducted in Europe (the Netherlands and UK), one in the USA and one in Canada. This highlights a lack of replication of studies within the same school systems.

Across the four studies, of ten cognitive assessment outcomes – compared to controls – there were two positive, five no difference and three mixed outcomes. There were no negative outcomes. The two positive outcomes were observed when testing protocols did not control for day-to-day variation

Table 15.1 Descriptive analysis of studies examining acute classroom-based movement breaks on cognition

Study, country, age, design	Physical activity bout	Control	Duration/intensity	Cognition test time
(1) van den Berg et al. (2016) Netherlands, age: 10–13 years, RCrT	12 minutes, whole class: aerobic exercise with easy repetitive movements ($n = 66$, girls = 47%)	12 minutes, whole class: sedentary lesson on exercise and movement ($n = 66$, girls = 47%)	HR assessed: of the main body, 10 minutes, 39.5% (3.95 minutes) in MVPA (64–94% HRmax)	Pre Post @ 0 minutes
	12 minutes, whole class: coordination exercise with complex bilateral and movements crossing midline ($n = 71$, girls = 44%)	12 minutes, whole class: sedentary lesson on exercise and movement ($n = 71$, girls = 44%)	HR assessed: of the main body, 10 minutes, 14.1% (1.41 minutes) in MVPA (64–94% HRmax)	Pre Post @ 0 minutes
	12 minutes, whole class: strength-based dynamic and static body weight exercises ($n = 47$, girls = 49%)	12 minutes, whole class: sedentary lesson on exercise and movement ($n = 47$, girls = 49%)	HR assessed: of the main body, 10 minutes, 18.1% (1.81 minutes) in MVPA (64–94% HR_{max})	Pre Post @ 0 minutes
(2) Howie et al. (2015) USA, age: 9–12 years, RCrT (Latin square)	5 minutes, whole class: Brain Bites aerobic exercise involving marching, jumping and running on the spot @ MVPA intensity, 150 bpm ($n = 96$, girls = 65%)	10 minutes, whole class: sedentary lesson on exercise science ($n = 96$, girls = 65%)	SOFIT assessed: average PA intensity 4 out of 5	Pre Post unreported
	10 minutes, whole class: Brain Bites aerobic exercise involving marching, jumping and running on the spot @ MVPA intensity, 150 bpm ($n = 96$, girls = 65%)	10 minutes, whole class: sedentary lesson on exercise science ($n = 96$, girls = 65%)	SOFIT assessed: average PA intensity 4.35 out of 5	Pre Post unreported

(continued)

Table 15.1 (continued)

Study, country, age, design	Physical activity bout	Control	Duration/intensity	Cognition test time
	20 minutes, whole class: Brain Bites aerobic exercise involving marching, jumping and running on the spot @ MVPA intensity, 150 bpm (n = 96, girls =65%)	10 minutes, whole class: sedentary lesson on exercise science (n = 96, girls = 65%)	SOFIT assessed: average PA intensity 4.26 out of 5	Pre Post unreported
(3) Ma et al. (2015) Canada, age: 8–11 years, RCrT	10 minutes (4 minutes of activity), whole class: FUNterval aerobic exercise involving jumping jacks, scissor kicks, jumping and running on the spot. High-intensity intervals: 20 seconds exercise, 10 seconds rest (n = 88, girls = 50%)	10 minutes, whole class: sedentary lesson on kinesiology (n = 88, girls = 50%)	No assessment	No pre Post @ 10 minutes
(4) Hill et al. (2010) UK, age: 8–11 years, RCrT	10–15 minutes, whole class: 'classroom exercise programme' aerobic exercise involving stretching, running and hopping on the spot to music @ MPA intensity (n = 1224, no gender data)	10–15 minutes, whole class: normal classroom session (n = 1224, no gender data)	Teacher reported students out of breath and starting to perspire	No pre Post @ 60 minutes

RCrT, randomized cross-over trial; HR, heart rate; HR$_{max}$, maximum heart rate; MVPA, moderate-to-vigorous physical activity; MPA, moderate-intensity physical activity; PA, physical activity; SOFIT, System for Observing Fitness Instruction Time.

in cognition; this would be furnished by including pre-intervention measures (Hill et al., 2010; Ma et al., 2015). More recent studies using pre–post
designs concluded no change in cognition. Treatment fidelity was difficult
to ascertain; no studies accounted for variability of individual engagement
within the session. Two studies reported group-level engagement: one
via HR (van den Berg et al., 2016) and the other through direct observation using System for Observing Fitness Instruction Time (SOFIT: Howie,
Schatz, & Pate, 2015). Two studies provided no assessment of the resulting
duration and intensity of the exercise (Hill et al., 2010; Ma et al., 2015).
Superficially, the strength of evidence suggests CEBs do not lead to improvements in cognition, but there are important issues with treatment fidelity.
Current CEB study designs may not elicit sufficient exposure to MVPA to
generate improvements in cognition; papers often claim higher exposure
than was confirmed by evidence of engagement.

Detail emerging from Table 15.1

Exercise breaks within the classroom (CEB) have varied in duration from 4
(Ma et al., 2015) to 20 minutes (Howie et al., 2015). Activities focused on
aerobic – on-the-spot – activity involving marching with arm movements,
jogging, running, jumping and hopping. The activities seem to be quantitative
in nature, simple and repetitive with a low cognitive load (Pesce, 2012). Only
one study expanded beyond an aerobic focus to look at three different intervention types: aerobic, strength and coordination (van den Berg et al., 2016).

   Selective attention was the most commonly assessed cognitive process, followed by information processing, working memory and planning. Assessed
across three studies, selective attention showed positive change (Hill et al.,
2010), no change (van den Berg et al., 2016) and mixed results (Ma et al., 2015).
Following a 10–15-minute CEB, Hill et al. (2010) assessed selective attention
using the digit symbol-coding task, finding improvements in the second week
of testing. In contrast, van den Berg et al. (2016) found no change in overall
selective attention (assessed by the d2 test) following three separate 12-minute
bouts of exercise. In comparison, Ma et al. (2015) reported that 4 minutes of
high-intensity interval exercise improved accuracy on the d2 test, although the
total number of items processed by participants decreased. Unfortunately, no
data were presented to account for the speed–accuracy trade-off, which limits
our ability to make direct comparisons. The two studies which assessed information processing found no change in speed or accuracy immediately after
physical activity (van den Berg et al., 2016) or after a 60-minute delay (Hill
et al., 2010), as measured by the letter digit substitution test and the paced
serial addition task, respectively.

   Working memory – assessed immediately after a 5-, 10- or 20-minute
CEB – showed no change when assessed by the digit recall test (Howie et al.,
2015). Further, in Hill et al. (2010), after a 60-minute delay postexercise,

no improvements were observed in a size-ordering task. In the same study, positive improvements were observed in the listening span and digit span backwards tests. Only Howie et al. (2015) assessed planning ability using the Trail-Making Task; no change was observed in performance between conditions.

In summary, recent studies have demonstrated some improvements in cognition in association with CEB, principally in selective attention. Some of these effects have been observed immediately postexercise and after extended delays. The majority of evidence shows no change, meaning we should currently be cautiously optimistic about the benefits of such active breaks. One reason for optimism stems from our understanding of CEB. While the prescribed duration and intensity of the breaks are *theoretically* sufficient to lead to changes in cognition, more evidence needs to be presented to confirm the treatment fidelity of the intervention, especially given that laboratory-based studies dominate this area. The only study to confirm engagement showed that children were active for 40% or less of the session duration (van den Berg et al., 2016). Future studies must confirm exposure to the active components of CEBs using more accurate methods. In addition, a wider array of cognitive domains should be examined. So far, no studies have assessed inhibition, updating, shifting, reaction time or recall.

Aerobic exercise outside of the classroom

Summarizing Table 15.2

Thirteen peer-reviewed papers examined the impact of an acute bout of aerobic activity outside of the classroom on cognition (Table 15.2, studies 5–17). Across the 13 papers, sample size varied from 33 (Etnier, Labban, Piepmeier, Davis, & Henning, 2014) to 234 (Jäger et al., 2015), with a mean of 93 participants (girls = 50%) per study. All studies focused on children aged 8–14 years. Ten studies were conducted in Europe: three in Italy (Gallotta et al., 2012, 2015; Pesce, Crova, Cereatti, Casella, & Bellucci, 2009), two in the Netherlands (Altenburg et al., 2016; Janssen et al., 2014), two in Germany (Kubesch et al., 2009; Niemann et al., 2013), two in the UK (Cooper, Bandelow, Nute, Morris, & Nevill, 2012; Pirrie & Lodewyk, 2012) and one in Switzerland (Jäger et al., 2015). Of the remaining studies, two were conducted in the USA (Etnier et al., 2014; Tine & Butler, 2012) and one in China (Chen et al., 2014).

Across the studies, of 39 cognitive assessment outcomes there were seven positive, 23 no difference, nine mixed and zero negative when comparing aerobic exercise outside of the classroom to control conditions. Seven studies, the majority, assessed treatment fidelity at the group level, presenting mean HR data and/or the percentage of time spent in activity thresholds (Chen et al., 2014; Cooper et al., 2012; Gallotta et al., 2012, 2015;

Table 15.2 Descriptive analysis of studies examining an acute bout of aerobic exercise outside of the classroom environment on cognition.

Study, country, age, design	Physical activity bout	Control	Duration/intensity	Cognition test time
(5) Jäger et al. (2015), Switzerland, 10–12 years, RCT	20 minutes, groups of 4: games requiring running (n = 62, girls = 45%)	20 minutes, groups of 4: seated cognitively engaging card game, average HR 94.52 ± 8.71 bpm (n = 60, girls = 50%) 20 minutes, groups of 4: seated story and questions, average HR 81.93 ± 10.13 bpm (n = 58, girls = 57%)	HR assessed: average 150.76 ± 15.14 bpm	Pre Post @ 0 minutes
(6) Gallotta et al. (2015), Italy, 8–11 years, RCT	50 minutes, whole class; aerobic exercise circuit involving continuous walking, running and skipping @ HR >139 bpm (n = 31, no gender data)	50 minutes, whole class: seated lesson on humanistic subject (n = 39, no gender data)	HR assessed: during main component of 30 minutes, average 146.56 ± 14.09 bpm	Pre Post @ 0 minutes Post @ 50 minutes
(7) Altenburg et al. (2016), Netherlands, 10–13 years, RCT	20 minutes, whole group: aerobic dance video at beginning (C1) and halfway (C2) through morning @ MPA intensity, 40–60% HR (n = 20, girls = 45%)	20 minutes, whole group: simulated school tasks (A + B) (n = 36, girls = 47%) (T0–T2) 200 minutes, whole group: simulated school tasks (A) (n = 19, girls = 63%) (T0–T4)	No analysis, researchers checked HR monitors during session to encourage MPA, non-compliers removed from analysis	Pre (T0) Post @ 90 minutes (T2) Post @ 200 minutes (T4)
(8) Janssen et al. (2014), Netherlands, 10–11 years, RCrT	15 minutes, whole class: aerobic exercise involving walking, jogging, dribbling and passing football @ MPA intensity (n = 123, girls = 50%)	15 minutes, whole class: no break, continued classroom lesson (n = 123, girls = 50%) 15 minutes, whole class: break in provision for seated story time (n = 123, girls = 50%)	Accelerometers assessed: MPA intensity @ 2000 cpm. Participants with <12 minutes excluded from analysis	Pre Post unreported (immediate)

(continued)

Table 15.2 (continued)

Study, country, age, design	Physical activity bout	Control	Duration/intensity	Cognition test time
	15 minutes, whole class: aerobic exercise involving running jumping and skipping @ VPA intensity ($n = 123$, girls = 50%)	15 minutes, whole class: no break, continued classroom lesson ($n = 123$, girls = 50%) 15 minutes, whole class: break in provision for seated story time ($n = 123$, girls = 50%)	Accelerometers assessed: MPA intensity @ 3000 cpm. Participants with <12 minutes excluded from analysis	Pre Post unreported (immediate)
(9) Etnier et al. (2014), USA, 11–12 years, RCT	7 minutes 2 seconds–13 minutes 46 seconds, whole class: jogging warm up followed by PACER maximal aerobic exercise test ($n = 19$, no gender data)	No detail on control condition prior to completing the memory test ($n = 24$, no gender data)	No assessment	No pre Post @ 0 minutes
(10) Chen et al. (2014), China, 8–11 years, RCT	30 minutes, whole class: steady-state jogging @ 60–70% of HR_{max} ($n = 44$, girls = 48%)	30 minutes, whole class: seated independent reading task ($n = 39$, girls = 54%)	HR assessed: third grade, average 64.29% HR_{max}, fifth grade: average 64.40% HR_{max}	Pre Post @ 20–25 minutes
(11) Niemann et al. (2013), Germany, 9–10 years, RCT	12 minutes, whole group: steady-state running @ 85–90% of HR_{max}, 180–190 bpm ($n = 21$, girls = 48%)	12 minutes, whole group: seated watching *Happy Feet* video ($n = 21$, girls = 47%)	No assessment, during session HR monitor feedback to participant	Pre Post @ 5 minutes
(12) Tine and Butler (2012), USA, 10–13 years, RCT	12 minutes, whole class; steady-state running @ 70–80% of HR_{max} ($n = 86$, girls = 53%)	12 minutes, whole class: seated watching video on exercise ($n = 78$, girls = 51%)	No assessment, Participants not achieving set intensity in session, data withdrawn	Pre Post @ 1 minute
(13) Pirrie and Lodewyk (2012), UK, 9–10 years, within subjects	60 minutes, whole class: Heart Smart PE lesson focused on active games using activities including hopping and running @ MVPA intensity for minimum of 20 minutes ($n = 40$, girls = 45%)	60 minutes, whole class: seated classroom reading ($n = 40$, girls = 45%)	HR assessed: range 27.89–31.0 minutes in MVPA	No pre Post varied 10, 25 or 40 minutes

Study	Intervention	Comparison/control	HR assessment	Timing
(14) Gallotta et al. (2012), Italy, 8–11 years, RCrT	50 minutes, whole class: aerobic exercise circuit involving continuous walking, running and skipping @ HR >139 bpm (n = 138, no gender data)	50 minutes, whole class: seated classroom lesson on humanistic subject (n = 138, no gender data)	HR assessed: average 146.56 ± 14.09 bpm	Pre Post @ 0 minutes
(15) Cooper et al. (2012), UK, 12–13 years, RCrT	10 minutes, whole group: aerobic shuttle runs @ 8 kph, 10 sets, 7 reps, 20 metres distance, 30 seconds rest between sets (n = 45, girls = 67%)	No detail. Presume normal school morning (n = 45, girls = 67%)	HR assessed: average 172 ± 17bpm	Pre Post @ 45–60 minutes
(16) Pesce et al. (2009), Italy, 11–12 years, within subjects counterbalanced order	38 minutes, whole class: aerobic circuit. no interaction with peers (n = 52, no gender data)	No control condition, baseline control test undertaken at start of school day (n = 52, no gender data)	HR assessed: average 146 ± 19bpm, 54.2% of lesson in MVPA, 20.6 minutes	No pre Post @ 5–8 minutes
(17) Kubesch et al. (2009), Germany, 13–14 years, RCrT	30 minutes, whole class: continuous running and jumping over benches followed by core exercises (n = 45, girls = 42%)	30 minutes, whole class: seated listening to audio book (n = 45, girls = 42%)	No assessment	Pre Post @ 0 minutes Post after following lesson
	5 minutes, whole class: 'virtual Berlin Marathon' running on the spot with integrated movements (n = 36, girls = 42%)	5 minutes, whole class: watched virtual Berlin Marathon session (n = 36, girls = 42%)	No assessment	Pre Post @ 0 minutes Post after following lesson

RCT, randomized controlled trial; RCrT, randomized crossover trial; HR, heart rate; HR_{max}, maximum heart rate; MVPA, moderate-to-vigorous physical activity; MPA, moderate-intensity physical activity; PE, physical education; VPA, vigorous-intensity physical activity; PACER, progressive aerobic cardiovascular endurance run.

Jäger et al., 2015; Pesce et al., 2009; Pirrie and Lodewyk, 2012). Two studies did not record the intensity and/or duration of the physical activity bout (Etnier et al., 2014; Kubesch et al., 2009). Three studies attempted to control for individual variation in engagement during the acute bout: one provided feedback through HR monitors to participants during the bout (Niemann et al., 2013) and two withdrew participants from their analysis who did not meet the required HR intensity (Altenburg et al., 2016; Tine & Butler, 2012). The final study assessed engagement through accelerometry. Participants who accumulated <12 minutes MVPA were withdrawn from the analysis, ensuring treatment fidelity at the individual level (Janssen et al., 2014). A range of activities were used to elicit a moderate-to-high intensity; examples included: running games (Jäger et al., 2015), steady-state jogging (Chen et al., 2014), maximal tests (Etnier et al., 2014), dance videos (Altenburg et al., 2016) and aerobic circuits (Gallotta et al., 2015; Pesce et al., 2009).

Detail emerging from Table 15.2

A range of cognitive domains were tested directly after the exercise bout, the most common being inhibitory control and selective attention. Beginning with inhibitory control, two studies reported conflicting results. After a 30-minute PE session on aerobic exercise, Kubesch et al. (2009) revealed a significant improvement in immediate inhibitory control performance assessed by the flanker test, but not when assessed by the dots test. In contrast, Jäger et al. (2015) reported no change in immediate flanker test performance after 20 minutes of running games, regardless of fitness level or academic ability. Studies which delayed the postexercise test found differing results. Ten minutes after the session, no change was found in inhibitory control assessed by the Stroop test after a heart-smart aerobically focused PE lesson (Pirrie & Lodewyk, 2012). After 25 minutes, following 30 minutes of continual jogging, an improvement in inhibitory control processing speed was found on a flanker test (Chen et al., 2014). An extended delay of 45 minutes or more found no difference in scores between aerobic shuttle runs and an aerobic exercise group compared to sedentary control conditions (Cooper et al., 2012; Kubesch et al., 2009). In summary, improvements in inhibition following aerobic exercise are mixed, some suggesting increased performance and others no difference.

A similar pattern emerges for selective attention. Twelve minutes of high-intensity running (Niemann et al., 2013; Tine & Butler, 2012) and 15 minutes of moderate, but not vigorous, aerobic activity (Janssen et al., 2014) improved immediate selective attention on the d2 and sky search tests respectively. Yet, contrary to these observed improvements, a 50-minute aerobic circuit elicited no change in immediate performance on the d2 test (Gallotta et al., 2015). Two studies assessed selective attention after an extended delay following the acute bout. Gallotta et al. (2015) assessed selective attention again following a 50-minute delay. Overall improvement did not differ from that of control conditions, yet the percentage error rate increased slightly, suggesting a reduction in performance following this extended delay. In contrast, after two repeat 20-minute bouts of exercise conducted during a simulated school morning, sky search test performance was highest in the intervention group at 90 and 200 minutes postexercise (Altenburg et al., 2016). This suggests that acute exercise repeated across a school morning can improve selective attention of children when placed between learning activities.

Further cognitive processes have been investigated in relation to acute aerobic exercise. Working memory assessed through the n-back test (Chen et al., 2014) and Sternberg test (Cooper et al., 2012) found improvements in processing speed after delays of 25 and 45 minutes, respectively. The exercise mode, intensity and duration varied greatly from 30 minutes of continuous jogging (Chen et al., 2014) to 10 minutes of repeated shuttle running (Cooper et al., 2012), suggesting that exercise volume (duration × intensity) may play a role in promoting cognitive benefits. This same study also investigated the impact of exercise on shifting, assessed by a more-odd task, finding that processing speed improved with no differences in accuracy. The only other study to investigate changes to shifting found no significant changes on a modified flanker test (Jäger et al., 2015). Two studies have investigated the effects of acute aerobic exercise on the higher-order executive function, planning. Both studies used an aerobically focused PE lesson, where a 60-minute lesson led to increased performance on the Trail-Making Test (Pirrie & Lodewyk, 2012), while a 30-minute lesson showed no change in performance either immediately after exercise or after the following maths lesson on the dots task (Kubesch et al., 2009). In summary, there is emerging evidence to support the positive impact of acute exercise on working memory. Currently, the findings for shifting and planning are equivocal, and warrant further investigation.

A small number of studies have investigated wider cognitive abilities, including information processing, reaction time and immediate/delayed recall. For instance, Cooper et al. (2012) reported that information-processing speed improved 45 minutes after completing a 10-minute bout of shuttle running, although a significant reduction in accuracy was observed, suggesting a speed–accuracy trade-off. Kubesch et al. (2009) recorded no changes in reaction time, assessed by the dots task, immediately after exercise and following an extended delay.

For immediate recall, conflicting results have been found. Pirrie and Lodewyk (2012) observed no improvements in a sentence repetition test following aerobic exercises. In contrast, Pesce et al. (2009) found improvements in primary and recency effects but not overall performance on an immediate free-recall memory test. Following a 12-minute discussion, delayed recall was then assessed. Significant improvements were observed in recency effects but not primary or overall effects. Similarly, Etnier et al. (2014) reported a significant improvement in immediate Rey Auditory Verbal Learning Test (RAVALT) performance following a progressive aerobic cardiovascular endurance run (PACER) test. These improvements were maintained in delayed recall 12 minutes after the initial test, but not 24 hours later.

Cognitively enhanced physical activity outside of the classroom

Summarizing Table 15.3

Seven peer-reviewed papers examined the impact of an acute bout of CEPA-OC on cognition (Table 15.3, studies 5, 6, 14, 16, 18–20). Sample size varied from 52 (Pesce et al., 2009) to 234 (Jäger et al., 2015), with a mean of 115 participants (girls = 46%) per study. Participants within these studies were predominantly aged 8–12 years (Gallotta et al., 2012, 2015; Jäger et al., 2015; Pesce et al., 2009; Schmidt et al., 2015), although one study included younger children aged 6–8 years (Jäger et al., 2014), and another young people aged 15 years (Budde et al., 2008). All studies were conducted in Europe: three in Switzerland (Jäger et al., 2014, 2015; Schmidt et al., 2015), three in Italy (Gallotta et al., 2012, 2015; Pesce et al., 2009) and one in Germany (Budde et al., 2008).

Across the seven studies, of 17 cognitive assessment outcomes – compared to controls – two were positive, nine showed no difference, one was negative and five mixed. Treatment fidelity was difficult to ascertain: studies only reported mean group HRs, meaning that full engagement of each participant could not be confirmed. Furthermore, the duration of the bouts varied widely; short sessions lasted <10 minutes (Budde et al., 2008) while other sessions lasted up to 50 minutes (Gallotta et al., 2012, 2015). In addition, the type of cognitively engaging physical activity varied widely, with examples including bilateral coordinate exercises (Budde et al., 2008), cooperative and competitive games requiring executive function (Jäger et al., 2014, 2015), team games (Pesce et al., 2009), cognitively demanding exercise circuits (Schmidt et al., 2015) and movement-based problem-solving and decision-making tasks (Gallotta et al., 2012, 2015). Given all these factors, all related interpretations and conclusions require due caution.

Detail emerging from Table 15.3

Selective attention, consistently assessed by the d2 test, was the most commonly examined cognitive process. The first study in the field assessed the impact of bilateral coordinate exercise on selective attention (Budde et al., 2008). Findings showed that, compared to a moderately active control, speed

Table 15.3 Descriptive analysis of studies examining an acute bout of cognitively enhanced physical activity outside of the classroom environment on cognition

Study, country, age, design	Physical activity bout	Control	Duration/intensity	Cognition test time
(18) Schmidt et al. (2015), Switzerland, age, 11 ± 0.6 years, RCT	45 minutes, whole class: cognitively demanding coordinate exercise circuit (n = 48, girls = 54%);	45 minutes, whole class: seated language session in mother tongue (n = 42, girls = 55%);	No assessment	Pre Post @ 0 minutes Post @ 90 minutes
(5) Jäger et al. (2015), Switzerland, age, 10–12 years, RCT	20 minutes, groups of four: cooperative and competitive games requiring executive function (n = 54, girls = 65%)	20 minutes, groups of four: seated cognitively engaging card game. Average HR 94.52 ± 8.71 bpm (n = 60, girls = 50%); 20 minutes, groups of four: seated story and questions. Average HR 81.93 ± 10.13 bpm (n = 58, girls = 57%)	HR assessed: average 147.79 ± 17.62 bpm	Pre Post @ 0 minutes
(6) Gallotta et al. (2015), Italy, age 8–11 years, RCT	50 minutes; whole class: movement-based problem solving using basketballs @ HR >139 bpm (n = 46, no gender data)	50 minutes, whole class: seated lesson on humanistic subject (n = 39, no gender data)	HR assessed: during main component of 30 minutes, average 147.25 ± 15.50 bpm	Pre Post @ 0 minutes Post @ 50 minutes
(19) Jäger et al. (2014), Switzerland, age 6–8 years, RCT	20 minutes, groups of four: cooperative and competitive games requiring executive function (n = 51, girls = 53%)	20 minutes, groups of four: seated story and questions. Average HR 89.66 ± 9.33 bpm (n = 53, girls = 57%)	HR assessed: average 156.6 ± 14.09 bpm	Pre Post @ 0 minutes Post @ 40 minutes
(14) Gallotta et al. (2012), Italy, age 8–11 years, RCrT	50 minutes, whole class: movement-based problem solving using basketballs @ HR >139 bpm (n = 138, no gender data)	50 minutes, whole class: seated classroom lesson on humanistic subject (n = 138, no gender data)	HR assessed: average 147.25 ± 15.5 bpm	Pre Post @ 0 minutes
(16) Pesce et al. (2009), Italy, age 11–12 years, within-subjects counterbalanced order	42 minutes, whole class: team games @ HR> 139 bpm, 54% of time interacting with peers (n = 52, no gender data)	No control condition, baseline control test undertaken at start of school day (n = 52, no gender data)	HR assessed average 137 ± 18 bpm; 43.3% of lesson in MVPA, 18.19 minutes	No pre Post @ 5–8 minutes
(20) Budde et al. (2008), Germany, age 15 years, RCT	10 minutes, whole class; bilateral-coordinate exercises in circuit, five exercise (n = 47, girls = 23%)	10 minutes, whole class: normal sport lesson with no formal direction @ MPA, average HR 121.96 ± 27.06 bpm (n = 57, girls = 15%)	HR assessed: average 122.30 ± 21.91 bpm	Pre after lesson week prior Post @ 0 minutes

RCT, randomized controlled trial; RCrT, randomized crossover trial; HR, heart rate; MVPA, moderate-to-vigorous physical activity; MPA, moderate-intensity physical activity,.

and accuracy significantly improved within CEPA-OC participants immediately after exercise. In contrast, more recent research found a 45-minute cognitively demanding exercise circuit showed no immediate improvements in selective attention (Schmidt et al., 2015). Yet, after a delay of 90 minutes, the intervention group, compared to sedentary controls, improved their attention scores for speed only, as well as combined speed and accuracy scores. The first of two studies by Gallotta et al. (2012) found no change in selective attention immediately following movement-based problem-solving and decision-making tasks. In a follow-up study, focused on immediate and delayed cognition, mixed results were found. Immediately postintervention, speed decreased, with accuracy and combined speed remaining consistent. After a 90-minute delay, the combined speed and accuracy remained consistent but accuracy decreased (Gallotta et al., 2015).

Conflicting results were reported within a series of studies investigating the impact of a cooperative and competitive games session requiring executive function on inhibition control, updating and shifting (Jäger et al., 2014, 2015). In the first study, compared to sedentary controls, CEPA-OC resulted in improved inhibitory control immediately postexercise, with no change observed in updating or shifting (Jäger et al., 2014). To identify whether this improvement was due to the quantitative characteristics or the cognitively engaging activity, a four-arm follow-up study was conducted. This study compared aerobic exercise, cognitively challenging physically active games, a cognitively challenging sedentary session and a non-cognitively engaging sedentary session (Jäger et al., 2015). Immediately after exercise, inhibition and shifting improved across all conditions, although no differences were observed between groups. Refined analysis revealed that students with higher fitness and academic achievement levels improved their updating scores compared to less fit individuals or lower academic achievers. This suggests that exercise may have differing effects on cognition due to personal characteristics. Follow-up studies are required to confirm that these effects truly exist.

Finally, Pesce et al. (2009) investigated the impact of team games on immediate and delayed recall. Immediately following team games, significantly higher rates of primacy and recency but not total number of recalled items were observed compared to the sedentary control condition, with no difference found for aerobically based exercise. For delayed recall (i.e. 12 minutes postsession), both team games and aerobic exercise elicited improvements in recency items but not primacy or overall effects.

In summary, while the positive effects of CEPA-OC appear limited, beneficial effects have been observed. The strongest positive outcomes are found within selective attention, mainly due to the volume of research being conducted within this cognitive domain (Budde et al., 2008; Schmidt et al., 2015). Inhibitory control has been seen to improve immediately after exercise, although these benefits were not sustained 45 minutes later (Jäger et al., 2014) or confirmed in a follow-up study (Jäger et al., 2015).

Implications and future directions

We are confident in making the following recommendations precisely because the studies pool the recent evidence established using powerful research designs. Given the translational nature of the data, the strengths and limitations are so tightly intertwined that they relate to both research and implementation. The key issues will now be addressed.

What is common?

Task impurity affects the assessment of both cognition and of physical activity. Within different cognitive assessments it is likely that more than one cognitive process is being measured. While researchers would be wise not to elevate an outcome from one measure (e.g. inhibition control–Stroop task) to claim 'improved executive functioning', a nod should be made to other cognitive domains that may have been challenged within the test. Within physical activity, there was high variability in the activity that was completed, despite authors' claims for uniformity. Handling the variability inherent to each component of the FITT-VP framework illustrates the scale of the challenge here.

Few studies are replicated within school systems. Obviously, this field of research examining cognition, within the school environment, in children and young people is still in its infancy. At present, studies are spread across countries with little replication within country. For example, in Table 15.1, of only four studies, each was conducted in a different country and therefore, in widely differing school systems. Confirmatory studies are needed to establish outcomes. With proof of concept, international studies should be conducted.

What is specific to the physical activity experience?

Confirming the dose establishes face validity of both the treatment and the control conditions. Currently, due to measurement issues, studies over-report the duration and intensity of physical activity within acute bouts. Therefore, confident conclusions cannot be drawn from *theoretically* doing 10 minutes of physical activity when only a proportion of children *actually* did this; most did far less. Assessment methods need to report clearly the number of minutes of physical activity performed at a moderate to vigorous intensity. Where necessary, non-compliance should be addressed in the outcome analysis.

Address the interindividual variability in the dose–response. As outlined, not all individuals engage in equal measures within real-world physical activity opportunities. Therefore, all individuals may not achieve advertised cognitive benefits because their involvement did not meet thresholds for duration and intensity. Practitioners need to create physical activity environments that maximize the engagement of all individuals within the session.

Researchers need to assess accurately interindividual variability using measurement tools appropriate to the activity context and paediatric population (Corder et al., 2008). To enable accurate assessment of cognitive outcomes, minimum thresholds for activity should be used to identify participants who qualify to be included in the analysis (Janssen et al., 2014).

Classroom control conditions favour what the teachers are likely to consider the alternative to being physically active. The majority of control conditions utilize seated or sedentary control conditions. First, it is inherently unhelpful to endorse to teachers, whether implicitly or explicitly, an activity–sedentary dichotomy. Where no cognitive improvements are attributable to exercise conditions, the research incidentally endorses sedentary learning. Studies should have multiple comparison groups to enable the identification of successful active ingredients (Jäger et al., 2015). Equally, designing studies with more physically active control conditions is justified. In addition, future studies should look to assess physically active learning that has been confirmed within laboratory-based experiments (Vazou & Smiley-Oyen, 2014).

Specific issues affecting cognitive assessment

Assess a wider range of cognitive domains. To develop the evidence base, studies should strive to assess a wider range of cognitive domains. Care must be taken to structure appropriately larger cognitive assessment batteries to control time-dependent effects of acute physical activity on cognition and minimize test-induced fatigue. Within the current review, 50% of the studies assess a single cognitive outcome, limiting understanding of the potential impact of exercise on cognition. Further, within the current literature, there is a skewed distribution of cognitive domains assessed, with a dominant focus on selective attention, closely followed by inhibition. By extending the scope of experimental designs to incorporate a broader range of cognitive domains, researchers and practitioners stand to benefit from evidence that offers a deeper comprehension of the complex relationship that exists between exercise and cognition. Due to time-dependent effects of acute physical activity on cognition, care should be taken to limit the range of cognitive tests included within testing batteries.

Cognitive tasks must use age-appropriate stimuli and instructions. Studies and interventions need to detail the selection criteria for the testing battery, clearly outlining the validity of the test adopted for use with children and young people. Specifically, stimuli and instructions utilized within research and practice should be specific to the age of the participants, ensuring that cognitive maturation is accounted for as explicitly as physical capability.

Chronological age groups should be underpinned by relevant theory, and not based solely on opportunistic sampling. Building upon the above conclusion, it is crucial that sampling methods go beyond mere convenience.

Future interventions and research studies should make greater efforts to develop and justify robust participant recruitment strategies to ensure effective alignment between population samples and the protocols deployed. To this end, it is important that appropriate theories, models and frameworks are utilized in the development of research questions and evaluation methods.

Final conclusions

Based on our review, we suggest cautious optimism regarding claims for the impact of acute bouts of physical activity on cognition within the school environment. To be more confident would require further studies that address the depth of the problem in confirming the benefits of physical activity – within the school context – on cognition. Many of the shortcomings affecting the current evidence base arise from the complexity inherent to all the possible combinations of FITT-VP, the cognitive processes and how they are observed. Within the current literature, the physical activity bout is generally defined as a common experience, whereas the observation data indicate a highly variable experience. To progress the field, researchers need to define clearly the physical activity provision and confirm levels of individual engagement.

Further, to progress more systematically, there is need for researchers to manipulate single components of the FITT-VP framework within each experimental study, assessing the alteration against each cognitive outcome. To aid these developments, multidisciplinary research teams together with context-relevant practitioners need to design interventions that optimize the physical activity that can be achieved while assessing the impact on a range of cognitive outcomes.

References

ACSM. (2014). *ACSM's guidelines for exercise testing and prescription* (9th revised North American ed.). Baltimore, MD: Lippincott Williams and Wilkins.

Altenburg, T. M., Chinapaw, M. J. M., & Singh, A. S. (2016). Effects of one versus two bouts of moderate intensity physical activity on selective attention during a school morning in Dutch primary schoolchildren: A randomized controlled trial. *Journal of Science and Medicine in Sport / Sports Medicine Australia, 19*(10), 820–824.

Awh, E., & Pashler, H. (2000). Evidence for split attentional foci. *Journal of Experimental Psychology. Human Perception and Performance, 26*, 834–846.

Baddeley, A. D. (2012). Working memory: Theories, models, and controversies. *Annual Review of Psychology, 63*, 1–29.

Baddeley, A. D., & Hitch, G. (1974). Working memory. In G. H. Bower (Ed.), *Psychology of learning and motivation* (Vol. 8, pp. 47–89). New York: Academic Press.

Bailey, R. C., Olson, J., Pepper, S. L., Porszasz, J., Barstow, T. J., & Cooper, D. M. (1995). The level and tempo of children's physical activities: An observational study. *Medicine and Science in Sports and Exercise, 27*, 1033–1041.

Budde, H., Voelcker-Rehage, C., Pietrabyk-Kendziorra, S., Ribeiro, P., & Tidow, G. (2008). Acute coordinative exercise improves attentional performance in adolescents. *Neuroscience Letters, 441,* 219–223.

Chang, Y. K., Labban, J. D., Gapin, J. I., & Etnier, J. L. (2012). The effects of acute exercise on cognitive performance: A meta-analysis. *Brain Research, 1453,* 87–101.

Chen, A.-G., Yan, J., Yin, H.-C., Pan, C.-Y., & Chang, Y.-K. (2014). Effects of acute aerobic exercise on multiple aspects of executive function in preadolescent children. *Psychology of Sport and Exercise, 15,* 627–636.

Cooper, S. B., Bandelow, S., Nute, M. L., Morris, J. G., & Nevill, M. E. (2012). The effects of a mid-morning bout of exercise on adolescents' cognitive function. *Mental Health and Physical Activity, 5,* 183–190.

Corder, K., Ekelund, U., Steele, R. M., Wareham, N. J., & Brage, S. (2008). Assessment of physical activity in youth. *Journal of Applied Physiology, 105,* 977–987.

Defeyter, M. A., Russo, R., & McPartlin, P. L. (2009). The picture superiority effect in recognition memory: A developmental study using the response signal procedure. *Cognitive Development, 24,* 265–273.

Diamond, A. (2013). Executive functions. *Annual Review of Psychology, 64,* 135–168.

Donnelly, J. E., Hillman, C. H., Castelli, D., Etnier, J. L., Lee, S., Tomporowski, P., . . . Szabo-Reed, A. N. (2016). Physical activity, fitness, cognitive function, and academic achievement in children: A systematic review. *Medicine and Science in Sports and Exercise, 48,* 1223–1224.

Eriksen, C. W., & St James, J. D. (1986). Visual attention within and around the field of focal attention: A zoom lens model. *Perception and Psychophysics, 40,* 225–240.

Etnier, J., Labban, J. D., Piepmeier, A., Davis, M. E., & Henning, D. A. (2014). Effects of an acute bout of exercise on memory in 6th grade children. *Pediatric Exercise Science, 26,* 250–258.

Furley, P., & Wood, G. (2016). Working memory, attentional control, and expertise in sports: A review of current literature and directions for future research. *Journal of Applied Research in Memory and Cognition, 5*(4), 415–425.

Gallotta, M. C., Emerenziani, G. P., Franciosi, E., Meucci, M., Guidetti, L., & Baldari, C. (2015). Acute physical activity and delayed attention in primary school students. *Scandinavian Journal of Medicine and Science in Sports, 25,* e331–e338.

Gallotta, M. C., Guidetti, L., Franciosi, E., Emerenziani, G. P., Bonavolontà, V., & Baldari, C. (2012). Effects of varying type of exertion on children's attention capacity. *Medicine and Science in Sports and Exercise, 44,* 550–555.

Hill, L., Williams, J. H. G., Aucott, L., Milne, J., Thomson, J., Greig, J., . . . Mon-Williams, M. (2010). Exercising attention within the classroom. *Developmental Medicine and Child Neurology, 52,* 929–934.

Hillman, C. H., Pontifex, M. B., Raine, L. B., Castelli, D. M., Hall, E. E., & Kramer, A. F. (2009). The effect of acute treadmill walking on cognitive control and academic achievement in preadolescent children. *Neuroscience, 159,* 1044–1054.

Howie, E. K., Schatz, J., & Pate, R. R. (2015). Acute effects of classroom exercise breaks on executive function and math performance: A dose–response study. *Research Quarterly for Exercise and Sport, 86,* 217–224.

Jäger, K., Schmidt, M., Conzelmann, A., & Roebers, C. M. (2014). Cognitive and physiological effects of an acute physical activity intervention in elementary school children. *Frontiers in Psychology*, 5, 1473.

Jäger, K., Schmidt, M., Conzelmann, A., & Roebers, C. M. (2015). The effects of qualitatively different acute physical activity interventions in real-world settings on executive functions in preadolescent children. *Mental Health and Physical Activity*, 9, 1–9.

Janssen, M., Chinapaw, M. J. M., Rauh, S. P., Toussaint, H. M., van Mechelen, W., & Verhagen, E. A. L. M. (2014). A short physical activity break from cognitive tasks increases selective attention in primary school children aged 10–11. *Mental Health and Physical Activity*, 7, 129–134.

Kubesch, S., Walk, L., Spitzer, M., Kammer, T., Lainburg, A., Heim, R., & Hille, K. (2009). A 30-minute physical education program improves students' executive attention. *Mind, Brain and Education: The Official Journal of the International Mind, Brain, and Education Society*, 3, 235–242.

Ma, J. K., Le Mare, L., & Gurd, B. J. (2015). Four minutes of in-class high-intensity interval activity improves selective attention in 9- to 11-year-olds. *Applied Physiology, Nutrition, and Metabolism = Physiologie Appliquée, Nutrition et Metabolisme*, 40, 238–244.

Miyake, A., Friedman, N. P., Emerson, M. J., Witzki, A. H., Howerter, A., & Wager, T. D. (2000). The unity and diversity of executive functions and their contributions to complex "frontal lobe" tasks: A latent variable analysis. *Cognitive Psychology*, 41, 49–100.

Niemann, C., Wegner, M., Voelcker-Rehage, C., Holzweg, M., Arafat, A. M., & Budde, H. (2013). Influence of acute and chronic physical activity on cognitive performance and saliva testosterone in preadolescent school children. *Mental Health and Physical Activity*, 6, 197–204.

Pesce, C. (2012). Shifting the focus from quantitative to qualitative exercise characteristics in exercise and cognition research. *Journal of Sport and Exercise Psychology*, 34, 766–786.

Pesce, C., Crova, C., Cereatti, L., Casella, R., & Bellucci, M. (2009). Physical activity and mental performance in preadolescents: Effects of acute exercise on free-recall memory. *Mental Health and Physical Activity*, 2, 16–22.

Pirrie, A. M., & Lodewyk, K. R. (2012). Investigating links between moderate-to-vigorous physical activity and cognitive performance in elementary school students. *Mental Health and Physical Activity*, 5, 93–98.

Posner, M. I. (1980). Orienting of attention. *The Quarterly Journal of Experimental Psychology*, 32, 3–25.

Rowlands, A. V., & Eston, R. G. (2007). The measurement and interpretation of children's physical activity. *Journal of Sports Science and Medicine*, 6, 270–276.

Schmidt, M., Egger, F., & Conzelmann, A. (2015). Delayed positive effects of an acute bout of coordinative exercise on children's attention. *Perceptual and Motor Skills*, 121, 431–446.

Shephard, R. J., & Balady, G. J. (1999). Exercise as cardiovascular therapy. *Circulation*, 99, 963–972.

Steinmayr, R., Ziegler, M., & Träuble, B. (2010). Do intelligence and sustained attention interact in predicting academic achievement? *Learning and Individual Differences*, 20, 14–18.

Tine, M. T., & Butler, A. G. (2012). Acute aerobic exercise impacts selective attention: An exceptional boost in lower-income children. *Educational Psychology Review, 32,* 821–834.

Tomporowski, P. D., McCullick, B., Pendleton, D. M., & Pesce, C. (2015). Exercise and children's cognition: The role of exercise characteristics and a place for metacognition. *Journal of Sport and Health Science, 4,* 47–55.

van den Berg, V., Saliasi, E., de Groot, R. H. M., Jolles, J., Chinapaw, M. J. M., & Singh, A. S. (2016). Physical activity in the school setting: Cognitive performance is not affected by three different types of acute exercise. *Frontiers in Psychology, 7,* 723.

Vazou, S., & Smiley-Oyen, A. (2014). Moving and academic learning are not antagonists: Acute effects on executive function and enjoyment. *Journal of Sport and Exercise Psychology, 36,* 474–485.

Chapter 16

The effect of teaching methodologies in promoting physical and cognitive development in children

Patrizia Tortella and Guido Fumagalli

Introduction

Mens sana in corpore sano. This quotation from the Roman poet Juvenal summarizes the common belief that a bond between physical health and cognition exists. Even though the link between body and mind has been one of the enduring legacies of *Some Thoughts Concerning Education* (Locke's treatise on philosophy of education that has provided the basis for future development of pedagogy as science), the scientific effort to demonstrate the reality of this connection has been slow to build up.

Indeed, the scientific literature on issues concerning physical activity has grown continuously only in the last decades and most of it was due to interest in health. A search on PubMed for the items 'physical activity human' shows that in 1985 the number of published papers was 1,366 but increased to 23,353 in 2015. Within these numbers, the publications addressing 'physical activity cognition' were just 32 in 1985 and 1,026 in 2015. Based on these studies, a large consensus has been reached on the role of physical activity in reducing preventable and avoidable mortality and disability due to non-communicable diseases, such as cardiovascular and chronic respiratory diseases, cancer and diabetes (Katzmarzyk, Church, Craig, & Bouchard, 2009; Tremblay, Colley, Saunders, Healy, & Owen, 2010). Accordingly, most of the international organizations concerned with health (World Health Organization, National Association for Sport and Physical Education, American Academy of Pediatrics, American Heart Association) have published recommendations to encourage health by preventing sedentary behaviour and promoting the practice of physical activity (Tremblay et al., 2012). In contrast, no clear recommendations (or no recommendations at all) have been issued for exploiting physical activity to stimulate cognition.

The interest in the relation between physical activity and cognition started to grow when scientists first examined motor development. As stated by Karen Adolph (Adolph & Berger, 2015), the idea that development was mostly driven by the genetic programme and 'maturation' of brain and muscles had limited scientific curiosity. It was only around the 1970s that the role of the environment (at large) and experience were recognized as funda-mental determinants of motor development.

Development is a continuous phenomenon that occurs mostly during the early years of human life. Indeed, adult human beings are continuously built on what had been layered during their own development and the early years of life are the most relevant and sensitive in this respect. Knowing how motor competences and other human capacities are built, and how this pro-cess reflects on adult life, implies that the centre of scientific interest must be shifted from adulthood to childhood. This shift has occurred only recently, as indicated by the still relatively low number of scientific publications found in MedLine for the item 'physical activity children' in 2015 (from 23,353 items dedicated to physical activity, only 2,839 concern children).

A growing mass of evidence has identified modes and determinants of motor development. The relationships between development of basic motor skills, motor competences and fitness call for consideration on the educational strategies that must be put in place to promote persistency of physically active lifestyles. In addition, the recognition that emotional and cognitive components accompany motor development (Stodden et al., 2008) had provided the final push for the scientific interest in the links between physical activity and cognition. Accordingly, physical education adapted to children has emerged from the mud of the cultural 'obviousness' that fre-quently hinders the development of scientific knowledge and the elaboration of evidence-based educational strategies.

In this chapter, we will analyse the recent indications emerging from the scientific literature linking physical activity and cognition. In particular, we will focus on executive functions, a group of interrelated and prefrontal cortex-linked processes relevant for school and social achievements; we will discuss how physical education may participate in promoting executive functions along with motor development and health.

The changing view on development and the link between motor activities and cognition

As mentioned above, the 'maturational perspective' of development domi-nated the first half of the 20th century; development was considered an internal or innate process guided by a biological and genetic clock control-ling maturation of the central nervous system and development of the mus-culoskeletal system (Gesell, 1933; Shirley, 1933). The adult/educator had mostly the role of the attending person, accompanying the child along the path of new knowledge, with minimal methodological distinction between educational strategies for acquisition of cultural knowledges or motor com-petences. Cross-cultural studies have highlighted the differences in patterns of cultural and motor development in early childhood among populations from different parts of the world, and have been instrumental in modifying views on child development leading to the definition of the 'ecological perspective'. As for many aspects of social sciences, Bronfenbrenner's (1979) bioecological theory has been dominant in guiding research on motor development, which is now considered the result of the development of multiple and connected systems, each limited by constraints. Since constraints change throughout life, development is a lifelong process.

The theoretical picture of child development predicted by the dynamical system theory proposed by Ester Thelen (Kamm, Thelen, & Jensen, 1990) has relevant and practical implications. As development is dependent on experience and constraint, education becomes an important aspect and the role of teacher (referring to both professional and parents) needs to be reconsidered. Indeed, different behaviours of caregivers might influence different motor and cognitive development, as suggested by cross-cultural studies (Keller, 2007; Kolling et al., 2014; Yen-Tzu et al., 2008). The adult is not only the provider of conditions for new cultural and motor experiences; he/she must also comply with constraints and create the conditions that promote the increasing acquisition of skills and competencies for each child/individual. In this integrated view, motor development becomes tightly integrated with the psychological, sociological and cognitive aspects of the subject's life (Diamond, 2000, 2007, 2014). As pointed out by Kamm et al. (1990), the mind is firmly coupled with the body, and the development of motor competencies involves psychological processes including individual perception of capacity (Stodden et al., 2008).

Executive functions and physical activities

This new view of motor development has spurred interest in the links with cognition. The term has a very broad meaning, yet in this review we will limit our analysis to executive functions, a set of cognitive processes mostly linked to the prefrontal cortex which have been found to be predictors of academic achievements (Blair & Razza, 2007; Hughes & Ensor, 2008; Morrison, Ponitz, & McClelland, 2010).

Executive functions are a group of interrelated top-down mental processes responsible for selection, scheduling, coordination and monitoring of goal-directed processes regulating perception, memory and action (Donnelly et al., 2016). Inhibitory control, working memory and cognitive flexibility are considered 'high-order' core functions used to build up reasoning, problem solving and planning (Collins & Koechlin, 2012; Diamond, 2013; Diamond & Ling, 2016; Lehto, Juujärvi, Kooistra, & Pulkkinen, 2003; Lunt et al., 2012; Miyake et al., 2000).

Inhibitory control is critical for social life, because it regulates the capability to wait and think before acting, to resist temptations, to resist doing illegal acts, to be able to stay focused. In a longitudinal study, children with a good level of inhibitory control (those able to wait their turn, more resistant to distractors, more persistent on tasks, less impulsive) on an age range between 3 and 11 years old were found to be in better physical and mental health when checked 30 years later (Moffitt et al., 2011). They were also less likely to be overweight, to use drugs, to commit a crime; they earned more and were happier compared to children in the control group.

Working memory is important to hold information in our mind, to do one or more mental operations, to solve problems. Working memory and inhibitory control have been shown to predict maths and reading competence from kindergarten to university (Borella, Carretti, & Pelgrina, 2010). Cognitive flexibility helps to approach problems, to change perspectives, to switch easily from one task to another.

Executive functions are relevant in every aspect of life (Diamond, 2013) and several studies have confirmed that they are predictive of social, professional and scholastic achievements (Blair & Razza, 2007; Hughes & Ensor, 2008), mental (Baler & Volkow, 2006; Lui & Tannock, 2007) and physical health (Crescioni et al., 2011; Miller, Barnes, & Beaver, 2011), wealth and quality of life (Brown & Landgraf, 2010; Davis, Marra, Najafzadeh, & Lui-Ambrose, 2010). In this respect, high levels of executive functions appear to be better predictors than IQ or socioeconomic status.

A relevant aspect of executive functions is that their levels are not innate and can be improved from infants to elders (Kovács & Mehler, 2009; Williams & Lord, 1997). The interest has grown on possible modulators. Among these, physical activity has been thoroughly examined. In a recent extensive review of the literature, Donnelly et al. (2016) report that the majority of the published data suggest that cognitive functions, as well as brain structure, benefit from physical fitness and from the practice of physical activity; a lower level of consensus links physical activity with scholastic achievements. On the other hand, as pointed out by the authors of the review, most of the studies do not meet the methodological criteria that usually characterize clinical studies; among limitations, the most common appear to be lack of randomization or lack of controls, low statistical power, low level of definition/characterization of inclusion criteria of participants, poor definition of physical practices, lack of double-blind approaches to data collection and management. In conclusion, new, larger and better-designed studies are needed to define whether a clear and direct correlation between physical activity and executive functions really exists.

In a literature review produced by Adele Diamond (Diamond & Ling, 2016), the analysis aimed to identify patterns of physical activity and/or physical education that may positively influence development of executive functions. It appeared that these functions and motor competences share similar properties. For both, (1) transfer is limited (training a basic motor skill such as balance does not improve another basic skill such as running; similarly, training working memory does not improve self-control); (2) gains depend on the amount of time spent practising; (3) persistence is limited and requires continuous training/exercising; and (4) improvements are higher when initial competences are low.

On the other hand, executive function improvement is obtained when additional specific and more stringent criteria are met. First, children must enjoy the activity they are doing and the gain in executive functions is dependent on the way the activity is presented and conducted; second, the activity must always be challenging to induce cognitive improvement (not a requirement for most forms of resistance training). Thus the personal characteristics of both the educators (responsible for how an activity is presented and conducted) and of the participants are relevant to induce benefits for both motor and cognitive functions.

Interesting information on the role of teaching methodology was provided by a study by Trulson (1986), where three groups of 13–17-year-old juvenile delinquents received two different trainings of taekwondo, a martial art, for 1 hour three times a week for 6 months. The first group practised a traditional version of the art, with emphasis on the psychological/philosophical aspects; the second group received a more modern instruction with no attention to those traditional aspects; and the third group did not practise the art at all. The results showed that only the first group obtained a positive outcome in executive functions, resulting in decreased aggressiveness, lowered anxiety and increased social adroitness and value orthodoxy. The second group instead showed an increased tendency towards delinquency.

In a more recent study comparing one group of randomly selected preschool children trained in a traditional martial art and another group trained in school physical education, the authors (Lakes & Hoyt, 2004) found a greater capacity of self-regulation in children practising martial arts than in those from the second group. This possibly indicates that martial arts could increase the learning of children toward a higher self-awareness, an expanded ability to evaluate intentions and actions, and to a better adaptation to different life situations.

Finally, additional data to be considered by educators suggest that a continuous increment in difficulty levels for one activity in association with high variety/level of cognitive engagement would benefit the development of both motor competencies and executive functions (Blumenthal et al., 1989; Davis et al., 2011; Ericsson & Towne, 2010; Etnier, Nowell, Landers, & Sibley, 2006; Kramer & Erickson, 2007).

Executive functions are embedded in the prefrontal cortex and other interconnected regions (Aron, Behrens, Smith, Frank, & Poldrack, 2007). The functioning of these areas seems to be negatively modulated by conditions such as stress (Arnsten, 1998), sadness, solitude, loneliness and poor health; Diamond and Ling (2016) suggest that conditions reducing these negative aspects may improve the mental processes. Indeed, beneficial influences could be achieved by situations that promote health and fitness (such as physical activities), social support (Cacioppo & Patrick, 2008) and joy

(Gable & Harmon-Jones, 2008; Hirt, Devers, & McCrea, 2008) and that satisfy emotional and physical needs (Etnier et al., 2006; Jing, Zhang, Wolff, Bilkey, & Liu, 2013).

Enjoyment of the activities performed, as well as self-confidence and self-efficacy, are also very important for the optimal functioning of mental processes (Bandura, 1994). Feeling confidence in our ability to succeed and trusting that through our own efforts we can improve are key components for success. The same occurs when the subject feels that errors and failed attempts are learning opportunities. These are conditions that lead to successful improvement of motor and cognitive skills (Bandura, 1994; Murphy & Dweck, 2010). Self-confidence and feelings of self-efficacy, together with expectations, have a strong effect on capacity to accomplish a task (Good, Aronson, & Harder, 2008). Perception of competence is in relation to task difficulty (Eccles & Harold, 1991) and can influence children's engagement in physical activity (Stodden et al., 2008); positive perception leads to more engagement in the exercise with effects on amount, intensity and level of physical activity and thus, improvement of motor skill (Stodden et al., 2008). As suggested above, positive experiences are conditions that positively modulate executive functions as well.

The role of educators in linking physical activity and executive functions

Reviews from both Donnelly et al. (2016) and Diamond and Ling (2016) emphasize the need for appropriate and stringent study design when addressing questions related to the link(s) between physical activity and executive functions. Even more relevant is the consideration that games based on movement can be important instruments to foster executive functions in children together with physical fitness. In this regard, it is vital for educators to be able to create appropriate conditions for the development of both motor and executive functions.

An important aspect regarding the activities organized by educators is that they must meet the peculiar characteristics of each child. Indeed, it is the presence of appropriate and multiple conditions for practising that affects level of competence and the personal perception of it (Goodway & Smith, 2005). It should also be considered that the level of motor competence is fundamental to predict present and future (in adulthood) engagement in physical activities (Clark & Metcalfe, 2002; Haywood & Getchell, 2014; Malina, 1996).

Children's perception of competence encourages or discourages the practice of physical activity (Stodden et al., 2008). Welk et al. (2010) suggest that the perceptions of competence overshadow the actual competence of a person. Self-efficacy and perception of competence thus emerge as important components of the learning process that drives a subject to reach new levels of competence. These aspects should receive attention when children are engaged in sports or games performed in groups or when a child is exposed to a challenging condition. This is the typical situation with traditional games/sports or, at school, when the educator defines the rules of the game/activity and expects all children to act as requested. In most cases, only part of the group will be able to perform as requested, leading to a separation into two subgroups: the successful ones will feel high levels of competence and the others will be highly frustrated. The typical outcome of this condition is that the successful children will practise further and gain advantage from the physical activities, while the frustrated children will withdraw from the task (Tortella & Fumagalli, 2014).

As for executive functions, practice, training and motivation are fundamental to improve motor skill and acquire motor competence (Clark & Metcalfe, 2002). The strategies to increase efficacy of practice and, in turn, perceived success and motivation have been investigated only recently. As stated above, development of both motor skills and level of executive functions occurs when children are pushed to challenge with very difficult levels of skills, near the limit of competence (Davis et al., 2011; Diamond, Barnett, Thomas, & Munro, 2007). This is a 'learning condition' defined by Vygotsky (1986) as 'zone of proximal development'; it is a situation that is beyond the 'comfort space' of the subject, a level that can be reached only with a limited/little help from someone else.

The role of scaffolding by teachers and expert peers is fundamental in every child to promote the possibility of increasing motor and cognitive skills, feeling joy and pride during the activity, looking for repetition and thus achieving consolidation of the skill. In a study with preschoolers attending a playground designed to promote their motor development (Tortella, Haga, Loras, Sigmunsson, & Fumagalli, 2016), we have demonstrated that a limited experience (1 hour/week for 10 weeks) on a difficult motor task with a programme of structured activity in Vygotsky's zone of proximal development led to improvement of both motor skills and executive functions (Tortella & Fumagalli, 2014, 2016); children not trained in the zone of proximal development did not improve in motor and cognitive skills. Interestingly, the group of successful (scaffolded) children spontaneously continued to train by themselves outside the lesson, even after the initial negative results. Motivation was high in this group, as indicated by their usual sentences during their autonomous trials: 'I can. I know that if I train, I will learn'.

The above example underscores the need for teachers to regulate levels of scaffolding individually in order to give all children the opportunity to develop motor competence. The contribution of Vygotsky's theory to our understanding of development of executive functions is very important. Working in the zone of proximal development, with scaffolding provided by the adult, is the appropriate condition to avoid boredom and to motivate children to improve (Davis et al., 2011; Diamond, 2007; Manjunath &

Telles, 2001). Practical elaboration with translation of the theoretical key issues in daily practice is present in Tools of the Mind (Bodrova & Leong, 2007), a school programme for enhancing executive functions.

The educator should also consider that the positive emotion of enjoyment is a strong motivation to practise physical activity (Scanlan, Carpenter, Lobelm, & Simons, 1993; Brustad, 1993); indeed, when children have good actual motor competence and perception of competence (intrinsic motivation), they feel joy. Other elements to promote enjoyment during physical activities are movement sensations, social recognition and interactions, feeling appreciated, making new friends and staying with friends (Wankel & Kreisel, 1985a, b).

Diamond (2000, 2007, 2014) suggests that the different components of the human being are interrelated with each other and recommends examining the way a teacher communicates and relates to children as an important factor for the development of executive functions. The experiences of well-being at school together with perceived emotional engagement in the peer group and teacher–student interaction contribute to students' perceived cognitive engagement and school achievement (Pietarinen, Soini, & Pyhältö, 2014). The teacher's instructional behaviour and support (Skinner, Furrer, Marchand, & Kindermann, 2008), together with other components of the student–teacher relationship, contribute to student emotional and cognitive engagement, self-confidence in own abilities, future academic achievement and social and behavioural outcomes (Gest, Welsh, & Domitrovich, 2005; Hughes & Kwok, 2006; Li & Lerner, 2012; Walg & Holcombe, 2010). Preliminary data from a recent study on children engaged in a difficult task indicate that the combination of physical and emotional scaffolding induced both improvements in motor skills and executive functions, whereas physical scaffolding alone improved motor skills but not executive functions (Tortella & Fumagalli, 2016).

A final consideration that should be taken into account when planning activities to increment motor skills and/or executive functions is that both are very task-specific. From a teacher perspective, this indicates that learning objectives must be abundant and differentiated to cover the high spectrum of motor skills and executive functions. In addition, it may sometimes be difficult to design activities intended to lead to improvement of both types of skills. Clear understanding and definition of the teaching objectives and of the methods to tailor activities on individual properties of the child are thus prerequisite for new and modern teaching of physical education.

Conclusions

The practice of physical activity is believed to lead to improvement of motor skills and competencies with several beneficial effects on present and future health, as well as on psychological constraints of the child. However, no extensive data are available on the relationships between changes induced by motor activities on motor skills and executive functions. On the other hand, the data that have been accumulating in recent years indicate that the (psychological) conditions that lead to improvement of executive functions can be easily applied to the context of organized motor activities. Teaching methodologies of physical activity rather than the activity itself appears to be relevant to enhance this important set of cognitive processes. From the educational perspective and considering the appreciation of movement-based games among children, these conclusions highlight the potential significance of a revisited physical education in scholastic curricula for all ages.

References

Adolph, K.E., & Berger, S.E. (2015). Physical and motor development. In M.H. Bornstein & M.E. Lamb (Eds.), *Developmental science: An advanced textbook* (7th ed., pp. 261–333). New York: Psychology Press/Taylor & Francis.

Arnsten, A.F.T. (1998). The biology of being frazzled. *Science (New York, N.Y.), 280* (5370), 1711–1712. doi: 10.1126/science.280.5370.1711.

Aron, A.R., Behrens, T.E., Smith, S., Frank, M.J., & Poldrack, R.A. (2007). Triangulating a cognitive control network using diffusion-weighted magnetic resonance imaging (MRI) and functional MRI. *Journal of Neurosceince, 27*(14), 3743–3752. doi: 10.1523/JNEUROSCI.0519-07.2007.

Baler, R.D., & Volkow, N.D. (2006). Drug addiction: The neurobiology of disrupted self-control. *Trends in Molecular Medicine, 12, 559–566.* doi: 10.1016/j. molmed.2006.10.005.

Bandura, A. (1994). Self-efficacy. In V.S. Ramachaudran (Ed.), *Encyclopedia of human behavior, Vol. 4* (pp. 71–81). New York: Academy Press (reprinted in H. Friedman [Ed.]. *Encyclopedia of mental health.* San Diego, CA: Academic Press, 1998).

Blair, C., & Razza, R.P. (2007). Relating effortful control, executive function, and false-belief understanding to emerging math and literacy ability in kindergarten. *Child Development, 78, 647–663.* doi: 10.1111/j.1467-8624.2007.01019.x.

Blumenthal, J.A., Emery, C.F., Madden, D.J., George, L.K., Coleman, R.E., Riddle, M.W., . . . Williams, R.S. (1989). Cardiovascular and behavioral effects of aerobic exercise training in healthy older men and women. *The Journal of Gerontology, 44*(5), M147–M157. doi: 10.1093/geronj/44.5.M147.

Bodrova, E., & Leong, D.J. (2007). *Tools of the mind: The Vygotskian approach to early childhood education.* Upper Saddle River, NJ: Pearson Education.

Borella, E., Carretti, B., & Pelgrina, S. (2010). The specific role of inhibition in reading comprehension in good and poor comprehenders. *Journal of Learning Disabilities, 43, 541–552.* doi: 10.1177/0022219410371676.

Bronfenbrenner, U. (1979). *The ecology of human development: Experiments by nature and design.* Cambridge, MA: Harvard University Press.

Brown, T.E., & Landgraf, J.M. (2010). Improvements in executive function correlate with enhanced performance and functioning and health-related quality of life: Evidence from 2 large, double-blind, randomized, placebo-controlled trials in ADHD. *Postgraduate Medicine, 122, 42–51.* doi: http://dx.doi.org/10.3810/pgm.2010.09.2200.

Brustad, R.J. (1993). Youth in sport: Psychological consideration. In R.N. Singer, M. Murphy, and L.K. Tennant (Eds.), *Handbook of research on sport psychology* (pp. 695–717). New York: Macmillan.

Cacioppo, J., & Patrick, W. (2008). *Loneliness: Human nature and the need for social connection.* New York: W. W. Norton.

Clark, J.E., & Metcalfe, J.S. (2002). The mountain of motor development: A metaphor. In J.E. Clark & J. Humphrey (Eds.), *Motor development: Research and reviews, Vol. 2* (pp. 163–190). Reston, VA: NASPE Publication.

Collins, A., & Koechlin, E. (2012). Reasoning, learning and creativity: Frontal lobe function and human decision-making. *PLoS Biology, 10*(3), e1001293. doi: 10.1371/journal.pbio.1001293.

Crescioni, A.W., Ehrlinger, J., Alquist, J.L., Conlon, K.E., Baumeister, R.F., Schatschneider, C., & Dutton, G.R. (2011). High trait self-control predicts positive health behaviors and success in weight loss. *Journal of Health Psychology, 16*(5), 750–759. doi: 10.1177/1359105310390247.

Davis, J.C., Marra, C.A., Najafzadeh, M., & Lui-Ambrose, T. (2010). The independent contribution of executive functions to health-related quality of life in older women. *BMC Geriatrics, 10,* 16–23. doi: 10.1186/1471-2318-10-16.

Davis, C.L., Tomporowski, P.D., McDowell, J.E., Austin, B.P., Miller, P.H., Yanasak, N.E., . . . Naglieri, J.A. (2011). Exercise improves executive function and achievement and alters brain activation in overweight children: A randomized controlled trial. *Health Psychology, 30*(1), 91–98. doi: 10.1037/a0021766.

Diamond, A. (2000). Close interrelation of motor development and cognitive development and of the cerebellum and prefrontal cortex. *Child Development, 71,* 44–56. doi: 10.1111/1467-8624.00117.

Diamond, A. (2007). Interrelated and interdependent. *Developmental Science, 10*(1), 152–158. doi: 10.1111/j.1467-7687.2007.00578.x.

Diamond, A. (2013). Executive functions. *Annual Review of Psychology, 64,* 135–168. doi: 10.1146/annurev-psych-113011-143750.

Diamond, A. (2014). Want to optimize executive functions and academic outcomes? Simple, just nourish the human spirit. *Minnesota Symposia on Child Psychology, 37,* 203–230.

Diamond, A., Barnett, W.S., Thomas, J., & Munro, S. (2007). Preschool program improves cognitive control. *Science (New York, N.Y.), 318*(5855), 1387–1388. doi: 10.1126/science.1151148.

Diamond, A., & Ling, D.S. (2016). Conclusions about interventions, programs, and approaches for improving executive functions that appear justified and those that, despite much hype, do not. *Developmental Cognitive Neuroscience, 18,* 34–48. doi: 10.1016/j.dcn.2015.11.005.

Donnelly, J.E., Hillman, C., Castelli, D., Etnier, J.L., Lee, S., Tomporowski, P., . . . Szabo-Reed, A.N. (2016). Physical activity, fitness, cognitive function, and academic achievement in children: A systematic review. *Medicine and Science in Sports and Exercise, 48*(6), 1223–1224. doi: 10.1249/MSS.0000000000000901.

Eccles, J.S., & Harold, R.D. (1991). Gender differences in sport involvement: Applying the Eccles' Expectancy-Value Model. *Journal of Applied Sport Psychology, 3,* 7–35. doi: 10.1080/10413209108406432.

Ericsson, K.A., & Towne, T.J. (2010). Expertise. *Wires Cognitive Science, 1*(3) 404–416. doi: 10.1002/wcs.47.

Etnier, J.L., Nowell, P.M., Landers, D.M., & Sibley, B.A. (2006). A meta-regression to examine the relationship between aerobic fitness and cognitive performance. *Brain Research Reviews, 52*(1), 119–130. doi: 10.1016/j.brainresrev.2006.01.002.

Gable, P.A., & Harmon-Jones, E. (2008). Approach-motivated positive affect reduces breadth of attention. *Psychological Science, 19*(5), 476–482. doi: 10.1111/j.1467-9280.2008.02112.x.

Gesell, A. (1933). Maturation and the patterling of behavior. In C. Murchison (Ed.), *A handbook of child psychology* (2nd ed., Vol. 1, pp. 209–235). New York: Russell & Russell/Atheneum Publishers.

Gest, S.D., Welsh, J.A., & Domitrovich, C.E. (2005). Behavioral predictor of changes in social relatedness and liking school in elementary school. *Journal of School Psychology, 43*, 281–301. doi: 10.1016/j.jsp.2005.06.002.

Good, C., Aronson, J., & Harder, J.A. (2008). Problems in the pipeline: Stereotype threat and women's achievement in high-level math courses. *Journal of Applied Developmental Psychology, 29*(1), 17–28. doi: 10.1016/j.appdev.2007.10.004.

Goodway, J.D., & Smith, D.W. (2005). Keeping all children healthy: Challenges to leading an active lifestyle for preschool children qualifying for at-risk programs. *Family and Community Health, 28*(2), 142–155.

Haywood, K., & Getchell, N. (2014). *Life span motor development, 6th edition, with web study guide.* Champaign, IL: Human Kinetics.

Hirt, E.R., Devers, E.E., & McCrea, S.M. (2008). I want to be creative: Exploring the role of hedonic contingency theory in the positive mood-cognitive flexibility link. *Journal of Personality and Social Psychology, 94*(2), 214–230. doi: 10.1037/0022-3514.94.2.94.2.214J.

Hughes, J., & Kwok, O. (2006). Classroom engagement mediates the effects of teacher student support on elementary students peer acceptance: A prospective analysis. *Journal of School Psychology, 43*(6), 465–480. doi: 10.1016/j.jsp.2005.10.001.

Hughes, C., & Ensor, R. (2008). Does executive function matter for preschoolers' problem behaviors? *Journal of Abnormal Child Psychology, 36*, 1–14. doi: 10.1007/s10802-007-9107-6.

Jing, Y., Zhang, H., Wolff, A.R., Bilkey, D.K., & Liu, P. (2013). Altered arginine metabolism in the hippocampus and prefrontal cortex of maternal immune activation rat offspring. *Schizophrenia Research, 148*(1–3), 151–156. doi: 10.1016/j.schres.2013.06.001.

Kamm, K., Thelen, E., & Jensen, J.L. (1990). A dynamical system approach to motor development. *Physical Therapy, 70*, 763–775. Retrieved from http://ptjournal.apta.org/content/70/12/763.

Katzmarzyk, P.T., Church, T.S., Craig, C.L., & Bouchard, C. (2009). Sitting time and mortality from all causes, cardiovascular disease, and cancer. *Medicine and Science in Sports and Medicine, 41*(5), 998–1005. doi: 0.1249/MSS.0b013e3181930355.

Keller, H. (2007). *Cultures of infancy.* Mahwah, NJ: Lawrence Erlbaum.

Kolling, T., Lamm, B., Vierhaus, M., Knopf, M., Lohaus, A., Fassbender, I., . . . Keller, H. (2014). Differential development of motor abilities in western middle-class and Cameroonian Nso infants. *Journal of Cross-Cultural Psychology, 45*(9), 1502–1508. doi: 10.1177/0022022114542976.

Kovács, A.M., & Mehler, J. (2009). Cognitive gains in 7-month-old bilingual infants. *Proceedings of the National Academy of Sciences of the U.S.A., 106*(16), 6556–6560. doi:10.1073/pnas.0811323106.

Kramer, A.F., & Erickson, K.I. (2007). Capitalizing on cortical plasticity: Influence of PA on cognition and brain function. *Trends in Cognitive Sciences, 11*(8), 342–348. doi: 10.1016/j.tics.2007.06.009.

Lakes, K.D., & Hoyt, W.T. (2004). Promoting self-regulation through school-based martial arts training. *Journal of Applied Developmental Psychology, 25,* 283–302. doi: 10.1016/j.appdev.2004.04.002.

Lehto, J.E., Juujärvi, P., Kooistra, L., & Pulkkinen, L. (2003). Dimensions of executive functioning: Evidence from children. *British Journal of Developmental Psychology, 21,* 59–80. doi: 10.1348/026151003321164627.

Li, Y., & Lerner, R.M. (2012). Interrelations of behavioral, emotional, and cognitive school engagement in high school students. *Journal of Youth and Adolescence, 42,* 20–32. doi: 10.1007/s10964-012-9857-5.

Locke, J. (1996). *Some Thoughts Concerning Education and of the Conduct of the Understanding.* R.W. Grant & N. Tarcov (Eds.). Indianapolis, IN: Hackett.

Lui, M., & Tannock, R. (2007). Working memory and inattentive behaviour in a community sample of children. *Behavioral and Brain Functions, 3,* 12. doi: http://doi.org/10.1186/1744-9081-3-12.

Lunt, L., Bramham, J., Morris, R.G., Bullock, P.R., Selway, R.P., Xenitidis, K., & David, A.S. (2012). Prefrontal cortex dysfunction and 'Jumping to Conclusions': bias or deficit? *Journal of Neuropsychology, 6*(1), 65–78. doi: 10.1111/j.1748-6653.2011.02005.x.

Malina, R.M. (1996). Tracking of physical activity and physical fitness across the lifespan. *Research Quarterly for Exercise and Sport, 67*(3 Suppl), S48–S57. doi: 10.1080/02701367.1996.10608853.

Manjunath, N.K., & Telles, S. (2001). Improved performance in the Tower of London test following yoga. *Indian Journal of Physiology and Pharmacology, 45*(3), 351–354.

Miller, H.V., Barnes, J.C., & Beaver, K.M. (2011). Self-control and health outcomes in a nationally representative sample. *American Journal of Health Behavior, 35,* 15–27. doi: https://doi.org/10.5993/AJHB.35.1.2.

Miyake, A., Friedman, N.P., Emerson, M.J., Witzki, A.H., Howerter, A., & Wager, T.D. (2000). The unity and diversity of executive functions and their contributions to complex "frontal lobe" tasks: A latent variable analysis. *Cognitive Psychology, 41,* 49–100. doi: 10.1006/cogp.1999.0734.

Moffit, T.E., Arseneault, L., Belsky, D., Dickson, N., Hancox, R.J., Harrington, H., . . . Caspi, A. (2011). A gradient of childhood self-control predicts health, wealth, and public safety. *Proceedings of the National Academy of Sciences of the U.S.A., 108*(7), 2693–2698. doi: 10.1073/pnas.1010076108.

Morrison, F.J., Ponitz, C.C., & McClelland, M.M. (2010). Self-regulation and academic achievement in the transition to school. In S.D. Calkins & M.A. Bell (Eds.), *Child development at the intersection of emotion and cognition* (pp. 203–224). Washington, DC: American Psychological Association, x, 261. doi: 10.1037/12059-011.

Murphy, M.C., & Dweck, C.S. (2010). A culture of genius: How an organization's lay theories shape people's cognition, affect, and behavior. *Personality and Social Psychology Bulletin, 36,* 283–296. doi: 10.1177/0146167209347380.

Pietarinen, J., Soini, T., & Pyhältö, K. (2014). Student's emotional and cognitive engagement as the determinants of well-being and achievement in school.

International Journal of Educational Research, 67, 40–51. doi: 10.1016/j.ijer.2014.05.001.

Scanlan, T.K., Carpenter, P.J., Lobelm, M., & Simons, P. (1993). Sources of enjoyment for youth sport athletes. *Pediatric Exercise Science, 5,* 275–285. doi: 10.1123/pes.5.3.275.

Shirley, M.M. (1933). Locomotor and visual manual functions in the first two years. In C. Murchison (Ed.), *A handbook of child psychology, Vol. 1, 2nd ed.* (pp. 236–270). New York: Russell & Russell/Atheneum Publishers.

Skinner, E.A., Furrer, C., Marchand, G., & Kindermann, T. (2008). Engagement and disaffection in the classroom: Part of a larger motivational dynamic? *Journal of Educational Psychology, 100*(4), 765–781. doi: 10.1037/a0012840.

Stodden, D.F., Goodway, J.D., Langendorter, S.J., Roberton, M.A., Rudisill, M.E., Garcia, C., & Garcia, L.E. (2008). A developmental perspective on the role of motor skill competence in PA: An emergent relationship. *Quest, 60,* 290–306.

Tortella, P., & Fumagalli, G. (2014). Difficult motor skill acquisition in 5 years old children can be modulated by educators. *Science and Sports, 29*(Suppl), S49–S50. doi: 10.1016/j.scispo.2014.08.099.

Tortella, P., & Fumagalli, G. (2016). The role of scaffolding in physical activity in development of motor and cognitive skills. *Journal of Sport and Exercise Psychology, 38*(Suppl), S20.

Tortella, P., Haga, M., Loras, H., Sigmunsson, H., & Fumagalli, G. (2016). Motor skill development in Italian pre-school children induced by structured activities in a specific playground. *PLOS One, 11*(7), e0160244.

Tremblay, M.S., Colley, R.C., Saunders, T.J., Healy, G.N., & Owen, N. (2010). Physiological and health implications of a sedentary lifestyle. *Applied Physiology, Nutrition, and Metabolism, 35*(6), 725–740. doi: 10.1139/H10-079.

Tremblay, M.S., LeBlanc, A.G., Carson, V., Choquette, L., Connor Gorber, S., Dillman, C., . . . Canadian Society for Exercise Physiology. (2012). Canadian PA guidelines for the early years (aged 0–4 years). *Applied Physiology, Nutrition, and Metabolism, 37*(2), 345–369. doi: 10.1139/h2012-018.

Trulson, M.E. (1986). Martial arts training: A novel "cure" for juvenile delinquency. *Human Relations, 39,* 1131–1140. doi: 10.1177/001872678603901204.

Vygotsky, L.S. (1986). *Thought and language.* Cambridge, MA: MIT Press.

Walg, M., & Holcombe, R. (2010). Adolescents' perceptions of school environment, engagement and academic achievement in middle school. *American Educational Research Journal, 47,* 633–662. doi: 10.3102/0002831209361209.

Wankel, L.M., & Kreisel, P.S.J. (1985a). Factors underlying enjoyment of youth sports: Sport and age group comparisons. *Journal of Sport and Exercise Psychology, 7,* 51–64. doi: 10.1123/jsp.7.1.51.

Wankel, L.M., & Kreisel, P.S.J. (1985b). Methodological considerations in youth sport motivation research: A comparison of open-ended and paired comparison approaches. *Journal of Sport and Exercise Psychology, 7,* 65–74. doi: 10.1123/jsp.7.1.65.

Welk, G.J., Jackson, A.W., Morrow, J.R., Jr, Haskellm, W.H., Meredith, M.D., & Cooper, K.H. (2010). The association of health-related fitness with indicators of academic performance in Texas schools. *Research Quarterly for Exercise and Sport, 81*(3 Suppl), S16–S23. doi: 10.1080/02701367.2010.10599690.

Williams, P., & Lord, S.R. (1997). Effects of group exercise on cognitive function-ing and mood in older women. *Australian and New Zealand Journal of Public Health, 21*(1), 45–52. doi: 10.1111/j.1467-842X.1997.tb01653.x.

Yen-Tzu, W., Tsou, K., Hsu, C., Fang, L., Yao, G., & Jeng, S. (2008). Brief report: Taiwanese infants' mental and motor development 6–24 months. *Journal of Pediatric Psychology, 33*(1), 102–108. doi: 10.1093/jpepsy/jsm067.

Chapter 17

Different solutions from Finnish and Danish school systems for increasing school-day physical activity and supporting learning

A top-down or bottom-up approach?

Tuija Tammelin, Heidi Syväoja, Anna Bugge and Karsten Froberg

Introduction

The health benefits of regular physical activity (PA) are well known and recognized (WHO, 2010). The school setting is an essential arena for impacting the development of a physically active lifestyle, especially among the least active and unfit children, because all children can be reached at school regardless of their earlier experiences with, motivation and attitude toward, PA. In addition to the impact on health and overall well-being, PA has been shown to have both long-term (e.g. Davis et al., 2011; Hillman et al., 2014; Kamijo et al., 2011; Tuckman & Hinkle, 1986) and acute (e.g. Budde et al., 2008; Caterino & Polak, 1999; Hillman et al., 2009) effects on children's cognitive functions and academic achievement. Especially, PA seems to induce functional (Chaddock-Heyman et al., 2013; Davis et al., 2011) and structural (Chaddock et al., 2010a, b) changes in subcortical structures subserving executive functions and memory, such as the hippocampus and the basal ganglia, increase levels of brain-derived neurotrophic factor, which support cellular processes important for learning and memory (Hopkins et al., 2012) and enhance cerebrovascular function (Davenport et al., 2012). Furthermore, there is now sufficient evidence to conclude that increased school-day PA does not compromise or disturb academic performance (Bangsbo et al., 2016; Donnelly et al., 2016). Given that only one-third of children are sufficiently physically active based on current recommendations (Ekelund, Tomkinson, & Armstrong, 2011), PA promotion that benefits both health and learning is becoming an important part of education.

In Finland, national PA recommendations for school-aged children state that:

> All 7- to 18-year-olds should be physically active for at least one to two hours daily, continued periods of sitting for more than 2 hours at a time should be avoided, and screen time with entertainment media should be limited to 2 hours per day.
>
> (Ministry of Education and
> Young Finland Association, 2008)

In Denmark, the National Board of Health recommends that all children 5–17 years of age should be active at a moderate to high level of intensity for at least 60 minutes per day. Furthermore, engagement in high-intensity PA at least three times per week, to maintain or improve physical fitness and muscle strength, is recommended (Danish Health Authority, 2014). Based on the Health Behaviour in School-aged Children study (Inchley et al., 2016), the proportions of Finnish girls and boys reporting at least 1 hour of moderate-to-vigorous intensity PA daily was 34% and 47%, respectively, at age 11, but as low as 13% and 22% at age 15. Similar proportions were even lower among Danish girls and boys, with 11% and 19%, respectively, at age 11, and 7% and 16%, at age 15.

Finland and Denmark have chosen different ways of enhancing PA in the school context at the national level. In Finland, a national action programme, Finnish Schools on the Move (FSM), aims to establish a physically active culture in comprehensive schools. Schools and municipalities participating in the programme implement their own individual plans to enhance PA during the school day. This provides insight into a bottom-up approach to increasing PA in schools. In Denmark, the government implemented a comprehensive school reform; both the length of the school day and the amount of teaching in general (in mathematics, literature and foreign languages) were increased, and the decision was made to increase the amount of PA to 45 minutes every school day for all children in public schools. Physical education (PE) lessons were also increased by one extra hour in fifth and sixth grades. This top-down approach was initiated to make a fast and comprehensive change in the Danish school system (Folketinget, 2014).

This chapter presents these two different ways of increasing school-day PA by using a bottom-up approach in Finland and a top-down approach in Denmark. We briefly describe the school systems in the two countries with a special emphasis on opportunities for PA and PE, and the solutions implemented to make the school day more physically active. We finally discuss the strengths and weaknesses of these implementation methods based on research results and experiences from the field.

School systems in Finland and Denmark

The Finnish school system

The Finnish education system consists of several levels: voluntary pre-primary education; a 9-year basic education for all age groups (including compulsory education, starting at the age of 7 years); upper secondary education, comprising general education and vocational education and training; and higher education, provided by universities and polytechnics. Education is free at all levels, from pre-primary through to higher education, and most of the education is publicly funded. The Ministry of Education and Culture and the Finnish

National Board of Education develop educational objectives, content and methods, whereas local authorities are responsible for the practical arrangements, effectiveness and quality of the education provided. Local authorities also determine how much autonomy is passed on to schools, and, usually, budget management, acquisitions and recruitment are the responsibility of the schools. The schools can also decide their own timetables. In addition, teachers have pedagogical autonomy, including decision making regarding teaching methods, textbooks and materials (Finnish Ministry of Education, the National Board of Education (Finland), & CIMO, 2012; Finnish National Board of Education, 2016a, b; Ministry of Education and Culture, Finland, 2016).

Quality assurance

Educational activities are guided by the national core curricula, qualification requirements and objectives laid down in legislation. Schools' quality is assured through the self-evaluations of schools/education providers and regular sample-based national evaluations of learning outcomes. There are no national tests for pupils in basic education, but instead, the system relies on the proficiency of teachers; on the basis of the objectives included in the curriculum, teachers assess the learning outcomes in their respective subjects, including PE. Every pupil is assessed continuously during the course of studies and via a final assessment. All teachers in Finland, including PE teachers, have a Master's degree, which is seen as a necessity, since Finnish teachers are professionally autonomous. The first 6 years of basic education are taught by generalists, or class teachers, whereas the next years are taught by subject specialists, or subject teachers (Finnish Ministry of Education, the National Board of Education (Finland), & CIMO, 2012).

The school day

The number of lessons provided in Finnish schools is 19–30 per week, depending on the grade and number of optional subjects taken (Grades 1–2: a maximum of five lessons/day, Grades 3–9: a maximum of seven lessons/day). One lesson is 60 minutes in length; at least 45 minutes are used for teaching, and at least 10 minutes (usually 15 minutes) are devoted to recess. A meal is served during students' 30-minute lunch break. There are approximately two PE lessons per week per year in Grades 1–9 (Finnish National Board of Education, 2016a, b).

The Danish school system

The Danish education system consists of pre-primary education (pre-schools and preschool classes, called '0-classes'), primary and secondary education (Grades 1–9/10; compulsory education grades 0–9); upper secondary education, comprising general education (high school) and vocational education and training; and higher education, provided by universities, university colleges and polytechnics. Children typically start school the year they turn 6. Education is free at all levels. The Ministry for Children, Education and Gender Equality is primarily responsible for education policy (Folketinget, 2014; Ministry for Children, Education and Gender Equality, Denmark, 2016a).

Quality assurance

Danish schools' quality assurance comprises different tools. The school staff must produce a written lesson plan for all public school pupils from 0-class through to seventh grade. Pupils in eighth and ninth grades must have a written lesson and education plan used for evaluative purposes, and to help pupils to choose their scholastic and vocational education path after ninth grade. A national test system has been developed and gradually implemented in the last 10 years. As of 2016, compulsory tests are given in the following subjects: Danish, with an emphasis on reading in Grades 2, 4, 6 and 8; English, in Grade 7; mathematics, in Grades 3 and 6; geography, in Grade 8; biology, in Grade 8; and physics/chemistry, in Grade 8. Upon the completion of ninth grade, pupils must take two examinations, one in Danish and another covering each of the following subjects: mathematics, English and physics/chemistry. In addition, each pupil must take two examinations in two other subjects (beginning in summer 2015, this could include PE); these subjects are chosen by drawing lots. Every year, all pupils in Danish schools also complete a well-being survey, which asks about their enjoyment of school, relations with classmates and teachers, mental well-being and so on (Folketinget, 2014; Ministry for Children, Education and Gender Equality, Denmark, 2016b, c, d).

The school day

As part of the Danish school reform of 2014, it was decided that school days should be longer for all pupils in Grades 0–9. Weekly teaching time, including recesses, is mandated at 30 hours for Grades 0–3, at least 33 hours for Grades 4–6 and at least 35 hours for Grades 7–9. Each lesson is 45 minutes long, and lessons are often paired in a 90-minute delivery format. Usually, there is a short break after the first two lessons (10–20 minutes) and a longer lunch break of 20–35 minutes during the day. There are a minimum of two mandatory PE lessons per week in Grades 1–3, three lessons per week in Grades 4–6 and two lessons per week in Grades 7–9 (Folketinget, 2014, Ministry for Children, Education and Gender Equality, Denmark, 2016a, b).

Different solutions for increasing physical activity in the school day

Finland's way of promoting physical activity in schools

The FSM programme began in 2010. The programme coordinates actions aiming to establish a physically active culture in all Finnish comprehensive schools (Grades 1–9). FSM has been funded by the Ministry of Education and Culture and organized by the Board of Education, regional state administrative agencies and various other organizations (Finnish Schools on the Move, 2016). At first, in 2010, one of the main aims of the programme was to implement new national PA recommendations for school-aged children (launched in 2008) in all Finnish comprehensive schools, and thereby encourage children to be physically active in accordance with the recommendations during, before or after school. In the next phase, from 2012 onward, the goal has focused on creating a more active and pleasant school day through PA. Key themes include PA, student participation and learning. In addition to the promotion of PA, the aim has been to decrease excessive and continuous sedentary time.

During the first phase (pilot phase, 2010–2012), the programme comprised 21 local regional projects, including 45 schools and 10,000 students in Grades 1–9 throughout Finland. During the second phase (2012–2015), the programme expanded. By May 2015, 31% of schools (817) were registered in the programme. During the third phase (2015–2018), the goal is to get all comprehensive schools involved in the programme, and 21 million euros have been allocated to support the municipalities via the FSM programme for 2016–2018. Currently, the FSM programme is part of the government programme and is one of the key projects for developing learning environments in basic education (stated in May 2015): "The Schools on the Move project will be expanded across the country to ensure school children one hour of physical activity each day" (Prime minister's office, Finland, 2015). As of May 2016, 62% of schools (1,564 out of 2,523) were registered with the programme.

The schools and municipalities that participate in the programme can implement their own individual plans to enhance PA and diminish students' sedentary time during the school day. Schools have not been required to implement certain specific actions, but many have chosen to increase and promote PA during recesses, lessons and before and after school. Actions to increase PA during recess have been a key element for schools. In many of them, students have been educated to act as 'recess activators', to organize and instruct PA among their peers during recess times. Concrete actions in schools have also included investments in equipment and facilities to motivate recess activities, the change of the school-day structure to allow for prolonged recess periods with organized activities, active breaks during school lessons and the use of physically activating teaching methods.

The programme supports schools and teachers alike by disseminating ideas and practices regarding how to make the school day more physically active, and schools can access ideas by participating in local and national seminars. In addition, the programme provides materials and information about the latest research results and proven practices on its website. Schools also have the opportunity to get help from a local mentor, who offers support with the process, aiming to promote PA in schools. The programme also provides Schools on the Move educational programming for students in teacher education programmes at universities throughout Finland. Furthermore, to help schools implement their unique plans, a guide for how to become a School on the Move has been published, and a self-evaluation tool for PA promotion in schools was developed. The evaluation tool is an online survey consisting of nine sections: organizing actions, PA promotion, school staff participation, student participation, schoolyards and other facilities, educational methods and learning environments, active commuting to school, club activities and cooperation with other important actors (parents, school health services, other schools, municipalities, sports clubs, etc.). After completing the survey, schools get a visual summary of their answers, making them aware of their own courses of action and school culture in terms of PA promotion. It is recommended that schools evaluate the previous school year and then, based on the evaluation, develop action plans for the following year.

Denmark's way of promoting physical activity in schools

Denmark implemented a comprehensive school reform programme in 2014, including, among other things, PA requirements of approximately 45 minutes per day during the school day.

The acceptance of this change in the school system by both the Ministry for Children, Education and Gender Equality and the Danish Parliament can be explained by prior scientific and political discussions. As previously mentioned, the Danish health authorities revised their recommendations in 2013 based on growing scientific knowledge of the area. The new recommendations reaffirmed the importance of PA and fitness, including motor competences, as a tool for increasing students' health, cognition and academic performance (Kunststyrelsen, 2011). The recent recommendations from the World Health Organization on PA (WHO, 2010), and from the European Union on promoting health-enhancing PA across sectors (Council of the European Union, 2013), have also positively affected the general discussion about the role of PA and PE on students' health.

The PA requirements in the reform were quite simple, as mentioned: approximately 45 minutes per day PA must be included during the longer and more varied school day. PA may be included in the subject-divided lessons (e.g. PE and during assisted learning). This may be done by intro-ducing short periods of PA, such as a morning run, ball games or similar, or via other, longer-lasting and continual activities (e.g. in cooperation with local associations such as sports clubs, cultural centres, and so on), or by using PA as a pedagogical tool in working with the contents of the subjects. Focus could also be on increasing PA during recess or making PA at certain hours not connected to lessons. It is the duty of the headteacher to ensure that, within the overall teaching time, pupils participate in PA each day for an average of 45 minutes.

Top-down or bottom-up – results and experiences related to different solutions in Finland and Denmark

Results and experiences from the Finnish model for increasing physical activity in schools

The development of the FSM programme has been followed from the begin-ning of the programme by evaluation research funded by the Ministry of Education and Culture. Surveys and interviews with project coordinators and school staff have been used to monitor the progress of the local projects in schools and municipalities. At the student level, PA has been monitored by surveys and accelerometer measurements. Based on accelerometer meas-urements, students accumulated, on average, 20 minutes of moderate-to-vigorous PA (MVPA) during the school day. For the least active children, who accumulated less than 30 minutes' MVPA per day, PA during the school days comprised 42% of their total daily PA, while for children who accumulated more than the recommended 60 minutes' MVPA per day, PA during the school days comprised 32% of their total daily PA (Tammelin et al., 2016). Furthermore, PA during the school days decreased, and seden-tary time increased by age (Figure 17.1). During recess times, younger stu-dents at primary schools participated more frequently in physically active play and ball games, while older students spent their time mainly sitting and standing (Figure 17.2).

Results from four lower secondary schools between 2010 and 2012 showed that the proportion of students participating in physically active play during recess increased from 30% to 49%; in ball games, the increases were from 33% to 42% (Haapala et al., 2014). However, the increase was mostly observed among males. PA levels increased for females at recess in two schools that organized gender-specific activities or facilities for girls. Overall, organized recess activities, student recess activators (peers) and sports facility development positively impacted students' PA levels. A survey conducted at the end of the programme's pilot phase, in 2012, showed that half of primary

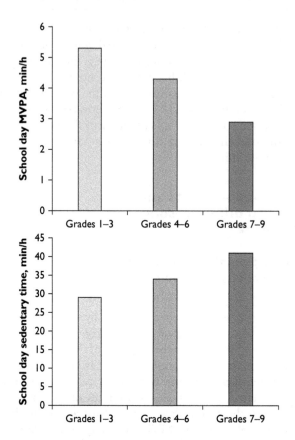

Figure 17.1 School day moderate-to-vigorous physical activity (MVPA) and sedentary time among Finnish students in Grades 1–9 between 2010 and 2015 (Tammelin et al., 2016).

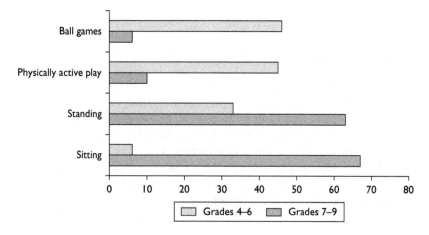

Figure 17.2 Physical activities during recess among Finnish students in Grades 4–9 (Tammelin et al., 2012).

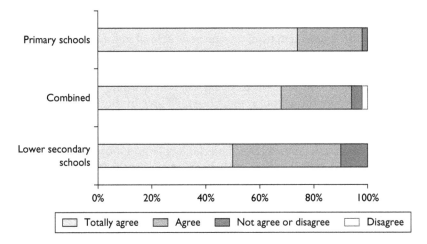

Figure 17.3 School staff answers in response to the statement, 'Physical activity during the school day increases satisfaction with school'. The survey in 2015 was conducted among school staff members at schools involved in the Finnish Schools on the Move programme (*n* = 374).

school students and one-third of lower secondary school students reported increased PA in various forms (Tammelin, Laine, & Turpeinen, 2012).

In 2012, school staff members answered a survey that included questions about their awareness of the programme's goals, students' PA recommendations, staff experiences regarding activities at their school and opinions on the school's role as a provider of PA (Kämppi et al., 2013). The experiences they reported were mostly positive. Most of the respondents believed that the pilot phase had introduced lasting changes in their schools, and most respondents agreed with the statements that PA during the school day had increased satisfaction with the school and that physically active recesses contribute to a peaceful learning environment. Similar results were obtained from a school staff survey in 2015 (Figure 17.3).

Popular reviews, articles, blog postings and short presentations on recent research results have been important tools for motivating school staff members to action; teachers are well educated and generally interested in research. In 2012, the National Board of Education published a literature review on the effects of PA on learning (Syväoja et al., 2012). In addition, published research reports of the follow-up study showing the students' PA levels, teachers' and school staff members' experiences with the programme, and children's participation rates in the planning of actions were all received with enthusiasm.

Results and experiences from the Danish model for increasing physical activity in schools

To monitor the implementation of its new school reform, the Danish Ministry of Education implemented an extensive follow-up and research programme. Furthermore, economic support was given to 11 research projects focusing on PA in relation to cognition and learning. These projects were initiated before the school reform began. Three of these projects were related to public schools, and their results are discussed in this section.

The results of about 3,000 teachers' and pedagogues' responses to a survey are reported in a status report regarding the longer and more varied school day (Jacobsen, Flarup, & Søndergaard, 2015). Among other things, teachers and pedagogues were asked how often they used PA in teaching Danish language and math lessons. The teachers reported using PA to a greater extent in 2015 (after implementation of the reform) compared to 2014 (before the reform). In 2015, 16% of teachers reported using PA every day in teaching, and 78% used it at least once a week. Only 2% reported never using PA during lessons. Teachers of the students' mother tongue, Danish, reported more frequent use of PA during lessons (85%, at least once a week) compared to mathematics teachers (69%). Furthermore, it was most common to use PA during lessons when teaching the youngest children, compared to older children (Figure 17.4). The majority (86%) of teachers in Grades 1–3 reported using PA at least once a week, while the numbers were 84% in Grades 4–6

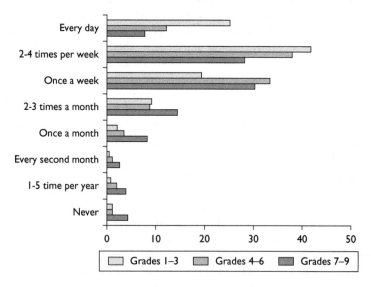

Figure 17.4 Danish teachers of Grades 1 through to 9 (*n* = 2,333) answered the question, 'How often do you use physical activity in your teaching of Danish or mathematics?'

and 66% in Grades 7–9. The difference was even larger when looking at teachers using PA at least twice a week: 67% did so in Grades 1–3, 50% in Grades 4–6 and 36% in Grades 7–9. Furthermore, 50% of teachers believed that students become more ready for learning when exposed to PA; however, 38% did not share this belief, and 12% reported no experience in that area (Jacobsen, Flarup, & Søndergaard, 2015).

The *Status Report Regarding the Pupils' Views on and Experiences with the New Public School* was based on roughly 16,300 students' answers (Nielsen, Hansen, Jensen, & Arendt, 2015). It found that younger children reported a greater amount of PA during school time than older school children (Figure 17.5), whereas no differences were found for leisure-time PA (not shown).

The LCoMotion study was a 20-week cluster randomized controlled trial including seven intervention and seven control schools (Bugge et al., 2014; Tarp et al., 2016). The intervention targeted PA during academic subjects, recess, active school transportation and leisure time (as PA homework). This intervention in many ways mirrored the new Danish school reform, in that schools endeavoured to activate students to be more physically active. Teachers reported an average of 24 minutes of classroom-based or scheduled recess activities per day during the intervention period. However, no significant changes were observed in students' PA levels, cognitive test results or mathematical skills between the intervention and control groups (Tarp et al., 2016). The study revealed some difficulties for teachers and other school staff in implementing PA on demand in the Danish context. This intervention was, like the reform itself, not based on either teachers' or pupils' views, and there was not a large allocation of resources. The lack of time to prepare and organize activities well was another of the problems teachers mentioned during qualitative interviews. In particular, when PA is integrated into academic subjects, it requires a lot of preparation, and, in this project,

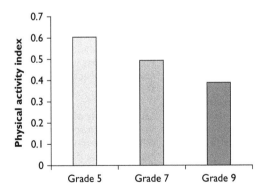

Figure 17.5 School time physical activity index (0 = no, 1 = high) among Danish students in Grades 5, 7 and 9 (*n* = 13,661).

the teachers did not feel that the aims of the project could mirror the actual time allocated for the preparation of their lectures (Bugge & Froberg, 2015).

Taken together, the results indicate that teachers reported more use of PA after the school reform (2015 vs. 2014), but there is still room for improvement when it comes to implementing PA during the school day, especially in the upper grades. The impact of increased PA on learning outcomes is, however, difficult to assess. A stronger emphasis on allocating time and resources for teacher upgrading and preparation should be recommended.

Discussion and directions for future studies

Both countries and approaches have some strengths, but there are also challenges related to promoting PA in school contexts, as presented in Table 17.1.

Certain elements of Finland's FSM programme may have contributed to its success as an initiative and can be considered a strength of this bottom-up approach (Table 17.1). Voluntary participation in the programme and

Table 17.1 Summary of the strengths and challenges of different approaches to increase physical activity during the school day

Approach, country	Strengths	Challenges
Bottom-up, Finland	• Participation is voluntary for schools • Schools can choose their own actions • Feeling of ownership of the process in schools at all levels • Broad and multidisciplinary approach taking into account school contentment, learning and well-being • Aiming toward permanent changes in school culture • Funding opportunities to begin and catalyse the programme's development • Strong political support – part of a government programme	• Change in school culture is relatively slow • Relatively small changes in physical activity levels at the student level • More cost-effective tools and means are needed in schools to activate students • Voluntary participation for students; no clear answers about how to motivate the least active students to participate • Involvement of all the school staff may be difficult, and key volunteers may become exhausted • Continuity of actions is not secured
Top-down, Denmark	• All public schools are included • Clear political support • Fast and comprehensive change • Different ways of increasing physical activity are possible • Autonomy is given to schools	• Lack of feeling of ownership of the process in schools by both school staff and students • Many teachers do not have the necessary competences to implement the programme • Lack of appropriate facilities and economic resources

the opportunity for each school to select and implement activities that are appropriate have appeared to enhance not only principals' and teachers', but also students', feelings of ownership of the process. Overall, the FSM has been perceived as a positive and successful programme among school staff. This might be due to the broad and multidisciplinary approach, which highlights the meaning of PA for learning and school contentment and shows the importance of student participation, the involvement of municipalities and the government. These actions have seemed to influence the introduction of long-lasting solutions and more permanent changes for PA in the schools' cultures.

Furthermore, the Finnish school system, featuring the autonomy of schools and teachers relative to timetables and teaching methods and the flexible structure of the school day, including recesses, has enabled the efforts to increase PA in schools.

Despite the above, it seems that the improvements in students' PA levels have been relatively small. Opportunities for increasing the amount of PA during the school day are limited when mandatory PE lessons are not added, but PA is added to recess time and academic lessons. It takes some time for the actions taken to manifest in schools, and as a result, long-term and systematic development work is required to increase children's PA during the school day. In addition, support for the volunteers and key persons at school sites should be guaranteed, and ways for motivating teachers and school staff not directly involved in the concept should be developed. There is a need for concrete and effective tools and means for schools to activate children, especially the least active children, and to improve student participation in the PA planning processes. Teachers, especially in lower secondary schools, feels that is not easy to get students to be active and it demands extra work. Therefore, actions directed toward older students, and support for their teachers, are needed.

Recent Danish reports have shown that it may be possible to implement more PA and movement in all public schools. The strengths of this top-down approach in Denmark have included clear and strong support from the government, which has guaranteed the involvement of all schools and fast and comprehensive change. In addition, schools have been given autonomy, enabling them to select and implement different activities that are appropriate for them to make school days more physically active. However, the challenges include both teachers and pupils feeling a lack of ownership of the process and a lack of appropriate PA facilities. Furthermore, many teachers may not have the necessary competences to activate children during the school day.

To rise above these challenges, it is recommended that the vision of more PA and movement in all types of schools be embedded in the institutions' strategies, along with the support of their boards, managers, teachers and parents. Involving pupils in the planning process can also have a positive impact on the implementation of PA sessions, especially when communication and relationship formation with peers are priorities in the activities.

It will be necessary to investigate whether teachers and education professionals have the adequate skills for using PA at school, and, if not, to support their acquisition of the necessary competences. It will also be essential to revise professional teacher training programmes to ensure they contain contents that offer new teachers necessary basic knowledge about the importance of PA for general health, cognition and learning outcomes and tools to implement this knowledge in practice.

There are still significant limitations to our knowledge about the types, amounts and intensities of activity that are most important for students' health and learning. We also lack knowledge about the best implementation methods in relation to the different age groups in schools. Hopefully, future research in this area can shed light on these issues.

The new Danish school reform provides a good basis from which to monitor the implementation and processes that will take place in various schools over the coming years. Now, given the opportunity through research grants to follow this development closely, it will also be possible within a few years to come up with qualified bids for the 'best and next practices' in relation to the implementation of PA and movement in Danish children's and young people's everyday lives. Similarly, the progress of the FSM programme and its development in different schools and municipalities will be evaluated in forthcoming years.

Even though the approaches for increasing PA in the school context have been different between Finland and Denmark, there are common strengths and challenges amid both approaches. Most probably, the best approach is to include elements from both top-down and bottom-up approaches. It is therefore recommended that other countries working for a successful implementation of PA during the school day focus on having strong political support, and also giving schools and teachers autonomy to choose their actions and the facilities and resources to carry out these actions. From the research point of view, in order to implement research results into practice, it is important that the development processes are evaluated and that research results are presented in a popular and inspiring way with a clear message. In addition, it is important to highlight those impacts of PA that have direct effects on the school day: learning, contentment and well-being among both students and teachers. The Danish school reform and the FSM programme will hopefully offer tools to increase the level of PA and establish physically active lifestyles in children in the years to come, and, in the process, improve their general health, cognition and academic achievements.

References

Bangsbo, J., Krustrup, P., Duda, J., Hillman, C., Andersen, L. B., Weiss, M., . . . Elbe, A-M. (2016). The Copenhagen Consensus Conference 2016: Children, youth, and physical activity in schools and during leisure time. *British Journal of Sports Medicine, 50*(19), 1177–1178.

Budde, H., Voelcker-Rehage, C., Pietraßyk-Kendziorra, S., Ribeiro, P., & Tidow, G. (2008). Acute coordinative exercise improves attentional performance in adolescents. *Neuroscience Letters, 441*(2), 219–223.

Bugge, A., & Froberg, K. (Eds.). (2015). *Learning by moving (Forsøg med Læring i Bevægelse)*. University of Southern Denmark. Retrieved from http://static.sdu.dk/mediafiles//C/E/E/%7BCEE2E548-DBAB-42EC-A284-7753E1C6EFD0%7DRapport_Fors%C3%B8g_L%C3%A6ring_i_Bev%C3%A6gelse_2015.pdf.

Bugge, A., Tarp, J., Østergaard, L., Domazet, S. L., Andersen, L. B., & Froberg, K. (2014). LCoMotion – Learning, cognition and motion: A multicomponent cluster randomized school-based intervention aimed at increasing learning and cognition – rationale, design and methods. *BMC Public Health, 14*, 967. doi: http://doi.org/10.1186/1471-2458-14-967.

Caterino, M. C., & Polak, E. D. (1999). Effects of two types of activity on the performance of second-, third-, and fourth-grade students on a test of concentration. *Perceptual and Motor Skills, 89*(1), 245–248.

Chaddock, L., Erickson, K. I., Prakash, R. S., VanPatter, M., Voss, M. W., Pontifex, M. B., . . . Kramer, A. F. (2010a). Basal ganglia volume is associated with aerobic fitness in preadolescent children. *Developmental Neuroscience, 32*(3), 249–256.

Chaddock, L., Erickson, K. I., Prakash, R. S., Kim, J. S., Voss, M. W., VanPatter, M., . . . Cohen, N. J. (2010b). A neuroimaging investigation of the association between aerobic fitness, hippocampal volume, and memory performance in preadolescent children. *Brain Research, 1358*, 172–183.

Chaddock-Heyman, L., Erickson, K. I., Voss, M., Knecht, A., Pontifex, M. B., Castelli, D., . . . Kramer, A. (2013). The effects of physical activity on functional MRI activation associated with cognitive control in children: A randomized controlled intervention. *Frontiers in Human Neuroscience, 7*, 72.

Council of the European Union. (2013). *Council recommendation on promoting health-enhancing physical activity across sectors*. Interinstitutional File: 2013/0291 (NLE). Brussels: Council of the European Union.

Danish Health Authority. (2014). *Recommendations for children and adolescents (5–17 years old)*. Retrieved from https://sundhedsstyrelsen.dk/en/health-and-lifestyle/physical-activity/recommendations/recommendations-for-children-and-adolescents.

Davenport, M. H., Hogan, D. B., Eskes, G. A., Longman, R. S., & Poulin, M. J. (2012). Cerebrovascular reserve: The link between fitness and cognitive function? *Exercise and Sport Sciences Reviews, 40*(3), 153–158.

Davis, C. L., Tomporowski, P. D., McDowell, J. E., Austin, B. P., Miller, P. H., Yanasak, N. E., . . . Naglieri, J. A. (2011). Exercise improves executive function and achievement and alters brain activation in overweight children: A randomized, controlled trial. *Health Psychology, 30*(1), 91.

Donnelly, J. E., Hillman, C. H., Castelli, D., Etnier, J. L., Lee, S., Tomporowski, P., . . . Szabo-Reed, A. N. (2016). Physical activity, fitness, cognitive function, and academic achievement in children. *Medicine and Science in Sports and Exercise, 48*(6), 1197–1222. doi: http://doi.org/10.1249/MSS.0000000000000901.

Ekelund, U., Tomkinson, G., & Armstrong, N. (2011). What proportion of youth are physically active? Measurement issues, levels and recent time trends. *British Journal of Sports Medicine, 45*(11), 859–865. doi: http://doi.org/10.1136/bjsports-2011-090190.

Finnish Ministry of Education, the National Board of Education (Finland), & CIMO. (2012). *Finnish education in a nutshell.* Espoo, Finland: Kopijyvä. Retrieved from http://www.oph.fi/download/146428_Finnish_Education_in_a_Nutshell.pdf.

Finnish National Board of Education. (2016a). *Basic education.* Retrieved from http://www.oph.fi/english/curricula_and_qualifications/basic_education.

Finnish National Board of Education. (2016b). *Education system.* Retrieved from http://www.oph.fi/english/education_system.

Finnish Schools on the Move. (2016). *Increasing physical activity and decreasing sedentary time among school-aged children.* Retrieved from http://www.liikku vakoulu.fi/in-english.

Folketinget (2014). *Folketinget 2013–14, Lovforslag nr. L 150. Forslag til Lov om ændring af lov om folkeskolen og forskellige andre love.* Fremsat den 27. februar 2014 af undervisningsministeren. [The National Parliament of Denmark (2014). The National Parliament of Denmark 2013–14, Bill # L 150. Bill regarding Law on changing the law on public schools and other laws. Proposed February 27, 2014 by the Minister of Education]. http://www.ft.dk/samling/20131/lovforslag/l150/index.htm.

Haapala, H. L., Hirvensalo, M. H., Laine, K., Laakso, L., Hakonen, H., Lintunen, T., & Tammelin, T. H. (2014). Adolescents' physical activity at recess and actions to promote a physically active school day in four Finnish schools. *Health Education Research, 29*(5), 1–13. doi: http://doi.org/10.1093/her/cyu030.

Hillman, C. H., Pontifex, M. B., Castelli, D. M., Khan, N. A., Raine, L. B., Scudder, M. R., . . . Kamijo, K. (2014). Effects of the FITKids randomized controlled trial on executive control and brain function. *Pediatrics, 134*(4), e1063–e1071.

Hillman, C. H., Pontifex, M. B., Raine, L. B., Castelli, D. M., Hall, E. E., & Kramer, A. F. (2009). The effect of acute treadmill walking on cognitive control and academic achievement in preadolescent children. *Neuroscience, 159*(3), 1044–1054.

Hopkins, M. E., Davis, F. C., VanTieghem, M. R., Whalen, P. J., & Bucci, D. J. (2012). Differential effects of acute and regular physical exercise on cognition and affect. *Neuroscience, 215*, 59–68.

Inchley, J., Currie, D., Young, T., Samdal, O., Torsheim, T., Augustson, L., . . . Barnekow, V. (Eds.). (2016). *Growing up unequal: Gender and socioeconomic differences in young people's health and well-being. Health Behaviour in School-aged Children (HBSC) study: International report from the 2013/2014 survey.* Copenhagen: WHO Regional Office for Europe (Health Policy for Children and Adolescents no. 7). Retrieved from http://www.euro.who.int/__data/assets/pdf_file/0003/303438/HSBC-No7-Growing-up-unequal-full-report.pdf?ua=1.

Jacobsen, R. H., Flarup, L. H., & Søndergaard, N. M. (2015). *A longer and more varied school day. En længere og mere varieret skoledag. [KORA, Det Nationale Institut for Kommuners og Regioners Analyse og Forskning].* Retrieved from http://www.uvm.dk/Uddannelser/Folkeskolen/Viden-og-kompetencer/Publika-tioner-fra-forskningsprojekter.

Kamijo, K., Pontifex, M. B., O'Leary, K. C., Scudder, M. R., Wu, C. T., Castelli, D. M., & Hillman, C. H. (2011). The effects of an afterschool physical activity program on working memory in preadolescent children. *Developmental Science, 14*(5), 1046–1058.

Kunststyrelsen. (2011). *Fysisk aktivitet og læring – en konsensuskonference, Kulturministeriets Udvalg for Idrætsforskning.* [Physical activity and learning – a consensus conference, Ministry of Culture, Committee for Sports Science Research]. Retrieved from http://kum.dk/uploads/tx_templavoila/Fysisk%20aktivitet%20og%20laring_KIF.pdf.

Kämppi, K., Asanti, R., Hirvensalo, M., Laine, K., Pönkkö, A., Romar, J. E., & Tammelin, T. (2013). *A more pleasant and peaceful learning environment – school staff's experiences and views on promoting a physical activity based operating culture in school.* LIKES Research Reports on Sport and Health 269. Jyväskylä, Finland: LIKES – Foundation for Sport and Health Sciences.

Ministry for Children, Education and Gender Equality, Denmark. (2016a). *The Folkeskole.* Retrieved from http://eng.uvm.dk/Education/Primary-and-lower-secondary-education/The-Folkeskole.

Ministry for Children, Education and Gender Equality, Denmark. (2016b). *Lifelong learning.* Retrieved from http://eng.uvm.dk/Education/General/Lifelong-learning.

Ministry for Children, Education and Gender Equality, Denmark. (2016c). *Timetal.* Retrieved from http://www.uvm.dk/Uddannelser/Folkeskolen/Fag-timetal-og-overgange/Timetal.

Ministry for Children, Education and Gender Equality, Denmark. (2016d). *Trivselsmåling.* Retrieved from http://www.uvm.dk/Uddannelser/Folkeskolen/Elevplaner-nationale-test-og-trivselsmaaling/Trivselsmaaling.

Ministry of Education and Culture, Finland. (2016). *Education system in Finland.* Retrieved from http://www.minedu.fi/OPM/Koulutus/koulutusjaerjestelmae/?lang=en.

Ministry of Education and Young Finland Association. (2008). *Recommendations for the physical activity of school-aged children.* (Finnish report, abstract in English). Helsinki: Reprotalo Lauttasaari.

Nielsen, C. P., Hansen, A. T., Jensen, V. M., & Arendt, K. S. (2015). *Status report regarding the pupils' views on and experiences with the new public school.* [Folkeskolereformen. Beskrielse af 2. dataindsamling blandt elever. SFI, Det Nationale Forskningscenter for Velfærd]. Retrieved from http://www.uvm.dk/Uddannelser/Folkeskolen/Viden-og-kompetencer/Publikationer-fra-forskningsprojekter.

Prime minister's office, Finland. (2015). *Finland, a land of solutions.* Strategic Programme of Prime Minister Juha Sipilä's Government. 29 May 2015. Government Publications 12/2015. Retrieved from http://vnk.fi/en/publication?pubid=6407.

Syväoja, H., Kantomaa, M., Laine, K., Jaakkola, T., Pyhältö, K., & Tammelin, T. (2012). *Physical activity and learning. Summary.* Status review, October 2012. Muistiot 2012: 5. Helsinki: National Board of Education. Retrieved from http://www.oph.fi/download/145366_Physical_activity_and_learning.pdf.

Tammelin, T., Kulmala, J., Hakonen, H., & Kallio, J. (2016). *School makes you move and sit still. Finnish Schools on the Move research results from 2010 to 2015.* Jyväskylä, Finland: LIKES – Research Center for Sport and Health Sciences / Finnish Schools on the Move programme.

Tammelin, T., Laine, K., & Turpeinen, S. (2012). *Final report on the Finnish Schools on the Move programme's pilot phase 2010–2012.* LIKES Research Reports on Sport and Health 261. Jyväskylä, Finland: LIKES – Foundation for Sport and Health Sciences.

Tarp, J., Domazet, S. L., Froberg, K., Hillman, C. H., Andersen, L. B., & Bugge, A. (2016). Effectiveness of a school-based physical activity intervention on cognitive performance in Danish adolescents: LCoMotion – Learning, Cognition and Motion – A cluster randomized controlled trial. *PLOS One, 11*(6), e0158087. doi: http://doi.org/10.1371/journal.pone.0158087.

Tuckman, B. W., & Hinkle, J. S. (1986). An experimental study of the physical and psychological effects of aerobic exercise on schoolchildren. *Health Psychology, 5*(3), 197.

WHO. (2010). *Global recommendations of physical activity for health*. Geneva: WHO Press.

Chapter 18

Science, pseudoscience and exercise neuroscience

Untangling the good, the bad and the ugly

Richard Bailey

Introduction

The chapters in this book have sought to review current state and status of exercise neuroscience, and particularly to examine how this rapidly developing field might inform decisions about educational practice. Some chapters are technical, and report on the results of scientific experimentation, whilst others are more applied. However, the contributions have been informed by a recognition of the need to move research beyond the ivory tower into real-life settings, addressing key questions about the ways in which the emerging knowledge of the brain can help teachers and other educational practitioners. This is likely to be an ongoing task, facilitated by a reciprocal interaction between scientific research and practical knowledge.

Recent years have seen new research methods that have led to remarkable progress in the understanding of the neurological basis of human cognition and learning. For example, in 2011, fewer than 750 published scientific articles used findings from functional magnetic resonance imaging (fMRI) on the human brain. By the beginning of 2017, there were 32,500 fMRI studies reported in the PubMed database. fMRI and other imaging techniques have allowed researchers to look inside the living brain, creating images that locate regions of activity associated with specific cognitive tasks, as well as revealing structural differences among individual brains (Passingham & Rowe, 2015). Detailed understanding of the biochemistry of brain, intracellular recording, pharmacological interventions and other technologies has also developed at an accelerated pace (Pokorski, 2015). Combined with psychological research, these studies have greatly improved the understanding of the basic processes that underlie capabilities such as numeracy, literacy, attention, memory and social interaction (Immordino-Yang, 2016; Mareschal, Butterworth, & Tolmie, 2014). Understandably, these advances have sparked a great deal of interest in the possibility of improving learning and education using brain research, especially among teachers (Pickering & Howard-Jones, 2007; Serpati & Loughan, 2012). In an era of evidence-based practice, the new educational neuroscience seems an enthralling prospect.

The authors of a highly influential report from the Organisation for Economic Co-operation and Development (OECD) interpreted the scientific basis as the neural base, and asked whether 'it is acceptable, in any reflection about education, not to take into consideration what is known about the learning brain' (OECD, 2007, p. 28). Scientists tend to be rather more cautious of making bold claims, preferring to wait for more and better evidence (e.g. Della Sala, 2009; Goswami, 2014). However, the excitement surrounding this area of research is palpable.

It may well be the case that the relationship between physical activity and educational performance is one area of research capable of generating genuine insights for practice (Bailey, 2016). This has been hinted at by authors from the broad field of educational neuroscience, within which exercise neuroscience could be partly located (e.g. Dekker, Lee, Howard-Jones, & Jolles, 2012). But here, as in other areas of applied neuroscience, there exists a perennial risk of the intrusion of dubious claims and practices. This chapter discusses the danger of the phenomenon of pseudoscience, which is ideas or practices that seek to resemble real science but which fail to follow its guiding principles. Specifically, this chapter focuses on the intrusion of pseudoscience into educationally orientated activities, including physical activity and movement. Pseudoscience shadows real science as bird excrement sticks to statues, and it is argued that it presents serious difficulties for those seeking to move towards evidence-based practice in schools.

One way of thinking about this situation is in terms of 'the good', 'the bad' and 'the ugly'. Good research follows the procedures of the scientific method, with its established methods, analyses, checks and balances. Bad research fails to follows the protocols of the scientific method in some significant ways. Ugly research is bad, but adds an important additional element: it harms the people exposed to it. The risk of ugly science in the context of health is obvious, leaving patients worse off or even dead as result of 'quack' treatments (Singh & Ernst, 2008), but there are serious risks in education, too. The presence of bad and ugly neuroscience in the classroom is problematic because it wastes money, time and effort which might be better spent on the development of evidence-based practices.

What is the appeal of so-called 'brain-based' claims for schools? Has the growth of brain-based theories and practices outside of mainstream academic science been a useful development, a harmless distraction or positively risky for children's education and well-being? In seeking out answers to these questions, this chapter examines some of the most popular brain-based ideas and products that are currently being used in schools around the world, focusing on those that include aspects of physical activity and movement. It asks whether there is sufficient quality evidence to justify their place, which requires some discussion about the nature of evidence, science and its unreliable alter ego, pseudoscience. The rise and spread of pseudoscience, it is argued, threaten the integrity and development of education, and are genuine causes for concern that requires addressing by teachers, scientists and policy makers. The chapter concludes by suggesting some strategies for addressing this problem, and to ensure that students in schools are exposed to ideas and practices based on science, not nonsense.

The appeal and danger of brain-based approaches in education

Historically, the relationship between educational practice and empirical science has been an uncomfortable one. Difficulties in making meaningful connections between practice and evidence are not restricted to education, of course, and numerous fields, from sports coaching to medicine, are struggling with similar concerns (see, for example, Fulford, 2008). This is not to suggest that there is not a broad consensus that these areas should be informed by evidence, but there appears to be much less agreement about what this means in practice. For example, there is widespread interest among teachers, parents and policy makers in the application of neuroscientific research findings in educational practice. One study found that almost 90% of teachers in the UK considered knowledge of brain functioning to be relevant for their work (Pickering & Howard-Jones, 2007). In some circles, interest has morphed into a 'neuromania' (Legrenzi & Umilta, 2011), or a general sense of optimism that understanding the brain will help solve many previously intractable educational and social problems.

It seems, though, that a general receptiveness to the idea of neuroscience has not yet translated into changes to practice in classrooms. More accurately, the combination of interest in all things 'neuro', and the persistent difficulty of finding meaningful connections between scientists and practitioners, have created a fertile space in which a plethora of so-called 'brain-based' products, of highly variable scientific quality, have flooded into schools (Coch & Ansari, 2012). Many teachers who have been exposed to such materials assume a direct link between their often-ambitious claims and genuine science (Goswami, 2014). However, unlike real science, pseudoscience typically offers simple solutions to problems that routinely challenge teachers in classrooms.

It is important to stress that these concerns are not merely academic. To claim that a theory or practice is scientific is to present it as possessing a degree of value and credibility. In practice, it means that there is an implication that those ideas have been rigorously debated, refined and tested, and that they have survived that process. The science writer, Carl Sagan (2011), captured the spirit of science when he wrote:

> At the heart of science is an essential balance between two seemingly contradictory attitudes – an openness to new ideas, no matter how bizarre or counterintuitive they may be, and the most ruthless sceptical

scrutiny of all ideas, old and new. This is how deep truths are winnowed from deep nonsense.

(Sagan, 2011, p. 304)

The label of science does not indicate certainty or proof, but it does point to a provisional survival of a process of repeated, critical discussions, and ruthless experimentation. Untested ideas that use the language and imagery of science seek to leech off the credibility of science.

The translation of scientific research into practice is always going to be a challenge. Science is not simplistically prescriptive; it is primarily *descriptive*. In order words, science seeks to learn the truth about the world as it exists independently of human observation (Psillos, 1999); it is not particularly qualified, not typically willing to, advise about the practical or moral implications of its findings. So, even the most valid and reliable research findings cannot be applied into schools without serious consideration of the multiple factors that influence student learning and the inherent social complexity of schooling (Bailey, 2016). A difficulty that is specific to the neurosciences is that adding even meaningless references to the brain makes claims more persuasive (Weisberg, Keil, Goldstein, Rawson, & Gray, 2008).

The field of neuroscience is complex and the accurate transfer of research findings to the classroom is often difficult (Devonshire & Dommett, 2010). This gap between neuroscience and education has enabled many misconceptions about scientific findings to occur (Goswami, 2006). In 2002, the OECD drew international attention to this phenomenon. The organization raised concerns with regard to the rapid proliferation of so-called 'neuromyths'. These were defined as 'a misconception generated by a misunderstanding, a misreading, or a misquoting of facts scientifically established (by brain research) to make a case for use of brain research in education and other contexts'. There is little doubt that neuromyths abound in education, and their popularity has proved a major obstacle for disseminating genuine neuroscience (Fischer, 2009).

Many neuromyths are patently absurd, such as the suggestion that people generally use only 10% of their brain's capacity (cf. Geake, 2008). Presumably, part of the appeal of such beliefs lies in their promise of extraordinary potential change. Indeed, numerous films have been premised on precisely this beguiling thought: if a way to use more of the brain could be discovered, lives would be transformed. That many people seem to believe such ideas says a great deal about the power of appealing ideas to trump awkward scientific details (people using 10% of their brains would be registered brain-dead). Indeed, an early study examining neuroscientific knowledge in the general population of Brazil reported that the 10% neuromyth was the most prevalent misconception among the public (Herculano-Houzel, 2002).

Likewise, the misinterpretation of laterality studies to produce so-called 'left- and right-brained thinking' appears to rely for its appeal on the potential benefits that would follow its realization. There are countless products currently being sold to schools and parents that promise to facilitate some sort of integration of the left and right hemispheres of the brain, and many of these involve movement-based practices (such as Brain Gym, which will be discussed later). However, these products are based on a serious misunderstanding. The original laterality studies were of patients who had the major communication tract between the two brain hemispheres, the corpus callosum, surgically severed to reduce life-threatening epilepsy. Over time, the predicament of these poor people has somehow become generalized to the claim that almost everyone's head contains two relatively independently operating brains, and suffers from a communication breakdown between these two hemispheres. Moreover, it is usually claimed, only some special technique can get the two brains talking to each other again. Scientific understanding of the brain continues to grow, but the brain does not consist of two hemispheres operating in isolation (Eagleman, 2015). In fact, the different specialties of the left and right hemisphere are so well integrated that processing problems almost never occur. Creative thinking, the most common context for discussions of left- and right-brained thinking, is particularly dependent on interaction of both sides, as neither one can operate in isolation from the other. In fact, connectivity, not isolation, best characterizes the operation of the normal human brain (Mayringer & Wimmer, 2002).

Another popular product is Neuro-linguistic Programming (NLP; Bandler & Grinder, 1979). As the name suggest, NLP clearly aspires to align itself to the neurosciences, despite the problematic detail that it was developed before the current understanding of the brain took shape, and has retained much of its original content. Bandler and Grinder were mathematics student and linguistics lecturer respectively, and their lack of background in any discipline connected to the scientific study of the brain is a further concern. Nonetheless, NLP is hugely popular, and its claims that eye movements give insight into thought processes, that certain language patterns can subliminally influence others' behaviour and that the skills of experts can be learned with relative ease by identifying and coding their unconscious thought processes have bled into sport psychology, teacher education, professional development, talent identification and other areas (Carey, Churches, Hutchinson, Jones, & Tosey, 2010; Hippolyte & Théraulaz, unknown[1]; Lazarus & Cohen, 2009). A survey of British national governing bodies for sport found that NLP content could be found on most coach education programmes (Bailey, 2013).

The scientific status of NLP is controversial, and this is largely due to a disjunction between the often extremely ambitious claims made on its behalf by advocates and the relative lack of serious research in support of those claims. The academic response to NLP has generally been either to dismiss or ignore it (Witkowski, 2010). Beyerstein (1990) wrote that, 'though it claims neuroscience in its pedigree, NLP's outmoded view of the relationship between cognitive style and brain function ultimately boils down to crude analogies' (p. 27). A Delphi study (a survey of experts' opinions) listed NLP among 'discredited psychological treatments' (Norcross, Koocher, & Garofalo, 2006) and NLP is frequently included in lists of questionable or pseudoscientific methods (e.g. Tardif, Doudin, & Meylan, 2015).

Some supporters have responded by claiming that the evidence base for NLP is much stronger than critics present. Perhaps the most noteworthy of these responses is the 'research paper' by Carey et al. (2010). Part of the interest in this document is that it was published by the Centre for British Teachers (CfBT) Education Trust, an organization that has been closely involved with the delivery of aspects of UK government educational policy. The report begins with what is erroneously called a systematic review of the literature (erroneous, because none of the standard protocols for this specific type of review are followed, including explicit inclusion/exclusion criteria and search strings, the use of multiple databases and independent validation).[2]

After dismissing the relevance of 'occasional critical academic commentaries', the authors summarize their sources:

- journal articles (including articles that were not peer-reviewed);
- conference papers;
- 'Articles which had some form of university affiliation and articles whose writers had some form of university affiliation or track record in research';
- papers connected to government programmes and which presented evaluation data;
- postgraduate-level research findings (at both Masters and Doctoral level);
- practitioner findings published in journal articles and papers with some element of university or recognized research organization affiliation.

The result of this search strategy is a collection of findings, the great majority of which have never been through standard peer review, and seems to bias the selection to the work of people with a personal commitment to the topic. The condition that sources need to be 'some form of university affiliation' does not contribute anything at all to the assurance of quality, as it would allow students at the very start of their academic careers, but also individuals with only the most marginal connection with academic research. Interestingly, the literature review includes no reference to the critical literature on NLP (e.g. Witkowski, 2010).

The rest of the report is dominated by '24 teacher-led action research case studies' (p. 6), in which teachers explored the use of NLP in their classrooms, following a short course. These case studies do not seem to follow any recognized method for either action research (e.g. McNiff, 2013) or for the generation of case studies (e.g. Yin, 2013). Instead, they amount to little more than anecdotal reports of 'positive impact', 'reduced misbehaviour', and improved understanding of the 'needs of pupils'. No measures are given to support these findings, but the authors of this report were nonetheless able to state confidently that 'The evidence . . . clearly suggests that this project had a significant impact for the teachers and the schools involved' (Carey et al., 2010, p. 26). It may be the case that these experiments led to some improvements for students. It might also be the case that they caused harm. In the absence of some objective measures, such claims are meaningless.

Brain Gym, or sometimes Educational Kinesiology, is a very popular commercial brain-based programme, founded on the premise that learning problems are caused when different sections of the brain and body do not work in a coordinated manner, thereby blocking a student's ability to learn. To overcome these learning blocks, 26 simple movements are prescribed that are designed to improve the integration of specific brain functions with body movements. Students are led through combinations of crawling, drawing, tracing symbols in the air and yawning (yawning is claimed to improve eyesight; Dennison & Dennison, 1994). Lying behind Brain Gym's activities are three main theoretical hypotheses that have been borrowed and adapted from older theories: neurological repatterning, cerebral dominance and perceptual–motor training (Dennison & Dennison, 1994). Neurological repatterning is based on the idea that children develop in a linear manner, and that they must acquire specific motor skills during different developmental stages. If the skills associated with any of the developmental stages are missed, then neurological development is hindered and learning abilities are limited (Crain, 2000). For example, an infant who walks before crawling will miss a critical step in motor development, which could account for future difficulties with more complex neurological processes, such as reading. The treatment for this problem, therefore, is to teach the child to crawl, with the idea that this would repattern the neurons, leaving the child neurologically intact and ready to acquire academic skills. Cerebral dominance maintains that students who do not have a dominant hemisphere of the brain have weaker cognitive abilities, specifically difficulties with reading (Howard-Jones et al., 2007). The exercises of Brain Gym are intended to improve this hemispheric control (Dennison, 2009). Finally, perceptual motor training traces specific learning problems to the poor integration of visual, auditory and movement skills. So, teaching certain perceptual skills will result in the improvement of learning.

None of the foundational principles, at least as they are interpreted in Brain Gym, have empirical support (Hyatt, 2007). The Committee on Children with Disabilities (1999) has repeatedly denounced neurological repatterning, expressing serious concerns with the procedures, the claims of successful interventions and the concomitant lack of empirical evidence.

Cummins' (1988) comprehensive analysis of the effectiveness of neurological repatterning found that results supporting its effectiveness come from a small number of poorly controlled studies, and that there was no further evidence in its favour since that time (Ruhaak & Cook, 2016). It seems likely that any improvements observed in children following the programme are attributable to increased activity levels and attention paid to them. The cerebral dominance hypothesis seems to be based on a misunderstanding of the neuroscientific concept of modality, the fact that some parts of the brain do seem to be more involved in specific activities and emotions (Eagleman, 2015). However, it does not follow, as Brain Gym assumes, that individual parts of the brain control different processes and movements. The relationship between the two hemispheres of the brain is extremely complex, but nothing in the current understanding supports cerebral dominance (Hausmann, 2017). Finally, despite its continued popularity in some quarters, the effectiveness of perceptual motor training as an academic intervention has never been demonstrated (Kavale & Forness, 1987; Ruhaak & Cook, 2016).

Despite its unstable foundations, Brain Gym supporters continue to promote its methods, and schools continue to include them in their curriculum (Tardif et al., 2015). In addition, academic papers continue to be produced claiming to support Brain Gym's claims (e.g. Donczik & Bocker, 2009; Brain Gym International, 2003). However, scrutiny of this literature gives rise to some concerns. The most obvious is that hardly any of this literature is published in peer-reviewed academic journals, but appears in the in-house *Brain Gym® Journal*. Brain Gym International (2003) explains this in terms of the mainstream scientific community's exclusive interest in studies that have been undertaken experimentally with control groups and demonstrating statistical significance. This is not true, nor is the claim that scientific journals will not publish research that has previously appeared in *Brain Gym® Journal*. Ironically, many of the articles compiled to demonstrate the effectiveness of Brain Gym still claim statistical significance and the use of experimental techniques (e.g. Donczik & Bocker, 2009). In many of these cases, the problems seem to arise not from the scientific establishment's exclusionary practices, but from quite fundamental errors in methodology, such as misinterpreting statistical significance, use of incomparable control groups, failing to account for maturational effects.

By far the most researched neuromyth is learning styles, and academic interest in this subject reflects its very widespread acceptance in many countries (cf. Dekker et al., 2012). In fact, the term learning styles embraces a varied set of claims, inventories and models for assessment (Coffield, Moseley, Hall, & Ecclestone, 2004), but each of these theories maintains that people learn in qualitatively different ways, and that formal experiences can be tailored to the individual learning style of the student. For example, a very common form of the theory promotes the 'VAK' model, in which some people learn best by observing ('visual learners'), some by listening ('auditory learners'), and some by doing and moving ('kinaesthetic learners'). Learning styles theory also maintains that difficulties in school can often be traced to a mismatch between the student's learning style and the ways in which information is presented by the teacher (Coffield et al., 2004).

The VAK version of learning styles offers an attractive alternative to more traditional approaches to teaching, combining a scientifically appearing, but simple, framework for learning with the promise of addressing perennial problems of learning difficulties and lack of motivation. It certainly seems to be the case that teachers are often inclined to accept its claims. A review of studies from the UK, the Netherlands, Turkey, Greece and China found that more than 90% of teachers agreed that students learn better when they receive information tailored to their preferred learning styles (Howard-Jones, 2014). Similar findings from studies with teachers and trainee teachers in Portugal (Rato, Abreu, & Castro-Caldas, 2013), Latin America (Gleichgerrcht, Lira Luttges, Salvarezza, & Campos, 2015), Turkey (Dündar, & Gündüz, 2016) and China (Pei, Howard-Jones, Zhang, Liu, & Jin, 2015) suggest that learning styles have a firm foothold in educational practice around the world.

These findings suggest that learning styles are generally accepted by both professionals and the general population, and the quantity of books, articles and websites on the subject might suggest that the hypothesis at the heart of the theory – that matching teaching style to students' learning style – leads to improved learning, has been well studied, but that conclusion would be incorrect (Rogowsky, Calhoun, & Tallal, 2014). In fact, there is no compelling evidence that matching formal instruction to individual perceptual strengths and weaknesses is any more effective than instruction which is not multisensory-specific (Rohrer & Pashler, 2012). Teaching according to an assumed preference may even cause harm, as learning is best promoted by taking students out of their comfort zone, not keeping them in it (Coffield et al., 2004). One reviewer of the claimed evidence wrote that 'very few studies have even used an experimental methodology capable of testing the validity of learning styles applied to education. Moreover, of those that did use an appropriate method, several found results that flatly contradict the popular meshing hypothesis' (Pashler, McDaniel, Rohrer, & Bjork, 2009, p. 105). Almost all of the evidence base claimed for learning styles is theoretical and descriptive in nature rather than empirical, and rarely appears in peer-reviewed journals. The studies that do follow typical scientific procedures, such as featuring a randomly assigned control group, do not support the learning styles hypothesis (Pashler et al., 2009). Even researchers inclined to accept the existence of learning styles have been unable to provide empirical support for the claims (Kozhevnikov, Evans, & Kosslyn, 2014).

Most of the pseudoscientific claims discussed here fall within the category of 'bad science' mentioned in the introduction to this chapter. Learning styles, and similar assessment methods, are different, as the use of spurious cognitive assessment methods can be harmful to students, since they can result in teachers erroneously labelling students as being of a certain 'type', and providing a range of restricted resources that are appropriate to that type. Thus, they are 'ugly science': in addition to a restriction of educational opportunities that is likely to follow from this labelling process, and the detraction from the use of techniques which are demonstrably effective (Willingham, Hughes, & Dobolyi, 2015), there is a real danger that students will internalize these labels and think of themselves as certain types of learners who should limit themselves to the diagnosed activities (Demos, 2004). Consequently, the intrusion of some of these pseudoscientific practices into classrooms can waste a lot more than merely time and money; they can harm students' learning and development.

The brain-based theories discussed in this section were selected because they all touch upon the central concerns of this book, and as the chapters and the rest of this volume demonstrate, there have been remarkable developments in the understanding of the relationships between physical activity, the brain and educational achievement in recent years. So, despite the different limitations of these alternative theories, they share the same kernel of truth. The problem is that they extrapolate far beyond the valid and reliable evidence base, or misunderstand the findings and their implications. But it does not follow that the stylized movements of Brain Gym result in the activation of particular areas in the brain. Likewise, it is almost certainly the case that some students prefer movement-based ways of learning over others. It does not mean, however, that these preferences have any link to innate differences in the brain, nor that matching those preferences with pedagogy will accelerate learning.

It might be asked if the distinction between science and pseudoscience matters. Perhaps the proliferation of neuromyths and other pseudoscientific ideas form a harmless tax on people's gullibility and scientific illiteracy? That might be true in some cases. Many worthless ideas circulate, and with extraordinary speed thanks to social media (Pentland, 2014). If people wish to take homeopathic remedies or vitamin tablets for minor ailments like colds, the effect is likely to be nothing more than a placebo effect and interestingly coloured urine (of course, if they take these tablets instead of actual medicine, the costs could be much more serious). However, as has been suggested earlier in this chapter, introducing pseudoscience into classrooms is rarely without harm. Educational systems have finite financial and time resources, and engagement with learning styles inventories or Brain Gym movements usually means fewer opportunities to participate in activities that are likely to prove more worthwhile. It is hardly surprising that many of these ideas are couched in the language of neuroscience as they feed on a tendency to accept almost any claim if it appears to be backed by neuroscience (Weisberg et al., 2008). Allowing such ideas into the classroom gives them a credibility that undermines a meaningful distinction between the hard-won evidence of scientific research and overblown claims of untested products.

So, untested, unregulated and unsupported scientific practices can be harmful. There are other dangers, too, as outlined by the philosopher and biologist Massimo Pigliucci, who claimed that debating and exposing pseudoscience is important for a number of reasons:

> The first is philosophical: demarcation is crucial to our pursuit of knowledge; its issues go to the core of debates on epistemology and of the nature of truth and discovery. The second reason is civic: our society spends billions of tax dollars on scientific research, so it is important that we also have a good grasp of what constitutes money well spent in this regard . . . Third, as an ethical matter, pseudoscience is not – contrary to popular belief – merely a harmless pastime of the gullible; it often threatens people's welfare, sometimes fatally so.
>
> (Pigliucci & Boudry, 2013, unpaged)

There is high risk that some of these myths will propagate among teachers and then to students, and it needs to be remembered that some of the consequences of these pseudoscientific ideas harm children. Teaching students that they have a specific learning style, or that their poor scores are due to faulty integration between the hemispheres of their brains based on no valid or reliable evidence, risks limiting their educational opportunities and damaging their long-term achievements. It is known that many teachers wish to build on knowledge generated from research in neuroscience (Pickering & Howard-Jones, 2007). However, without an ability to tell the difference between good, bad and ugly science, those teachers are vulnerable to becoming victims of professionally marketed fads and fashions. The extremely widespread acceptance of pseudoscientific beliefs among teachers (e.g. Dekker et al., 2012) is testament to this danger.

If the distinction between science and pseudoscience does matter, then it seems important to have some way of telling the difference. This has proved to be a challenging task, and is one that continues to generate debate among both theorists and practitioners. Some of the terms of this debate are discussed in the next section.

The demarcation problem

The previous section has shown that practitioners are bombarded with claims about various supposedly brain-based theories and products, and most of them are couched in impressive-sounding language and the signs of science, such as brain images. So, it is often difficult to tell the difference between those ideas that are based on real science and those that merely pretend to be scientific. This latter group of ideas is sometimes called pseudoscience, because they masquerade as science. Collins and Bailey (2013) offered an alternative terminology for theories and practices that look superficially like science – 'scienciness' – which they define as, 'the illusion of scientific credibility and validity that provides a degree of authority to otherwise dubious ideas. Scienciness is conveyed through, for example, esoteric language and complex statistical representations, and supplemented by association with an apparently successful foreign system' (p. 2). Scienciness is just a more graphic term for pseudoscience.

Although science has been defined in many ways, most people who have examined the subject agree it is ultimately not a body of knowledge, but a way of establishing and developing a body of knowledge (Shneider, 2009). The philosopher Karl Popper hinted at this view when he described science as a process of bold guessing, followed by rigorous testing. In other words, at the heart of science is criticism – self-criticism and the criticism of others. Popper (1994) said: 'What we call scientific objectivity is nothing more than the fact that no scientific theory is accepted as dogma, and that all theories are tentative and are open all the time to severe criticism' (p. 160). Pseudoscientific theories claim to conform to the norms of science, but, when judged impartially, the claims violate them (Koertge, 2013).

The challenge of telling the difference between science and pseudoscience is called the demarcation problem (Popper, 1934). One difficulty confronting anyone reflecting on these issues is that there are many different types of science (such as theoretical and applied), concerned with many different sorts of objects (including people, animals, plants and minerals), at different stages of disciplinary maturity (from emerging areas of research to well-established sciences). Consider, for example, some of the types of research reported in recent sport and exercise sciences journals:

- randomized controlled trials of the effectiveness of physical activity interventions;
- surveillance reports of sports participation around the world;
- analysis of specific groups' motivations to engage in exercise;
- systematic literature reviews and meta-analyses of various, narrowly defined topics;
- observational studies of sports coaches' behaviours;
- laboratory studies of oxygen uptake on a treadmill;
- brain scans of skilled practice.

Research methods used in any multidisciplinary field are likely to be diverse, since the methods of each of the parent disciplines can potentially be used, and this variety will only be multiplied when that field encompasses both theoretical and applied work, and populations ranging from shortly after birth to death. In fact, the range of methods used by sport and exercise scientists is even wider than that, since many methods regularly used have been imported from further afield. Systematic reviewing has origins in agricultural studies of seeds and fertilizers. Cluster analysis was first used by bacteriologists. And the detailed observational procedures used to track player behaviour during a game or session were imported from ethologists' studies of animals in the wild.

Karl Popper is the philosopher most associated with the problem of demarcation, He argued that a theory is scientific if it can be shown to be false. This is in contrast to the idea that science operates through the generation of confirmations of theories, which had previously dominated discussions of the scientific method (and sometimes, in various forms, to this day). Popper argued the relative power of positive and negative evidence is asymmetrical: no amount of confirmations can demonstrate a theory's value because it is always possible to find them; but a single falsification, he claimed, can kill a theory dead. The scientist (or at least the good scientist) does not search for evidence that seems to support a theory, but looks for ways in which it might be found to be mistaken. In other words, genuinely scientific theories include statements that could be shown to be false by empirical evidence; pseudoscientific theories do not. Popper (1934) used his famous 'black swan' argument to force through the distinction between the persuasive powers of positive and negative evidence, which is paraphrased below:

> For thousands of years, Europeans had observed millions of white swans. Because of this, they induced (generalized) the theory that 'all swans are white'. However, exploration of Australasia introduced Europeans to black swans. The theory that 'all swans are white' was dead.

Popper's motto is that no matter how many observations are made which confirm a theory, there is always the possibility that future falsifying observations refute it. The spirit of falsification continues to extend to the scientific community, where the 'friendly–hostile co-operation' of scientists (Popper, 1994) is expressed through mechanisms like peer review of articles.

Falsification as the criterion of demarcation continues to be influential among scientists, but philosophers have generally abandoned it as a sufficient standard for setting science apart from pseudoscience. There have been various criticisms of Popper's view, but the most damaging is the 'Quine–Duhem problem' (Hacking, 1999). This is based on the observation that when a scientist tests a theory, it is not in isolation from other assumptions and hypotheses. So, what appear to be observations that falsify a theory might be some other factors. Popper modified his theory in response to these criticisms, arguing that scientists should be explicit about both the theory and any associated assumptions and hypotheses that might affect it. This is a stronger position, since it means that the scientist is prepared to dictate more fully the theoretical and experimental conditions necessary for proper testing. However, it does not adequately deal with the Quine–Duhem problem, since it will never be possible to remove complicating variables completely.

While philosophers of science have tended to reject Popper's formal theory of falsifications, most broadly endorse its central tenets, such as the central importance of a critical approach, well-designed tests and a suspicion of an overreliance on confirming evidence. However, some philosophers have offered different theories of sciences. There is not enough room to review all of these theories (see, for example, Chalmers, 1999; Monton, 2013), and that is not necessary for present purposes. It is worth noting, however, that despite the sometimes fractious debates among philosophers, many philosophers would concur that, at least at the most general level, certain basic elements cut across most or all scientific disciplines. Specifically, different sciences, despite their diversity, are marked by a willingness to root out error in one's beliefs and the implementation of procedural safeguards against confirmation bias – the deeply ingrained tendency to seek out evidence consistent with one's hypotheses and to deny, dismiss or distort evidence that is not (Lilienfeld, 2012). So, despite the evident differences between the sciences, they all seem to share certain core characteristics, and pre-eminent among these is a commitment to criticizing and testing proposed ideas ruthlessly, and removing potential barriers to that criticism and testing. Moreover, there is a much greater degree of agreement about what pseudoscience looks like (e.g. Koertge, 2013; Lilienfeld, Lynn, & Lohr, 2015).

Unfalsifiability

Popper's early insights came from his observation that some theories are apparently impossible to prove mistaken, whether because they do not make clear hypotheses that could be tested, or that they interpret any criticism in terms of the malicious intent of the critic. The mixture of practices, including mystical constructs like Jung's personality theory, suggests that the Action Type Approach (see note 1) is difficult to falsify, or even measure.

Absence of self-correction

Despite the identification of flaws in their ideas, pseudoscientists often keep faith in the original. Consider the case of Brain Gym as a paradigm example of this phenomenon, in which every one of its foundational principles has been shown to be either false or misinterpreted, but the programmes continue to be sold regardless.

Overuse of ad hoc immunizing tactics designed to protect theories from refutation

It is common for promoters of pseudoscience to add supplementary ideas to deflect criticism. An example of this ploy is the claim by Carey et al. (2010) that the critical responses to NLP are invalid due to 'inaccurate application/

interpretation of NLP techniques' (p. 12), and that 'Only a small number of papers, from the 1980s, contain formal research evidence that is critical' (p. 12); the first claim might be true, if unlikely; the latter is simply false (cf. Witkowski, 2010).

Absence of connectivity with other domains of knowledge

Many pseudoscientific ideas seem to come from nowhere, and have little or no relationship with current scientific understanding of a topic. As other chapters in this book demonstrate, there is now persuasive evidence that aerobic exercise, classroom activity breaks and active play can enhance cognitive functioning, but none of this research has been properly integrated into the theorizing of Brain Gym, NLP or other self-described brain-based methods.

Use of obscurantist language

Social media is littered with products prefaced with 'neuro-', 'psych-', 'physio-', and using incomprehensible descriptions, clearly aspiring for some sort of 'science' legitimacy. The Myers-Briggs test tells people that they are 'ENFJ' (extraverted intuitive feeling judging), 'INTP' (introverted intuitive thinking perceiving), or another of the 16 types drawn from the inventory (Barbuto, 1997). Or consider this quotation from the Brain Gym teachers' guide, which combines vague references to neurological language with factually incorrect statements about learning:

> The Brain Gym Lengthening Activities help students to develop and reinforce those neural pathways that enable them to make connections between what they already know in the back of the brain and the ability to express and process that information in the front of the brain . . . The front portion of the brain, especially the frontal lobe, is involved in comprehension, motor control, and rational behaviours necessary for participation in social situations. The Lengthening Activities have been found to relax those muscles and tendons that tighten and shorten by brainstem reflex when we are in unfamiliar learning situations.
>
> (Dennison & Dennison, 1994, p. 16)

Overreliance on anecdotes and testimonials at the expense of systematic evidence

Two of the most reliable markers for pseudoscience are the use of statements of support from satisfied customers, and the absence of reference to actual science. Most of the websites discussed here contain enthusiastic statements of support for their products. Although the 'case studies' in Carey et al.'s

(2010) report on NLP offer no measures of improvement, they are littered with comments like, 'this has been a life-changing experience' (p. 59) and, 'The impact of the knowledge base has been immense. It has changed me as a person' (p. 94). To be clear, such statements are not presented as testimonies by the report authors, but explicitly as evidence for the effectiveness of NLP in schools (Carey et al., 2010, pp. 16–18).

Evasion of peer review

Pseudoscientific ideas are seldom presented for independent assessment. The use of the *Brain Gym® Journal*, self-publications and other in-house strategies for disseminating generally low-quality information is an example of this, as is the use of student essays and other unpublished, non-reviewed materials in Carey et al.'s (2010) review of the literature on NLP.

Contrast this with the scientific studies discussed elsewhere in this book. Figure 18.1 summarizes the most basic form of peer review.

Emphasis on confirmation rather than refutation

Since it is almost always possible to find positive evidence, no matter how implausible, it is quite a simple matter to compile confirmations of ideas. If, for example, I am wedded to the idea that middle-aged male academics have a uniquely appealing charm, I simply need to:

- pay particular attention to any especially charming middle-aged male academics I might come across as confirmatory instances;
- either ignore, or preferably interpret, non-charming behaviour from middle-aged academics, rather like the way TV audiences have apparently learned to admire the ignorant and boorish behaviour of 'talent show' judges!

The search strategy used in the report on the educational applications of NLP by Carey et al. (2010) results in a bias towards supportive findings. A more scientific approach would have compiled a list of inclusive criteria

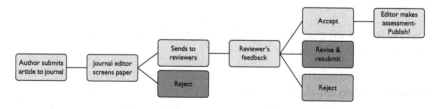

Figure 18.1 The basic peer review process.

before undertaking the search, and perhaps invited potential critics to comment on these criteria. Such inclusive criteria would probably not allow low-level resources to pass, such as student essays, and would insist on a standard for admission considerably higher than 'some form of university affiliation'.

Considered individually, these criteria are insufficient to indicate that a field is pseudoscientific or has cause for concern. None is sufficient to indicate pseudoscience. Conclusive falsification, as has been seen, is extremely difficult, and obscure language is hardly absent from scientific journals. In fact, many of these characteristics could be identified in the work of reputable scientists. The list also does not aim to show the necessary conditions for pseudoscience. The field is too complex and varied to be reduced to simple clues. The philosopher Ludwig Wittgenstein (1953) argued that some concepts do not have universally true features, but rather a patchwork of related family resemblances that may or may not fit to each application. Perhaps pseudoscience is one such concept; it is too fuzzy to succumb to a simple declination and requires, instead, ongoing discussion by theorists and practitioners about the nature of their work and the types of evidence that ought to inform it.

Despite the variations in its forms and the sometimes inaccessibility of its methodologies, science is ultimately a method of 'arrogance control' (Tavris and Aronson, 2007). The scientific method consists of a series of checks and balances that force scientists to doubt their most cherished and strongly held assumptions. Some of the pseudoscientific claims discussed in this chapter appear to be driven by the profit motive, but conversations with proponents of others make it clear that their commitments are often well-meaning. A recent online discussion (personal communication) with the inventor of a movement- and brain-based programme is revealing:

A: Could you please tell me about the evidence you have in support of this programme?

B: The thousands of children it has helped.

A: OK, but I meant, have you tested these benefits using scientific tests? For example, did you use control groups?

B: I don't have time for things like that! There are children in schools now who need [the programme].

A: But I still don't understand how you know it works. If you are relying on your own observations, surely that is limited? After all, it is your programme. You developed it, and have invested quite a lot of your own money in it. Aren't you worried that your subjective judgements could be unintentionally biased? You could be seeing what you want to see.

B: I've been working in schools for 30 years. I know what works! Anyway, the teachers tell me about the benefits.

A: But these teachers invited you into their classrooms, didn't they?

B: Yes, because they want the best for their children.

A: I have no doubt that is true. And I don't doubt you are convinced of the value of [the programme]. But what I am struggling with is the lack of objective measures. Without some sort of non-subjective assessment, I can't see how you can be so confident in your claims.

B: All I can say is that I have seen [the programme] improve children's performance. I have never seen a child fail with it. But I do intend to bring some researchers I've been working with. Because you are right, we need the numbers.

The social psychologist Timothy Wilson (2011) gathered evidence from studies measuring people's responses to programmes like those discussed above. His analysis shows how bad human beings are at knowing why they reacted to situations as they did. They tend to impose plausible explanations about the causes of those reactions, just as they do when trying to make sense of others' behaviours. This is especially true when they encounter novel situations, such as a new educational intervention, and have nothing with which to compare it. In fact, the problem of assessing effects of programmes is even worse. When people have gone through a programme designed to help those for whom they care, there is a tendency for them to misremember how things were before that programme began, therefore overestimating the effects of the intervention. Wilson (2011) advocates a 'don't ask, can't tell' policy – not asking people how much they benefited. Human beings are not very accurate at assessing the causes of their own feelings, attitudes, behaviour (p. 26). This advice does not dismiss the views of recipients of programmes from the research process. It is just a suggestion that it is unwise to rely too much on the recipients of an intervention to provide an accurate assessment of the nature and extent of influence on their behaviour or understanding. The various methods developed over the centuries by science have the significant advantage purely because they aim to be non-subjective and non-personal.

Conclusion

The American Nobel prize-winning physicist Richard Feynman (1974), in a speech at the Californian Institute of Technology, warned his audience of young science graduates about the dangers of 'cargo cult science':

In the South Seas there is a cargo cult of people. During the war they saw airplanes land with lots of good materials, and they want the same thing to happen now. So they've arranged to imitate things like runways, to put fires along the sides of the runways, to make a wooden hut for a man to sit in, with two wooden pieces on his head like headphones and bars of bamboo sticking out like antennas – he's the controller – and they wait for the airplanes to land. They're doing everything right. The form is perfect. It looks exactly the way it looked before. But it doesn't work. No airplanes land. So I call these things cargo cult science, because they follow all the apparent precepts and forms of scientific investigation, but they're missing something essential, because the planes don't land.

(Feynman, 1974, p. 11)

Feynman's point was that, while it might accord with human nature to engage in wishful thinking, good scientists learn not to fool themselves. Feynman's warning could well be applied to the myriad 'brain-based' strategies that pervade current educational thinking. Whereas it is commonly stated in such schemes that the brain is the most complex object in the universe, it is ironic that this assumption is then ignored in proposing pedagogies based on simplistic analyses of complex phenomena. The neurosciences are complex and the accurate transfer of research findings to the classroom is often difficult (Devonshire & Dommett, 2010). As has been seen in this chapter, the gap between neuroscience and education has enabled many misconceptions about scientific findings to arise.

Despite teachers' enthusiasm for what neuroscience might bring to education (Serpati & Loughan, 2012), there are currently few direct contributions that can be directly applied to the classroom, and the collaborative effort between the two disciplines should be considered a long-term process (Goswami & Szűcs, 2011). It has become commonplace in writing about the application of neuroscientific ideas to stress the need to explore ways of bridging the gap between scientists and practitioners (e.g. Howard-Jones, 2014), and there is little doubt that lack of communication between these groups has contributed to current levels of misunderstanding. While there is certainly a lot of truth in this account, there is also a danger that the way the problem is phrased might undermine efforts to address it. Neuroscience is still mainly a laboratory-based activity. Even with the best of intentions, extrapolations from the laboratory to the classroom need to be made with considerable caution. The scientist–practitioner gap, as it is often called in the literature (Cautin, 2011), assumes a clear disjunction between scientists, who gather evidence, and practitioners (in this case, teachers) who implement practices, whether based on that evidence or not. However, this dichotomy is both misleading and unhelpful. It is misleading because the lack of an understanding of basic scientific knowledge on the part of teachers should not be accepted as a given at a time of near-universal teacher education and professional development (Townsend, 2016). Nor should it be accepted that scientists, as a group, are unable to engage with teachers in meaningful terms (Goswami, 2006). That such blurring of the boundaries between scientists and practitioners happens too rarely does not mean that the boundaries cannot be transgressed.

	Science	Non-science
Research	Scientific researcher	Non-scientific researcher
Practice	Scientific practitioner	Non-scientific practitioner

Figure 18.2 The dimensions of science/non-science, research and practice.

Two conceptually distinct dimensions are at play here. The first is 'science/non-science'; the other is 'research/practice' (McFall, 1991). As Figure 18.2 shows, these dimensions generate four quadrants.

The difference between these distinctions and the standard scientist/practitioner gap is vital, because the former implicitly challenges the presumption that teachers should be recipients of research. Instead, it hints at the need to involve teachers much more fully in the production and application of science in education. This might mean the inclusion of neuroscience and psychology into initial teacher training and professional development courses (Pickering & Howard-Jones, 2007). More important, perhaps, would be a proper introduction to the scientific method, including ways of evaluating claims of scientific credibility. Teachers need to learn not just how to administer the ideas and practices presented to them, but also to become thoughtful and discerning consumers of proposed evidence (Lilienfeld, Ammirati, & David, 2012). In an era of evidence-based practice, this seems unarguable, not least because teachers are often the gatekeepers of new claims in the classroom.

The model offered above also acknowledges that not all research that seeks a place in classrooms is scientific, a point that should be amply clear from the earlier discussions of pseudoscience. The widespread acceptance of pseudoscientific claims about the brain and educational practice is serious cause for concern. The situation in education is of particular concern as it impacts on the life opportunities of children. Experimenting with children's lives without very good reasons, and without a clear awareness of the potential benefits and costs, is morally reprehensible, and is justifiably forbidden in many contexts. It is not obvious why children should not be protected from the endless stream of bad and ugly products and practices that continue to flood into classrooms. Many of these ideas have not been shown to work; others have been shown not to work. Yet they continue to find a place in classrooms around the world. This is not a call for the end of new ideas in education. On the contrary, such work is the life blood of evidence-based practice. But it is a call for caution about what is permitted to impact on children's learning and well-being, especially when what is being offered has no basis in science.

In late 2015, a psychological study made news headlines by bluntly demonstrating the human capacity to be misled by 'pseudo-profound bullshit' (Pennycook, Cheyne, Barr, Koehler, & Fugelsang, 2015). The authors, through a series of experiments, concluded that 'some people are more receptive to this type of bullshit and that detecting it is not merely a matter of indiscriminate skepticism but rather a discernment of deceptive vagueness in otherwise impressive sounding claims' (p. 549). Neuroscientific explanations are especially vulnerable to this tendency. Studies by Weisberg et al. (2008) show that even people with some neuroscientific knowledge (e.g. people who followed an introductory cognitive neuroscience class) can be fooled by neuroscientific explanations in the same way as laypeople. This reinforces the need for any professional education for teachers in neuroscience to be accompanied with information about how to evaluate claims, how to spot the markers of pseudoscience and how to make informed judgements about whether and how to implement new ideas and practices in their classrooms. In light of the time, energy and money that have already been lost due to the encroachment of pseudoscience into schools, as well as the potential harm that some of these can have on children's education, this is both a moral and professional necessity.

Notes

1 The last reference – from a soccer magazine – is one of the very few published sources on the Action Type Approach, a collection of supposedly brain-based practices, including the Myers-Briggs Type Indicator (MBTI), learning styles and movements reminiscent of 'educational kinesiology'. This model seeks to provide insight into the training of athletes 'to take it to the next level', by integrating on 'natural movement' (Action Types, 2013). As is common with such brain-based products, the claims made on behalf of the Action Type Approach are impressive, which might explain why it has been adopted by numerous elite sports groups, including the England cricket team and a number of international football clubs (Action Types, 2013). Unfortunately, not a single research article could be found on this method, and direct requests to the creators and leading advocates resulted in no other sources of research evidence.
2 The Evidence for Policy and Practice Information and Co-ordinating (EPPI) Centre at University College London Institute of Education, London, lists the key features of a systematic review:

- explicit and transparent methods are used;
- it is a piece of research following a standard set of stages;
- it is accountable, replicable and updateable;
- there is a requirement of user involvement to ensure reports are relevant and useful (https://eppi.ioe.ac.uk/cms/Default.aspx?tabid=56).

From the information provided in the CfBT report, it is not clear that any of these criteria were met.

References

Action Types (2013). *Action Types: move to your next level*. http://comingsoon.actiontypes.com (accessed 12/12/2013).
Bailey, R. P. (2013). The use of questionable methods in sports coach education in the UK. Unpublished manuscript.

Bailey, R. P. (2016). Sport, physical activity and educational achievement – towards an explanatory model. *Sport in Society*, 1–21. doi: doi.org/10.1080/17430437.2 016.1207756.

Bandler, R., & Grinder, J. (1979). *Frogs into princes*. Moab, UT: Real People Press.

Barbuto, J. E. (1997). A critique of the Myers-Briggs type indicator and its operationalization of Carl Jung's psychological types. *Psychological Reports, 80*(2), 611–625.

Beyerstein, B. L. (1990). Brainscams: Neuromythologies of the New Age. *International Journal of Mental Health, 19*(3), 2736, 27.

Brain Gym International (2003). *A chronology of annotated research study summaries in the field of educational kinesiology*. Ventura, CA: The Educational Kinesiology Foundation.

Carey, J., Churches, R., Hutchinson, G., Jones, J., & Tosey, P. (2010). *Neurolinguistic programming and learning: Teacher case studies on the impact of NLP in education*. Reading: CFBT.

Cautin, R. L. (2011). Invoking history to teach about the scientist–practitioner gap. *History of Psychology, 14*(2), 197–203.

Chalmers, A.F. (1999). *What is this thing called science?* Indianapolis, IN: Hackett Publishing.

Coch, C., & Ansari, D. (2012). Constructing connection: The evolving field of mind, brain and education. In S. D. Sala & M. Anderson (Eds.), *Neuroscience in education: The good, the bad and the ugly* (pp. 33–46). Oxford: Oxford University Press.

Coffield, F., Moseley, D., Hall, E., & Ecclestone, K. (2004). *Learning styles and pedagogy in post-16 learning. A systematic and critical review*. London: Learning and Skills Research Centre.

Collins, D., & Bailey, R. P. (2013). 'Scienciness' and the allure of second-hand strategy in talent identification and development. *International Journal of Sport Policy, 5*(2), 183–191.

Committee on Children with Disabilities. (1999). The treatment of neurologically impaired children using patterning. *Pediatrics, 104*(5), 1149–1151.

Crain, W. (2000). *Theories of development: Concepts and applications* (4th ed.). Upper Saddle River, NJ: Prentice Hall.

Cummins, R. A. (1988). *Neurologically impaired child: Doman-Delacato techniques reappraised*. Cheltenham: Nelson Thornes.

Dekker, S., Lee, N. C., Howard-Jones, P., & Jolles, J. (2012). Neuromyths in education: Prevalence and predictors of misconceptions among teachers. *Frontiers in Psychology: Educational Psychology, 3*(429), 1–8.

Della Sala, S. (2009). The use and misuse of neuroscience in education. *Cortex, 45*(4), 443.

Demos (2004). *About learning*. London: Demos.

Dennison, P. E. (2009). Research now validates movement-based learning. *Brain Gym Journal, 23*(1–2), 3.

Dennison, P. E., & Dennison, G. E. (1994). *Brain Gym® – Teacher's edition*. Ventura, CA: Edu-Kinesthetics.

Devonshire, I. M., & Dommett, E. J. (2010). Neuroscience: Viable applications in education? *The Neuroscientist, 16*(4), 349–356.

Donczik, J., & Bocker, I. (2009). Using Dennison laterality repatterning to increase mental speed. *Brain Gym Journal, 23*(1–2), 4–5.

Dündar, S., & Gündüz, N. (2016). Misconceptions regarding the brain: The neuro-myths of preservice teachers. *Mind, Brain, and Education, 10*(4), 212–232.

Eagleman, D. (2015). *The brain: The story of you.* New York: Pantheon.

Feynman, R. P. (1974). Cargo cult science. *Engineering and Science, 37*(7), 10–13.

Fischer, K. W. (2009). Mind, brain, and education: Building a scientific groundwork for learning and teaching. *Mind, Brain, and Education, 3*(1), 3–16.

Fulford, K. W. M. (2008). Values-based practice: A new partner to evidence-based practice and a first for psychiatry? *Mens Sana Monographs, 6*(1), 10–21.

Geake, J. (2008). Neuromythologies in education. *Educational Research, 50,* 123–133.

Gleichgerrcht, E., Lira Luttges, B., Salvarezza, F., & Campos, A. L. (2015). Educational neuromyths among teachers in Latin America. *Mind, Brain, and Education, 9*(3), 170–178.

Goswami, U. (2006). Neuroscience and education: From research to practice? *Nature Reviews Neuroscience, 7*(5), 406–413.

Goswami, U. (2014). Educational neuroscience: Bridging the gulf between basic research and implications for practice. In L. Florian (Ed.), *The Sage handbook of special education* (revised ed., Vol. 1) (pp. 315–332). London: Sage.

Goswami, U., & Szűcs, D. (2011). Educational neuroscience: Developmental mecha-nisms: towards a conceptual framework. *Neuroimage, 57*(3), 651–658.

Hacking, I. (1999). *The social construction of what?* Cambridge, MA: Harvard University Press.

Hausmann, M. (2017). Why sex hormones matter for neuroscience. *Journal of Neuroscience Research, 95*(1–2), 40–49.

Herculano-Houzel, S. (2002). Do you know your brain? A survey on public neu-roscience literacy at the closing of the decade of the brain. *Neuroscientist, 8*(2), 98–110.

Hippolyte, R., & Théraulaz, B. (unknown). The Action Types Approach (ATA): An insight into the power of preference. *On the Up, 7,* 78–81.

Howard-Jones, P. A. (2014). Neuroscience and education: Myths and messages. *Nature Reviews Neuroscience, 15*(12), 817–824.

Howard-Jones, P. A., Pollard, A., Blakemore, S.-J., Rogers, P., Goswami, U., Butterworth, B., . . . Kaufmann, L. (2007). *Neuroscience and education: Issues and opportunities.* Swindon: Economic and Social Research Council.

Hyatt, K. J. (2007). Brain Gym®: Building stronger brains or wishful thinking? *Remedial and Special Education, 28*(2), 117–124.

Immordino-Yang, M. H. (2016). *Emotions, learning, and the brain.* New York: W. W. Norton.

Kavale, K. A., & Forness, S. R. (1987). Substance over style: Assessing the efficacy of modality testing and teaching. *Exceptional Children, 54*(3), 228–239.

Koertge, N. (2013). Belief buddies versus critical communities: The social organiza-tion of pseudoscience. In M. Pigliucci & M. Boudry (Eds.), *Philosophy of pseu-doscience: Reconsidering the demarcation problem.* Chicago, IL: University of Chicago Press.

Kozhevnikov, M., Evans, C., & Kosslyn, S. M. (2014). Cognitive style as environ-mentally sensitive individual differences in cognition a modern synthesis and applications in education, business, and management. *Psychological Science in the Public Interest, 15*(1), 3–33.

Lazarus, J., & Cohen, R. (2009). Sport psychology and use of neuro linguistic programming (NLP) in sport. *Journal of Health, Social and Environmental Issues, 10*(1), 5–12.

Legrenzi, P., & Umilta, C. (2011). *Neuromania: On the limits of brain science*. Oxford: Oxford University Press.

Lilienfeld, S. O. (2012). Public skepticism of psychology: Why many people perceive the study of human behavior as unscientific. *American Psychologist, 67*(2), 111–129.

Lilienfeld, S. O., Ammirati, R., & David, M. (2012). Distinguishing science from pseudoscience in school psychology: Science and scientific thinking as safeguards against human error. *Journal of School Psychology, 50*(1), 7–36.

Lilienfeld, S. O., Lynn, S. J. E., & Lohr, J. M. (2015). *Science and pseudoscience in clinical psychology* (2nd ed.). New York: Guilford Press.

Mareschal, D., Butterworth, B., & Tolmie, A. (Eds.). (2014). *Educational neuroscience*. Chichester: Wiley-Blackwell.

Mayringer, H., & Wimmer, H. (2002). No deficits at the point of hemispheric indecision. *Neuropsychologia, 40*(7), 701–704.

McFall, R. M. (1991). Manifesto for a science of clinical psychology. *The Clinical Psychologist, 44*(6), 75–88.

McNiff, J. (2013). *Action research: Principles and practice*. London: Routledge.

Monton, B. S. (2013). Pseudoscience. In M. Curd & S. Psillos (Eds.), *The Routledge companion to philosophy of science* (pp. 469–478). London: Routledge.

Norcross, J. C., Koocher, G. P., & Garofalo, A. (2006). Discredited psychological treatments and tests: A Delphi poll. *Professional Psychology: Research and Practice, 37*(5), 515–522.

OECD (2002). *Understanding the brain: Towards a new learning science*. Paris: Organisation for Economic Cooperation and Development.

OECD (2007). *Understanding the brain: The birth of a learning science*. Paris: Organisation for Economic Cooperation and Development.

Pashler, H., McDaniel, M., Rohrer, D., & Bjork, R. (2009). Learning styles: Concepts and evidence. *Psychological Science in the Public Interest, 9*(3), 105–119.

Passingham, R. E., & Rowe, J. B. (2015). *A short guide to brain imaging: The neuroscience of human cognition*. Oxford: Oxford University Press.

Pei, X., Howard-Jones, P. A., Zhang, S., Liu, X., & Jin, Y. (2015). Teachers' understanding about the brain in East China. *Procedia-Social and Behavioral Sciences, 174*, 3681–3688.

Pennycook, G., Cheyne, J. A., Barr, N., Koehler, D. J., & Fugelsang, J. A. (2015). On the reception and detection of pseudo-profound bullshit. *Judgment and Decision Making, 10*(6), 549–563.

Pentland, A. (2014). *Social physics: How good ideas spread – the lessons from a new science*. New York: Penguin.

Pickering, S. J., & Howard-Jones, P. (2007). Educators' views on the role of neuroscience in education: Findings from a study of UK and international perspectives. *Mind, Brain, and Education, 1*(3), 109–113.

Pigliucci, M., & Boudry, M. (2013). The dangers of pseudoscience. *New York Times*. 10/10/13. https://opinionator.blogs.nytimes.com/2013/10/10/the-dangers-of-pseudoscience/? (accessed 10/10/15).

Pokorski, M. (Ed.). (2015). *Neurotransmitter interactions and cognitive function*. Berlin: Springer.

Popper, K. R. (1934). *Logik der Forschung: zur Erkenntnistheorie der moderner Naturwissenschaft*. Berlin: Springer.

Popper, K. R. (1994). *The myth of the framework: In defence of science and rationality* (Ed. M. A. Notturno). London: Routledge.

Psillos, S. (1999). *Scientific realism: How science tracks truth*. London: Routledge.

Rato, J. R., Abreu, A. M., & Castro-Caldas, A. (2013). Neuromyths in education: What is fact and what is fiction for Portuguese teachers? *Educational Research, 55*(4), 441–453.

Rogowsky, B. A., Calhoun, B. M., & Tallal, P. (2014). Matched learning style to instructional method. *Journal of Educational Psychology, 107*(1), 1–15.

Rohrer, D., & Pashler, H. (2012). Learning styles: Where's the evidence? *Medical Education, 46*(7), 634–635.

Ruhaak, A. E., & Cook, B. G. (2016). Movement as behavioral moderator: What does the research say? In B. Cook, M. Tankersley, & T. Landrum (Eds.), *Instructional practices with and without empirical validity* (pp. 111–134). Bingley: Emerald Group Publishing.

Sagan, C. (2011). *Demon-haunted world: Science as a candle in the dark*. New York: Ballantine Books.

Serpati, L., & Loughan, A. R. (2012). Teacher perceptions of neuro-education: A mixed methods survey of teachers in the United States. *Mind, Brain, and Education, 6*(3), 174–176.

Shneider, A. M. (2009). Four stages of a scientific discipline: Four types of scientist. *Trends in Biochemical Sciences, 34*(5), 217–223.

Singh, S., & Ernst, E. (2008). *Trick or treatment? Alternative medicine on trial*. London: Bentham.

Tardif, E., Doudin, P.-A., & Meylan, N. (2015). Neuromyths among teachers and student teachers. *Mind, Brain, and Education, 9*(1), 50–59.

Tavris, C., & Aronson, E. (2007). *Mistakes were made (but not by me): Why we justify foolish beliefs, bad decisions, and hurtful acts*. Orlando, FL: Harcourt.

Townsend, T. (Ed.). (2016). *International perspectives on teacher education*. London: Routledge.

Weisberg, D. S., Keil, F. C., Goodstein, J., Rawson, E., & Gray, J. R. (2008). The seductive allure of neuroscience explanations. *Journal of Cognitive Neuroscience, 20*(3), 470–477.

Willingham, D. T., Hughes, E. M., & Dobolyi, D. G. (2015). The scientific status of learning styles theories. *Teaching Psychology, 42*, 266–271.

Wilson, T. (2011). *Redirect: The surprising new science of psychological change*. London: Penguin.

Witkowski, T. (2010). Thirty-five years of research on neuro-linguistic programming. NLP research data base. State of the art or pseudoscientific decoration? *Polish Psychological Bulletin, 41*(2), 58–66.

Wittgenstein, L. (1953). *Philosophical investigations*. New York: Macmillan.

Yin, R. K. (2013). *Case study research*. Thousand Oaks, CA: Sage.

Index

task switching 194, 195, 197, 199
taxi drivers 37
Taylor, A. F. 198
teachers 25–6, 305, 307, 308–10;
    Denmark 326, 327–8, 329–30;
    educational neuroscience 337, 345,
    353, 355; Finland 319, 325, 329;
    pseudoscience 340–1, 343, 345,
    351–2, 355; scientist-practitioner
    gap 353–4
teaching methodologies 308–10, 311,
    321, 326, 343
team games 295, 296
temporal cortex 44–5
temporal processing 192–3
testimonials 349–50
testosterone 218–19, 220–1
thalamus 40–1, 43, 78, 95, 132
Thelen, Ester 305
Themanson, J. R. 147, 152
therapy 201, 205
Thernlund, G. 202
Thimas, E. 200
Thomas, A. G. 38
Thomas, R. 149
Thomson, J. 197
time see duration of physical activity
time point of assessment 145
timetabling 102, 318, 319, 320, 329
timing of physical activity 102,
    103, 281
Tine, M. T. 288, 290, 292
Tomporowski, Phillip 1–5, 32–62,
    92–4, 196, 247–74
Tonoli, Cajsa 2–3, 77–88
Tools of the Mind 310
Tortella, Patrizia 4, 303–16
track and field 200
transdisciplinary research 65, 67–8;
    see also multidisciplinary research
translational research 53, 54, 65, 261,
    277, 282, 297
treadmill walking 9, 10, 12, 144,
    180–3, 184; ADHD 196; dual-task
    effects 114, 115; duration of physical
    activity 16; neurotransmitters 79;
    see also walking
Trulson, M. E. 307
truth 338
Tsai, C. L. 117
Tsai, Y. J. 23
twin studies 216

types of physical activity 14, 23–5, 26,
    281, 283
tyrosine 77, 83, 90, 103

ultrafine particle (UFP) deposition 83,
    84–5
unfalsifiability 348
updating 279
urban environment 262

vagus nerve 95, 101–2
'VAK' model 342–3
van den Berg, V. 285, 287, 288
van Donkelaar, P. 118
Van Mier, H. 121
variability of practice 50, 254
vascular endothelial growth factor
    (VEGF) 138, 150, 172–3, 231–2
Vaynman, S. 232
Vazou, S. 15
VEGF see vascular endothelial growth
    factor
ventral striatum 92
verbal learning 48, 50
Verburgh, L. 215
Verghese, J. 168, 172
Verret, C. 199
Visser, J. 117
visual attention 280
visual cortex 40–1, 46
visuospatial sketchpad 97–8, 278–9
Voelcker-Rehage, Claudia 3,
    143–63, 219
Vogel, S. 134
Vygotsky, L. S. 309

walking 9–10, 12, 144, 152, 216–17,
    283; ADHD 196, 198; dual-task
    effects 113–17, 118–19; duration of
    physical activity 16, 19; laboratory
    studies 178–9, 180–3, 184;
    neurogenesis 81; neurotransmitters
    79; older people 169; school-based
    studies 289, 291
walking desks 66
Walter, Nadja 3, 178–90
water-based exercise 199
Wechsler Intelligence Scale for Children
    (WISC) 17–18, 20, 21–2, 23
Weden, S. 198
Wegner, Mirko 3–4, 148, 213–29
Weisberg, D. S. 355

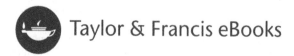